Physiological
Assessment
of
Human Fitness

Peter J. Maud, PhD
University of Texas, El Paso

Carl Foster, PhD
Milwaukee Heart Institute

LRC : Library

SOMERSET COLLEGE OF ARTS & TECHNOLOGY

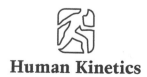

Human Kinetics

Library of Congress Cataloging-in-Publication Data

Physiological assessment of human fitness / Peter J. Maud, Carl
  Foster.
     p. cm.
  Includes bibliographical references and index.
  ISBN 0-87322-776-X (hbk.)
  1. Exercise--Physiological aspects. 2. Physical fitness--Testing.
3. Exercise tests.   I. Maud, Peter J., 1938- .   II. Foster, Carl.
QP301.P57   1995
613.7'028'7--dc20   94-40072
                                                      CIP

ISBN: 0-87322-776-X

Acquisitions Editor: Richard D. Frey, PhD
Developmental Editor: Holly Gilly
Assistant Editors: Kirby Mittelmeier, Ed Giles, Ann Greenseth
Copyeditor: Wendy Nelson
Proofreader: Karin Leszczynski
Indexer: Sheila Ary
Typesetting and Text Layout: Julie Overholt and Angela K. Snyder
Text Designer: Judy Henderson
Paste-Up: Denise Lowry
Cover Designer: Jack Davis
Photographer (cover): John Kelly
Printer: Braun-Brumfield

Printed in the United States of America

10 9 8 7 6 5 4 3 2 1

Human Kinetics
P.O. Box 5076, Champaign, IL 61825-5076
1-800-747-4457

Canada: Human Kinetics, Box 24040, Windsor, ON N8Y 4Y9
1-800-465-7301 (in Canada only)

Europe: Human Kinetics, P.O. Box IW14, Leeds LS16 6TR, England
(44) 532 781708

Australia: Human Kinetics, 2 Ingrid Street, Clapham 5062, South Australia
(08) 371 3755

New Zealand: Human Kinetics, P.O. Box 105-231, Auckland 1
(09) 309-2259

Contents

Chapter 10 The Measurement of Body Composition

Michael L. Pollock, James E. Graves, Linda Garzarella

Chapter 11 Anthropometry

Robert M. Malina

Chapter 12 Static Techniques for the Evaluation of Joint Range of Motion

Peter J. Maud, Miriam Y. Cortez-Cooper

CHAPTER 1

Parameters of Fitness Assessment

Peter J. Maud, PhD

University of Texas at El Paso

There appears to be no widely accepted definition of fitness, nor any agreement as to what specific components should comprise a fitness evaluation. Over 50 years ago Steinhaus (47), evidently viewing fitness from the perspective of the physiologist, defined it as distance from death, a description somewhat like that of many in the medical profession, who tend to regard physical fitness as absence of disease. Willgoose (49) has defined it as ''a capacity for sustained physical activity'' (p. 105). A more appropriate and universal definition of physical fitness, at least from a health perspective, is probably the one found in *Mosby's Medical and Nursing Dictionary* (31), which defines physical fitness as ''the ability to carry out daily tasks with alertness and vigor, without undue fatigue, and with enough reserve to meet emergencies or to enjoy leisure time pursuits'' (p. 880). Differences in interpretation of the term probably depend upon whether fitness is applied to health or relative to athletic competition. It is obvious that in the latter case, where successful, rewarding, and enjoyable participation in sport is desired, higher levels of fitness are necessary and more specific test items are required for measurement of fitness attributes. It is, therefore, necessary to attempt to define fitness parameters and to select those items appropriate for inclusion in a text primarily intended to discuss fitness from a physiological and physiologically related perspective. Consideration must also be given to techniques that allow determination of changes that result from different types of training programs, whether information so gained is useful for planning health enhancement programs or for improving fitness for sport participation. The purpose of this text is to provide a comprehensive coverage of the methods used for the evaluation of fitness from both physical health and athletic competition perspectives.

Fitness assessment may be viewed in different ways, including the determination of energy system utilization (which may be particularly important for sport participation), the evaluation of the perceptual motor domain and vision requirements, or the use of traditional component tests for sport fitness assessment and profiling. Additionally, study of the historical development of fitness testing is interesting and applicable to an understanding of current practices.

HISTORICAL PERSPECTIVES

Obviously it is beyond the scope of this chapter to include more than a few examples of the types of tests that have been used to assess fitness in earlier times. The tests described are not necessarily those that were the most universally accepted but rather serve as examples of what was thought to be current and appropriate at that time. Three general areas of fitness—anthropometry; muscular strength, endurance, and power; and cardiovascular fitness—received prime consideration.

Anthropometric Measurement

Some of the earliest tests used to evaluate or describe fitness were restricted to anthropometric measurement. An early pioneer of anthropometric assessment was Hitchcock of Amherst College, who measured such items as age, height, weight, chest girth, arm girth, forearm girth, and lung capacity, as described in the text that he coauthored with Seelye (19) in 1893 and in which he describes data collected approximately between the years 1861 and 1880. (Seaver [42] had, however, published *Anthropometry in Physical Education* in 1890 and thus is perhaps the first modern author in this area.) Description of body type can be traced back to Hippocrates, who recognized two basic body types, and later to Rostan, who in the late 19th century proposed a three–body type classification system. It was Sheldon, in association with Stevens and Tucker (43), who first made a serious attempt to further classify body types as having proportions that were a mixture of the three general classifications of ectomorph, mesomorph, and endomorph. The study of somatotype and anthropometry and the study of their relationship to human motion are still important today, as is illustrated by the rather recent formation in 1986 of a new association, the International Society for the Advancement of Kinanthropometry, whose purpose and function were recently described by Beunen and Borms (7).

Assessment of Muscular Strength, Endurance, and Power

The move to include strength tests as a major component of fitness evaluation was probably initiated by Sargent in about 1880. However, Kellogg (21) in 1896 described a "universal dynamometer" that made possible more accurate muscle strength testing. Sargent (40), in a 1921 journal article entitled "The Physical Test of Man," described the vertical jump test—or Sargent jump, as it is now popularly known—one of the first tests of muscular power. Rogers' (37) development of the strength index, which was considered a general test of athletic ability, and a physical fitness index, and which was derived by comparing the strength index to norms based upon gender, weight, and age, probably contributed more to the popularity of strength testing than any other individual during the earlier part of the century. Seven measurements were obtained, consisting of left and right handgrip strength, back strength, leg strength, strength of the arms and shoulder girdle as measured in men by dips on the parallel bars and by pull-ups with overhand grip, and forced vital capacity. Several modifications to this original test have been made, as for example by MacCurdy (22), who eliminated the endurance factors associated with the pull-up and dip tests by replacing them with static tests of arm strength using the back/leg dynamometer. McCloy (28) later eliminated the lung capacity test, arguing that it was not a test of muscle strength. Isometric tests as evaluated by the typical dynamometer are still in use, as are muscle endurance tests such as dips and push-ups. However, today measurement of dynamic strength such as by determination of maximum weight moved in one repetition (1RM), and isokinetic testing are far more likely to be found in the scientific literature.

Evaluation of Cardiovascular Fitness

There are many well-known tests of cardiovascular fitness that date back to the early 20th century. One of the first compared heart rate and systolic blood pressure responses between the horizontal and the standing position (12). It was believed that a fitter individual would exhibit a maximal rise in blood pressure with no change in heart rate, "evidencing such a complete working of the splanchnic mechanism that the heart would not be called to help raise blood-pressure" (29, p. 267). The Barach Cardio-Vascular Test (4), described in 1919, was another test that used blood pressure and heart rate to evaluate cardiovascular function. In this test, which was claimed to indicate the energy demands of the circulatory system, an index was obtained by adding systolic and diastolic pressures and then multiplying by heart rate. One of the earlier tests used to investigate the response of heart rate to exercise and recovery was the Foster Cardio-Vascular Test (16) published in 1914. Preexercise, immediate postexercise, and 45-s postexercise heart rates were obtained. These three heart rates comprised separate tests with norms established for all three conditions. The exercise component consisted of stepping up and down on the floor for 30 s at a rate of 180 steps per minute, with heart rate measured manually for a 5-s period. Lack of standardization of the stepping exercise and the potential for error in measurement of heart rate would tend to invalidate the test. Schneider (41) used a combination of pulse rate and blood pressure obtained in the horizontal and standing positions, and pulse rates taken immediately following 15 s of bench-stepping exercise and during recovery, to evaluate aviators during World War I. Tuttle's well-known pulse ratio test, using a bench 13.5 in. high, was described in 1931 (48). A 2-min pulse count obtained following standardized exercise was divided by a 1-min pretest resting rate. McCurdy and Larson (29) described a test of "organic efficiency" and provided comprehensive normative tables for males aged 18 to 80 years (p. 274). Test items included sitting diastolic pressure, breath-holding ability taken 20 s following 90 s of standardized bench-stepping exercise, the difference between preexercise standing pulse rate and pulse rate obtained 2 min following standardized exercise, standing pulse pressure, and vital capacity. More recent tests have included the renowned Harvard Step Test developed by Brouha (9) and other step tests that are still currently in use. Other exercise modalities, such as the treadmill and the bicycle ergometer, have replaced bench stepping in popularity, but heart rates taken during either exercise or recovery are still widely used to assess cardiovascular fitness.

Contribution of Technology to Fitness Assessment

Some of the most significant advancements in fitness assessment have been made possible by the development of sophisticated equipment and techniques. For example, in the assessment of metabolic response, although the Douglas bag and associated chemical evaluation for gas composition using Scholander equipment can be still found in some laboratory settings, it is far more common to find elaborate, on-line computer equipment capable of providing instantaneous feedback utilizing breath-by-breath analysis. Similarly, muscular strength, endurance, and power are also commonly evaluated in the laboratory by isokinetic methods with detailed computer analysis. Even heart rate measurement has been greatly facilitated and made more accurate by use of the ECG or small and simple, yet accurate, heart rate telemetry systems. Advanced techniques in body tissue analysis, and instruments like the electron microscope, have greatly enhanced our ability to evaluate fitness changes at the cellular and ultracellular levels. Certainly, therefore, from a historical perspective these advances have changed the ways fitness is assessed in the laboratory, although many techniques and methods used in earlier times are still appropriate, particularly in field-testing.

HEALTH FITNESS

Probably the most commonly accepted components of health fitness include cardiovascular endurance, body composition, flexibility, and muscular strength and endurance. However, these four components are not necessarily accepted as the only ones that need to be assessed. Medically oriented health fitness evaluation centers offer far more comprehensive programs that may include, for example, extensive cardiovascular evaluations with an ECG exercise tolerance test, blood chemistry analysis and blood count, maximum oxygen uptake measurement, pulmonary function tests, and orthopedic assessments (25). The American College of Sports Medicine (2) recommends that prior to commencement of a vigorous exercise training program, defined as requiring energy expenditure in excess of 60% of maximum oxygen uptake, apparently healthy men aged 40 and women aged 50 and above should receive a medical examination and a maximal ECG exercise tolerance test. It has also been recommended that younger individuals "with two or more major coronary risk factors and/or symptoms

suggestive of cardiopulmonary or metabolic disease" (p. 7) be similarly evaluated. However, the American College of Cardiology and the American Heart Association (1) generally do not consider diagnostic exercise testing to be of value to apparently healthy people. The necessity for extensive medical testing in the evaluation of fitness is, therefore, questionable but readily available. Blood chemistry and blood pressure screening are, however, invaluable when assessing health status and predisposition toward cardiovascular disease and diabetes (46).

THE ENERGY SYSTEMS APPROACH

Another approach to fitness evaluation is to base all tests on the energy systems used during physical activity. The contribution to the energy requirements by initial stores of adenosine triphosphate (ATP) present within the muscle and the subsequent restoration of these stores by creatine phosphate (CP), by the anaerobic breakdown of glycogen, or by aerobic utilization of glycogen, fat, and protein, would require assessment. Fox, Robinson, and Wiegman (17) classified activity by the prime source of energy being utilized and proposed four time periods. Period 1 comprised activities that lasted less than 30 s that they suggested depended primarily on the contribution of ATP and CP. Period 2, from 30 to 90 s, utilized mainly the phosphagens and anaerobic glycolysis. Period 3, lasting from 90 to 180 s, depended mainly upon anaerobic glycolysis and aerobic metabolism, and Period 4, consisting of exercise in excess of 180 s, was reported to be primarily aerobic in nature. Shephard (44) described another classification system using a similar approach but which had five phases. Phase 1 was a single maximum contraction; Phase 2 comprised very brief events that lasted less than 10 s; Phase 3 was for events that lasted 10 to 60 s; Phase 4 was for activity that lasted from 1 min to 1 hour; and Phase 5 was for prolonged events that lasted in excess of 1 hour. Skinner and Morgan (45) have proposed another four-period classification system based upon more recent research, particularly in the areas of power output and lactate tolerance. They suggested that it consist of an anaerobic power phase lasting 1 to 10 s, where initial stores of ATP and CP would be the main energy sources; an anaerobic capacity phase of 20 to 45 s, where anaerobic glycolysis, in addition to ATP and CP stores, would be the prime energy contributor; a lactic acid tolerance phase lasting 1 to 8 min; and an aerobic phase of 10 or more minutes, where aerobic metabolism would be the prime energy source.

Use of gas analysis during maximal work tests to derive a maximum oxygen uptake is well documented as being indicative of the aerobic system's contribution to fitness. However, methods for assessing other systems' contributions are far more controversial. Numerous tests have been devised to measure mechanical power output during time periods thought to represent the energy contribution phase. A short single contraction, as in the vertical jump test described by Sargent (40), would, if considered only from the perspective of the energy requirements for the activity, be indicative of the contribution of ATP stores. The 2 to 4 s required to complete the Margaria stair-run test (24) or the 5-s Wingate test (5,6) would be representative of peak anaerobic power where ATP and CP stores should be the main energy contributors. The 30-s Wingate test (6) measures mechanical mean anaerobic power output during the anaerobic glycolytic phase. However, there are many problems in assuming that the power output during specified time periods is in fact representative of specific energy contributions. Muscle biopsy techniques may allow quantification of ATP and CP stores, but the size, strength, and speed of contraction of the muscle, the predominant fiber type, the structural arrangement of the individual muscle, and coordination all affect power output. Because it is easy to measure, blood lactate is commonly used to predict anaerobic glycolytic ability, but diffusion of lactate into the blood does not provide an accurate assessment of individual muscle contribution. Further, motivation plays a very important role in tests requiring maximal effort. In the measurement of maximum oxygen uptake, parameters have been identified as denoting achievement of a true maximal effort, but measurable characteristics to identify maximal effort are less clearly defined for anaerobic testing.

THE PERCEPTUAL MOTOR DOMAIN

The performance of complex skills is dependent upon neuromuscular coordination produced in response to sensory feedback and its subsequent processing. Testing within this domain is fraught with problems mainly stemming from a lack of agreement as to the specific parameters that define the area.

Motor Ability

During the 1920s it was hypothesized that ability to perform motor tasks was an inherent characteristic much like intelligence. It was therefore believed that tests similar to those used to measure IQ could be developed to predict ability to perform the motor tasks involved

in sport and other complex movement patterns. Brace (8), in 1927, was one of the earliest researchers to develop such a test battery, comprising 20 different stunts designed to evaluate "inherent motor skill" ability. In 1929, Cozens (11) published a test which purported to identify "general athletic ability." This was followed by Johnson's test (20) in 1932 used to evaluate "native neuromuscular skill capacity." McCloy (27) then published a modification of the Brace test in 1937 in an attempt to evaluate "motor educability." Subsequently came the realization that there is no such thing as general motor ability but that there may be a number of rather broad, yet relatively independent, motor abilities as have been described by Fleishman (14). He used a two classification system to describe motor abilities, one consisting of perceptual motor abilities and the other of physical proficiencies. His tests of perceptual motor ability consisted of 11 items: "control precision, multilimb coordination, response orientation, reaction time, speed of arm movement, rate control (timing), manual dexterity, finger dexterity, arm-hand steadiness, wrist-finger speed, [and] aiming." The physical proficiency battery included "extent flexibility, dynamic flexibility, static strength, dynamic strength, explosive strength, trunk strength, gross body coordination, equilibrium, [and] stamina" (15, p. 1132). The purpose for inclusion of this brief discussion of motor abilities is to indicate that there are many traits that may contribute to fitness for athletic performance, particularly reaction time, balance, movement speed, agility, and coordination. These abilities, applicable to specific sports, need to be evaluated and do form a significant part of many fitness testing batteries.

Vision Testing

Whether vision testing should be separate from other sensory tests or from the psychomotor domain is debatable. However, vision certainly can affect athletic performance, and vision testing has comprised a part of the assessment of athletes in the sports medicine program at the USOC training center in Colorado Springs. In sports where aiming is a crucial skill component, as in archery and shooting, visual abilities are paramount; but vision testing in other sports has also been undertaken. Extensive evaluation of the visual abilities of athletes was conducted during the 1985 National Sports Festival held in Baton Rouge (13). A series of 23 vision tests was administered to 304 competitors in the sports of baseball, field hockey, team handball, volleyball, soccer, and archery. These tests were designed to evaluate such traits as visual acuity (the sharpness and clarity of vision), dynamic visual acuity (the ability to clearly see moving objects), vision pursuit (the ability to follow the pathway of moving objects), depth perception (the ability to judge distance and speed), and eye/hand/body coordination. If tests such as these do differentiate performance ability, then they should be a part of athletic fitness measurement, particularly if training can remedy any deficiencies.

FITNESS EVALUATION FOR ATHLETIC PARTICIPATION

A plethora of tests has been developed to evaluate the fitness of athletes representing a wide variety of sports and activities, and it would be a monumental task to review all athletic group fitness profiles or individual tests administered. Methods used to evaluate athletic fitness depend upon the requirements of the individual sport or event, the available equipment and facilities, the practicality of assessment, and the personal perspectives of the researcher. The following brief discussion of 12 studies representing a variety of sports and methodologies will indicate the commonalities and diversities of test items used.

Some investigators have evaluated cardiovascular fitness in rugby (26), football (50), soccer (36), lacrosse (51), field hockey (35), and tennis (10) participants by direct determination of maximum oxygen uptake. Others have assessed this parameter by indirect means, using a timed 15-min run for Australian football players (34); a 2-mi (30) or 1-mi (32) run for downhill skiers; a 15-mi run for racquetball players (39); and a 3,000-yd run for rugby players (38).

Anaerobic capacities have been evaluated by a 600-yd run for rugby players (38); by a 600-m (30) or 440-yd (32) run for downhill skiers; by the Wingate test for rugby (26), racquetball (39), and downhill skiing (30) athletes; by the Margaria stair-run test for lacrosse (51), field hockey (35), and tennis (10) players; and by postexercise blood lactate levels in lacrosse players (51).

Grip strength has traditionally been used as a general measure of muscular strength, as in rugby (26, 38), Australian football (34), tennis (10), and racquetball (39). Back (38) and leg (39) strength have also been evaluated, and isokinetic evaluation has been used to assess thigh strength (10, 30).

Field tests have commonly been used to assess muscular endurance. Five such tests were used in the Australian football study (34) and four in one of the rugby studies (38). Isokinetic endurance evaluation was undertaken in two studies (10, 30).

The vertical jump has been used to evaluate muscular power, one of the most important attributes for successful performance in many games and sports, in six of the studies (26, 30, 32, 34, 38, 39). Isokinetic evaluation,

as for muscular strength and endurance, was used for power evaluation of downhill skiers (30) and tennis players (10).

The sit-and-reach test has been the most widely used measure of flexibility, despite its controversial nature. The only other flexibility assessments used in the studies being examined were wrist and shoulder flexibility in racquetball players (39).

Skinfold measurement was the most prevalent method for estimating body composition (10, 26, 30, 34, 35, 51). Two of the studies (10, 30) also used the underwater weighing technique, and one study (10) also described skeletal widths and circumferences.

Other data collected to further describe athletic attributes have included measurement of speed by timing of a 40-yd dash (32, 35, 39) or, in the case of the Australian football study (34), by using 15-, 40-, and 55-m run times plus a 40-m run following a 15-m running start, and measurement of agility by shuttle runs (32, 38), agility runs (32, 35, 39), or hurdle jumps in the case of downhill skiing (30).

These examples illustrate the diversity of sports evaluated and assessment methods used.

RATIONALE FOR TEXT TEST ITEMS

Several authorities have suggested items that should be included in a typical fitness evaluation. For example, the Canadian Association of Sport Sciences recently had a text published (23) detailing areas of testing believed necessary to evaluate athletic performance potential. Specific test protocols are included. Test items cover evaluation of muscular strength and power; aerobic power (maximum oxygen uptake and lactate threshold); anaerobic power and capacity by measurement of mechanical power output; kinanthropometry (including anthropometry, somatotype, body composition, and maturation); static flexibility; and health status.

It has been noted by Åstrand and Rodahl (3) that many such test items "including evaluation of flexibility, skill, strength, etc., are related to special gymnastic or athletic performance" and "are not really suitable for an analysis of basic physiological functions" (p. 355). However, many of these items may have a profound effect upon physiological performance and, therefore, these tests should be included. In point of fact there should be little argument against the inclusion of such test items as cardiovascular fitness, muscular strength and endurance, flexibility, and body composition in tests of health status or athletic ability in that these items are crucial to both areas. All other areas covered can be justified by their importance either to athletic competition or to sport physiology research.

Probably one of the most often evaluated fitness parameters is maximum oxygen uptake, which has long been considered the "gold standard" for the evaluation of cardiorespiratory fitness. Direct assessment of this variable is preferred. Many tests have, however, been devised to estimate maximum oxygen uptake, or general cardiovascular condition, using indirect measures purported to correlate well with direct assessment. Such tests have included time taken to run a specific distance, distance run in a specific time, or heart rate response either during, or recovering from, standardized work.

Direct methods for determination of aerobic power are detailed in chapter 2 by Davis, who gives a historical overview of the open-circuit method of determination of maximum oxygen uptake, discusses currently used systems, exercise testing protocols, and criteria for the achievement of a maximum value, and provides normative data.

Lamarra and Whipp in chapter 3 discuss in great detail breath-by-breath measurement of pulmonary gas exchange. Included are outlines of methods currently available with discussion of the assumptions, implications, and associated sources of error. Application to exercise testing and evaluation is well covered. The highly technical nature of this chapter is necessary in order to prevent misinterpretations, with subsequent disastrous consequences.

In chapter 4, Ward, Ebbeling, and Ahlquist describe methods for the estimation of maximum oxygen uptake and provide detailed examples of specific protocols using both submaximal tests, maximal tests, and tests appropriate for the evaluation of children. A variety of exercise modalities is also included.

Determination of the lactate threshold, the critical exercise intensity above which an exponential increase of blood lactate occurs, is an important measure affecting aerobic power output. Typically blood samples are taken during an incremental exercise test and subsequently evaluated for lactate concentration, although ventilatory phenomena are often used to identify the approximate anaerobic threshold in order to avoid invasive techniques. Maximal lactic acid tolerance can also provide useful information for fitness evaluations for activities that depend heavily upon anaerobic glycolysis. This area is covered by Foster, Schrager, and Snyder in chapter 5.

In chapter 6, Foster, Hector, McDonald, and Snyder evaluate anaerobic performance and advocate the measurement of oxygen deficit rather than the indirect measurement of mechanical power output, which provides no physiological data. Discussion of several power output tests is, however, included.

Muscular strength, endurance, and power are requisites for most athletic events. Methods of assessment range from field tests to laboratory techniques. In chapter 7, Harman describes the measurement of human mechanical power and gives an excellent, yet readily understandable, review of the methodologies for recording mechanical power output. His discussion of specific technical requirements and techniques is of particular interest, especially to those with somewhat limited backgrounds in computer application fields.

Kraemer and Fry in chapter 8 provide a comprehensive review, and a very complete bibliography, of the strength-testing domain. Detailed methodologies for different modalities are provided with consideration given also to individual differences and specifics of performance method.

Evaluation of muscle tissue from muscle biopsy has been undertaken on numerous occasions (18), however, inclusion of a detailed chapter covering this area may be somewhat controversial in that, as expounded by Gollnick and Matoba (18), routine evaluation of muscle tissue for prediction of athletic success should probably not be recommended. However, it must be remembered that this text is designed also for research purposes where such information as obtained from muscle biopsy can be invaluable in the study of chronic exercise effects. Chapter 9, by Fink and Costill, provides an excellent introduction to and comprehensive coverage of muscle biopsy technique, histochemical preparation, fiber typing, and analysis of chemical composition of muscle tissue.

Body physique likewise is important when considering suitability for specific athletic events and also from a health fitness perspective. In chapter 10, Pollock, Graves, and Garzarella give very in-depth coverage of current body composition assessment techniques and very complete bibliographical references. Malina, in chapter 11, covers the application of anthropometry to sport science, and appropriate methodologies.

Flexibility is also important for many athletes, whether they view performance in terms of time, distance, speed, or aesthetics. It has also been advocated that flexibility is an important contributor to normal daily function from a health perspective. In chapter 12, Maud and Cortez discuss the limitations of certain measurement methods and provide details of preferred measurement methods. Also advocated is utilization of the contribution of limited range of motion to impairment for classification purposes rather than normative methods currently used.

Chapter 13, by Daniels and Foster, is devoted to the collection of physiological data in the field, a topic that certainly warrants attention in that all too often this area is neglected. Athletic performance does not take place in the laboratory, but rather in the field under a myriad of physical, environmental, sociological, and psychological conditions. Testing under these conditions certainly results in a more realistic exposure when considering athletic performance.

A comprehensive discussion of the appropriate use of statistical procedures for evaluation of fitness data is provided by Shultz and Sands in chapter 14. Obviously the accumulation of fitness assessment data is meaningless without appropriate use of the tools necessary to evaluate the effectiveness of training programs or other intervention strategies. This concluding chapter provides an excellent guide to statistical methods and interpretation.

EXCLUSIONS

Although a rationalization could be given for the inclusion of more comprehensive evaluations of cardiovascular function by use of such means as ECG exercise tolerance testing, particularly when health is the prime concern, and assessment of visual abilities when considering either health or athletic performance, tests such as these are not included due to their specialized nature and probable necessity for some form of medical supervision. Similarly, the perceptual motor domain is not included for, as already discussed, the generally held view is that there is no such thing as a general motor ability, but rather several rather broad and independent perceptual motor abilities and physical proficiencies that are usually applicable to specific athletic events.

CONCLUSION

Undoubtedly, athletic competition requires fitness beyond that necessary for optimal health. But the value of specific fitness test items to athletes and coaches, and the use that can be made of data collected, have been much debated (18, 33). Ultimately it becomes the responsibility of physiological fitness professionals to assess the value of the different areas that can be evaluated and the specific methods that can be used for those evaluations. Obviously, differing approaches will be made depending upon requirements, whether they be health related, for the evaluation of fitness necessary for successful athletic participation, or for research into the human body's response to varied exercise intensities and regimes.

REFERENCES

1. American College of Cardiology, & American Heart Association. (1986). Guidelines for exercise testing. *Circulation*, **74**, 653A-667A.
2. American College of Sports Medicine. (1991). *Guidelines for exercise testing and prescription.* Philadelphia: Lea & Febiger.
3. Åstrand, P.-O., & Rodahl, K. (1986). *Textbook of work physiology.* New York: McGraw-Hill.
4. Barach, J.H. (1919). The energy index (S.D.R.) of the cardiovascular system. *Archives of Internal Medicine*, **24**(5), 509.
5. Bar-Or, O. (1987). The Wingate anaerobic test. An update on methodology, reliability and validity. *Sports Medicine*, **4**, 381-394.
6. Bar-Or, O., Dotan, R., Inbar, O., Rothstein, A., Karlsson, J., & Tesch, P. (1980). Anaerobic capacity and muscle fiber type distribution in man. *International Journal of Sports Medicine*, **1**, 82-85.
7. Beunen, G., & Borms, J. (1990). Kinanthropometry: Roots, developments and future. *Journal of Sports Sciences*, **8**, 1-15.
8. Brace, D.K. (1927). *Measuring motor ability.* New York: Barnes.
9. Brouha, L. (1943). The step test: A simple method of measuring physical fitness for muscular work in young men. *Research Quarterly*, **14**, 31-36.
10. Carlson, J.S., & Cera, M.A. (1984). Cardiorespiratory, muscular strength and anthropometric characteristics of elite Australian junior male and female tennis players. *Australian Journal of Science and Medicine in Sport*, **16**(4), 7-13.
11. Cozens, F.W. (1929). *The measurement of general athletic ability in college men.* Eugene, OR: University of Oregon Press.
12. Crampton, C.W. (1913). Blood ptosis; A test of vasomotor efficiency. *New York Medical Journal*, **98**, 916-918.
13. Farnsworth, C.L. (1990). Personal correspondence.
14. Fleishman, E.A. (1964). *The structure and measurement of physical fitness.* Englewood Cliffs, NJ: Prentice Hall.
15. Fleishman, E.A. (1975). Toward a taxonomy of human performance. *American Psychologist*, **30**, 1127-1149.
16. Foster, W.L. (1914). A test of physical efficiency. *American Physical Education Review*, **19**, 632.
17. Fox, E., Robinson, S., & Wiegman, D. (1969). Metabolic energy sources during continuous and interval running. *Journal of Applied Physiology*, **27**, 174-178.
18. Gollnick, P.D., & Matoba H. (1984). The muscle fiber composition of skeletal muscle as a predictor of athletic success. *American Journal of Sports Medicine*, **12**(3), 212-216.
19. Hitchcock, E., & Seelye, H.H. (1893). *An anthropometric manual.* Amherst, MA: Carpenter & Morehouse.
20. Johnson, G.B. (1932). Physical skills test for sectioning classes into homogeneous units. *Research Quarterly*, **3**, 128-136.
21. Kellogg, J.H. (1896). *The value of strength tests in the prescription of exercise* (Vol. 2). Battle Creek, MI: Modern Medicine Library.

22. MacCurdy, H.L. (1933). *A test for measuring the physical capacity of secondary school boys.* Yonkers, NY: Author.

23. MacDougall, J.D., Wenger, H.A., & Green, H.J. (Eds.). (1990). *Physiological testing of the high-performance athlete.* Champaign, IL: Human Kinetics.

24. Margaria, R., Aghemo, P., & Rovelli, E. (1966). Measurement of muscular power (anaerobic) in man. *Journal of Applied Physiology*, **21**, 1662-1664.

25. Maud, P.J., & Longmuir, G.E. (1983). A survey of health-fitness evaluation centers. *Public Health Reports*, **98**, 30-34.

26. Maud, P.J., & Shultz, B.B. (1984). The U.S. national rugby team: A physiological and anthropometric assessment. *Physician and Sportsmedicine*, **12**(9), 86-99.

27. McCloy, C.H. (1937). An analytical study of the stunt type tests as a measure of motor educability. *Research Quarterly*, **8**, 46-55.

28. McCloy, C.H. (1939). *Tests and measurements in health and physical education.* New York: F.S. Croft.

29. McCurdy, J.H., & Larson, L.A. (1939). *The physiology of exercise.* Philadelphia: Lea & Febiger.

30. Morrell, R.W. (1990). Personal correspondence.

31. *Mosby's medical and nursing dictionary.* (1986). St. Louis: Mosby.

32. National Alpine Staff. (1990). *United States Ski Team training manual.* Park City, UT: United States Ski Team.

33. Noakes, T.D. (1988). Implications of exercise testing for prediction of athletic performance: A contemporary perspective. *Medicine and Science in Sports and Exercise*, **20**(4), 319-330.

34. Parkin, D. (1982). Fitness appraisal in Australian football. *Sports Coach*, **6**(1), 40-43.

35. Rate, R., & Pyke, F. (1978). Testing and training of women field hockey players. *Sports Coach*, **2**(2), 14-17.

36. Raven, P., Gettman, L., Pollock, M.L., & Cooper, K.H. (1976). A physiological evaluation of professional soccer players. *British Journal of Sports Medicine*, **10**, 209-216.

37. Rogers, F.R. (1927). *Tests and measurement programs in the redirection of physical education.* New York: Columbia University Bureau of Publications.

38. Rugby Football Union. (1978). *Fitness training for rugby.* Twickenham, England: Walker.

39. Salmoni, A.W., Guay, M., & Sidney, K. (1988). Skill analysis in racquetball. *Perceptual and Motor Skills*, **67**, 208-210.

40. Sargent, D.A. (1921). The physical test of man. *American Physical Education Review*, **25**, 188-194.

41. Schneider, E.C. (1920). A cardiovascular rating as a measure of physical fitness and efficiency. *Journal of the American Medical Association*, **74**(5), 1506-1507.

42. Seaver, J.W. (1890). *Anthropometry in physical education.* New Haven, CT: Tuttle, Morehouse and Taylor.

43. Sheldon W.H., Stevens, S.S., & Tucker, W.B. (1940). *The varieties of human physique.* New York: Harper and Brothers.

44. Shephard, R.J. (1978). Aerobic versus anaerobic training for success in various athletic events. *Canadian Journal of Applied Sport Sciences*, **3**, 9-15.

45. Skinner, J.S., & Morgan, D.W. (1984). Aspects of anaerobic performance. In *Limits of human performance* (American Academy of Physical Education Paper No. 18, pp. 31-44). Champaign, IL: Human Kinetics.

46. Smith, L.K. (1988). Health appraisal. In S.N. Blair, P. Painter, R.R. Pate, L.K. Smith, & C.B. Taylor (Eds.), *Resource manual for guidelines for exercise testing and prescription* (pp. 155-169). Philadelphia: Lea & Febiger.

47. Steinhaus, A.H. (1936). Health and physical fitness from the standpoint of the physiologist. *Journal of Health and Physical Education*, **7**(4), 224.

48. Tuttle, W.W. (1931). The use of the pulse rate test for rating physical efficiency. *Research Quarterly*, **11**(2), 5.

49. Willgoose, C.E. (1961). *Evaluation in health education and physical education.* New York: McGraw-Hill.

50. Wilmore, J.H., Parr, R.B., Haskell, W.L., Costill, D.L., Milburn, L.J., & Kerlan, R.K. (1976). Football pros' strengths—and CV weakness—charted. *Physician and Sportsmedicine*, **4**, 44-54.

51. Withers, R.T. (1978). Physiological responses of international female lacrosse players to pre-season conditioning. *Medicine and Science in Sports*, **10**(4), 238-242.

CHAPTER 2

Direct Determination of Aerobic Power

James A. Davis, PhD

California State University, Long Beach

The purpose of this chapter is to describe the direct determination of aerobic power, or maximal oxygen uptake ($\dot{V}O_2$max). First, several equipment configurations will be described. Second, exercise testing modes will be discussed. Third, the criteria for achievement of $\dot{V}O_2$max will be discussed. The last section of the chapter deals with normative data for $\dot{V}O_2$max.

There are four parameters of aerobic fitness: aerobic power, or maximal oxygen uptake ($\dot{V}O_2$max); work efficiency; time constant for $\dot{V}O_2$ kinetics; and the lactate threshold (1). Maximal oxygen uptake is an important parameter of human fitness because it represents the upper limit of aerobic exercise tolerance. Endurance activities are performed at some fraction of $\dot{V}O_2$max; if $\dot{V}O_2$max is abnormally low, then the level of endurance performance is necessarily constrained.

Whole-body oxygen uptake can be determined from cardiovascular measurements or from respiratory measurements, using equations based on the Fick principle. From cardiovascular measurements, $\dot{V}O_2$ = C.O. (CaO_2 − $C\bar{v}O_2$), where C.O. is cardiac output, CaO_2 is content of O_2 in arterial blood, and $C\bar{v}O_2$ is content of O_2 in mixed venous blood. From respiratory measurements, $\dot{V}O_2 = \dot{V}_A$ (F_IO_2 − $F_{\bar{A}}O_2$), where $\dot{V}_A$ is alveolar ventilation, F_IO_2 is the fraction of O_2 in inspired gas, and $F_{\bar{A}}O_2$ is the fraction of O_2 in the mean alveolar gas (this equation is not rigorous, because it does not account for the normally small differences between inspired and expired alveolar volumes). Thus, the determinants of $\dot{V}O_2$ are the heart (C.O.), the mechanical properties of

the lungs and the chest wall ($\dot{V}_A$), diffusion of O_2 from the alveolus into the pulmonary capillary blood ($F_{\bar{A}}O_2$ and CaO_2), and the extraction of O_2 from the capillary blood by the muscle cell ($C\bar{v}O_2$). A person with a high $\dot{V}O_2$max necessarily has good function in each of these determinants. Conversely, a sedentary person has relatively poor function for each determinant, which results in a low $\dot{V}O_2$max. If a person has pathology associated with any determinant (e.g., coronary artery disease, which would limit cardiac output during exercise), then $\dot{V}O_2$max will be very low. Hence, one of the important reasons for measuring $\dot{V}O_2$ during graded exercise testing (GXT) is to establish whether the $\dot{V}O_2$max is normal.

There are two controversies regarding the measurement of $\dot{V}O_2$max. The first is the criteria used to establish whether $\dot{V}O_2$max has been achieved during GXT. The most widely accepted criterion is that $\dot{V}O_2$ plateaus during the later stages of GXT as the work rate continues to increase. However, many subjects clearly reach their limit of tolerance during GXT without demonstrating a plateau in $\dot{V}O_2$. The second controversy is the recommendation that if a subject does not demonstrate a plateau in $\dot{V}O_2$, then the term should be $\dot{V}O_2$peak, not

$\dot{V}O_2$max. Both of these issues are discussed more fully later in the chapter.

EQUIPMENT CONFIGURATIONS

Over the years, $\dot{V}O_2$ during exercise has been measured by five open-circuit equipment configurations, which will be described chronologically. First the measurements that need to be made will be considered. The basic equation is as follows:

$$\dot{V}O_2 = \dot{V}_I F_I O_2 - \dot{V}_E F_{\bar{E}} O_2 \qquad (1)$$

However, it is generally assumed that inspired nitrogen ($\dot{V}_I F_I N_2$) equals expired nitrogen ($\dot{V}_E F_{\bar{E}} N_2$). Thus,

$$\dot{V}_I F_I N_2 = \dot{V}_E F_{\bar{E}} N_2$$

$$\dot{V}_I = \frac{\dot{V}_E F_{\bar{E}} N_2}{F_I N_2} \qquad (2)$$

$$\text{where } F_{\bar{E}} N_2 = 1 - (F_{\bar{E}} O_2 + F_{\bar{E}} CO_2)$$

Replacement of $\dot{V}_I$ with $\dfrac{\dot{V}_E F_{\bar{E}} N_2}{F_I N_2}$ in Equation 1 yields

$$\dot{V}O_2 = \left[\frac{\dot{V}_E F_{\bar{E}} N_2}{F_I N_2} \cdot F_I O_2 \right] - \dot{V}_E F_{\bar{E}} O_2 \qquad (3)$$

$$\dot{V}O_2 = \dot{V}_E \left[\frac{F_{\bar{E}} N_2 \cdot F_I O_2}{F_I N_2} - F_{\bar{E}} O_2 \right] \qquad (4)$$

Under normoxic (room air) conditions, dry $F_I O_2$ equals 0.2093 and dry $F_I N_2$ equals 0.7904. The ratio of dry inspired O_2 to dry inspired N_2 is 0.265. Hence, Equation 4 can be simplified to

$$\dot{V}O_2 = \dot{V}_E [F_{\bar{E}} N_2 (0.265) - F_{\bar{E}} O_2] \qquad (5)$$

Therefore, the quantities to measure for determination of $\dot{V}O_2$ at the mouth are $\dot{V}_E$, $F_{\bar{E}} O_2$, and $F_{\bar{E}} CO_2$.

Historical Development

One of the first open-circuit equipment configurations used to measure $\dot{V}O_2$ during exercise was the Tissot spirometer/volumetric gas analyzer system. Expired ventilation was measured by the Tissot spirometer. An aliquot sample of the mixed-expired gas was drawn from the spirometer and analyzed by a volumetric gas analyzer (e.g., a Haldane or Scholander) for fractional concentrations of O_2 and CO_2.

A slight variation of the Tissot spirometer/volumetric gas analyzer system was the Douglas bag/volumetric gas analyzer system. In later years, lightweight meteorological balloons replaced the heavy, bulky Douglas bags, and a gas meter replaced the Tissot spirometer for measurement of gas volume. In time, electronic gas analyzers replaced the volumetric gas analyzers. Thus, the meteorological balloon/electronic gas analyzer system was born.

The next development in equipment configuration was the semiautomated system (2). In this system, the subject's expired air went first into a mixing chamber and then into a gas meter. A pump pulled approximately 500 ml of gas per minute from the mixing chamber and sent it to a small anesthesia bag; a second pump pulled the gas from the anesthesia bag and sent it to the electronic analyzers for determination of $F_{\bar{E}} O_2$ and $F_{\bar{E}} CO_2$. There were three anesthesia bags in total. While the contents of one bag were being sampled by the gas analyzers, a second bag was being filled with gas from the mixing chamber, and a third bag was being evacuated. The bags were part of a spinner device that was manually rotated 120° each minute so that the previously evacuated bag would now be filling with gas from the mixing chamber, and so on. A problem with this mixing chamber system is that the measurements of ventilation and of the mixed-expired gas fractions are made at different times; ventilation is measured without any delay, but measurement of the mixed-expired gases is delayed because the gas must travel through tubing and the mixing chamber. Unless the mixed-expired gas fractions are not changing, the calculated $\dot{V}O_2$ will be in error. The magnitude of the error depends on the degree of temporal misalignment between the measurements of ventilation and the mixed-expired gas fractions. Fortunately, at heavy exercise, the ventilation is usually large enough to cause the temporal misalignment to be quite small, resulting in very little error in the calculated $\dot{V}O_2$max value.

Following the semiautomated system was the automated system—the Metabolic Measuring Cart (MMC)—developed by Beckman Instruments (3). This system measured ventilation with a turbine volume transducer (4), had a mixing chamber, and measured the mixed-expired gas fractions with O_2 and CO_2 electronic analyzers. The MMC did not have the anesthesia bag arrangement of the semiautomated system. The gas drawn from the mixing chamber was sent directly to the O_2 and CO_2 analyzers. A small computer was an attractive feature of the MMC. The analog signals from the turbine volume transducer and the electronic gas analyzers were sampled by the computer over a duration of typically 1 min. The computer then calculated the standard variables of interest (e.g., $\dot{V}O_2$, $\dot{V}CO_2$, and R, the respiratory exchange ratio), and outputted them via a printer a few seconds after the end of the sampling interval.

The MMC had many advantages over its predecessors. It eliminated the need to hand-calculate the variables of interest. There was no spinner device to manually turn after each sampling interval. It provided nearly on-line analysis of gas exchange (e.g., $\dot{V}O_2$ and $\dot{V}CO_2$). It did have one limitation: No attempt was made to temporally align ventilation and the mixed-expired gas fractions. However, the second generation of the MMC—the MMC

Horizon—was programmed to time-align these signals so that the accuracy of the computed $\dot{V}O_2$ and $\dot{V}CO_2$ would be independent of the ventilation magnitude (5).

The equipment configurations just described collected or sampled many breaths over some time interval, typically 1 min. The calculated $\dot{V}O_2$ represented the average $\dot{V}O_2$ during the sampling interval. These types of equipment configurations are sufficient for the measurement of $\dot{V}O_2$max. However, other parameters, most notably the time constant for $\dot{V}O_2$ kinetics, require a greater density of data. Hence, an equipment configuration was designed to provide on-line, breath-by-breath analysis of ventilation and gas exchange. A detailed description of the breath-by-breath measurement of pulmonary gas exchange is contained in the next chapter. Breath-by-breath systems became commercially available in the early 1980s.

Currently Used Systems

Of the five equipment configurations just described, three are routinely used today to measure $\dot{V}O_2$max. A description of two of these systems follows. The third system, which utilizes breath-by-breath measurements, is described in chapter 3.

The least sophisticated but perhaps the most practical system for measurement of $\dot{V}O_2$max consists of meteorological balloons and electronic O_2 and CO_2 gas analyzers. Fay et al. (6) recently used this system to measure the $\dot{V}O_2$max values of female distance runners. In their system, expired gas was directed through 3.175-cm ID smooth rubber tubing, corrugated plastic tubing, and a three-way, low-turbulence Collins valve into meteorological balloons. Expired gas was collected continuously in 30-s intervals after the subject indicated that she could run only 90 s longer. An aliquot sample was taken from each meteorological balloon and analyzed for fractional concentrations of O_2 and CO_2 with a Beckman E-2 analyzer and a Godart Capnograph, respectively. Reference gases for calibration of the electronic gas analyzers were verified with the Scholander apparatus. Expired gas volumes were measured with an American Meter Company dry gas meter (model 5-M-201). Oxygen uptake was calculated using Equation 5, presented earlier in the chapter.

The meteorological balloon/electronic gas analyzer system has become the gold standard against which other systems are validated. The validation of a system is typically done not at $\dot{V}O_2$max but instead at steady-state values for $\dot{V}O_2$ that represent a large physiological range. Test-retest reliability data are available for the $\dot{V}O_2$max measurement by the meteorological balloon/electronic gas analyzer system of McArdle, Katch, and Pechar (7). They performed duplicate cycle ergometer GXTs on 15 college-aged males. The mean ±SD $\dot{V}O_2$max values for the first and second tests were 4.157 ±0.445 and 4.146 ±0.480 L · min⁻¹, respectively. The standard error of estimate was low (0.094 L ·

min⁻¹) and the correlation coefficient was high (.959). Hence, the meteorological balloon/electronic gas analyzer system can provide excellent test-retest reliability.

The MMC Horizon (5) is an example of a widely used, contemporary mixing chamber system. It is an integrated instrument (see Figure 2.1) controlled by an INTEL 8085A microprocessor. The processor has 71K of random access memory and dual floppy disks for program and data storage; the processor controls a printer-plotter, an alphanumeric display, and a keyboard of alphanumeric and dedicated functions in addition to sensors, transducers, and sample-handling equipment. Expired gas travels through 1.8 m of 3.5-cm ID tubing connected to a 3-L mixing chamber. Gas is pulled from the mixing chamber at a rate of 0.5 L · min⁻¹ and sent to fast-responding, electronic O_2 and CO_2 analyzers. At the distal end of the mixing chamber, a turbine volume transducer measures the gas volume. Included as part of the MMC Horizon hardware are two E-size gas cylinders for calibration of the electronic gas analyzers; one is the zero gas and the other is the span gas. The processor controls an automatic calibration routine for the gas analyzers. Volume calibration requires the delivery of a 1-L volume of gas at three different flow rates using a manual pump. A time-alignment procedure is incorporated into the software to delay ventilation measurements and align them to the $F_{\bar{E}}O_2$ and $F_{\bar{E}}CO_2$ measurements.

The validity of $\dot{V}O_2$ measurements made by the MMC Horizon was investigated by Jones (5). He compared the $\dot{V}O_2$ measured in the steady state by the MMC Horizon to that measured by a reference system consisting of a dry gas meter (Parkinson-Cowan, CD4) and a mass spectrometer (Perkin Elmer, MGA 1100). Excellent agreement between the two systems was obtained and is shown in Figure 2.2. Davis et al. (8) examined the test-retest reliability of $\dot{V}O_2$max measurements made using a mixing chamber system. Thirty male subjects performed duplicate arm-cranking, leg-cycling, and treadmill-running GXTs. The test-retest correlation coefficients of $\dot{V}O_2$max for each of these GXT modes were .92, .94, and .96, respectively.

Whether one uses a meteorological balloon/electronic gas analyzer system or a mixing chamber system to measure $\dot{V}O_2$max, there are general features of any system that are desirable. First, the system should not have any leaks. Second, the resistance to inspiration or expiration caused by the system should be less than ±5 cm H_2O pressure at any ventilation. Third, the device used to measure gas volume should provide measurements to within 1% of the true value. Fourth, the device(s) used to measure fractional gas concentrations should be able to measure both O_2 and CO_2 to within 0.0003 of their true values.

EXERCISE TEST MODES

There are two popular exercise testing modes: the cycle ergometer and the motor-driven treadmill. On the

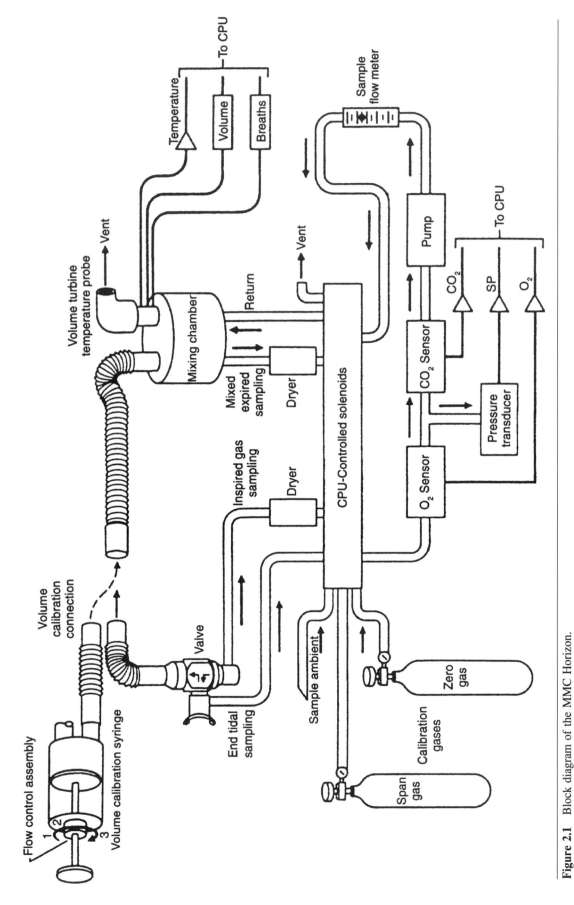

Figure 2.1   Block diagram of the MMC Horizon.

From "Evaluation of a Microprocessor-Controlled Exercise Testing System" by N.L. Jones, 1984, *Journal of Applied Physiology*, **57**, p. 1313. Copyright by American Physiological Society. Reprinted by permission.

Oxygen intake ml/min STPD

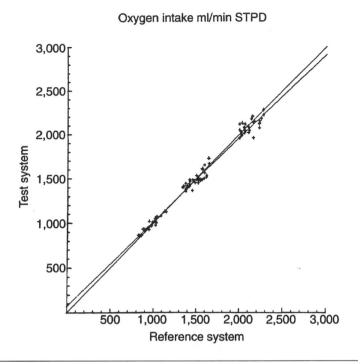

Figure 2.2   Validation of the $\dot{V}O_2$ measurement by the MMC Horizon during steady-state exercise. The regression of $\dot{V}O_2$ measured by the test system versus $\dot{V}O_2$ measured by the reference system was $Y = 0.945X + 72.7$ ml · min^{-1} with $r = 0.997$. From "Evaluation of a Microprocessor-Controlled Exercise Testing System" by N.L. Jones, 1984, *Journal of Applied Physiology*, **57**, p. 1316. Copyright by American Physiological Society. Reprinted by permission.

treadmill, the subject can be restricted to walking or to running. Maximal $\dot{V}O_2$ values are approximately 10% higher when measured during treadmill running, compared to cycle ergometry (9).

EXERCISE TESTING PROTOCOLS

The most widely used exercise testing protocols are continuous and graded. The study by Buchfuhrer et al. (10) will be reviewed before discussing specific GXT protocols. Buchfuhrer et al. examined the possibility that the $\dot{V}O_2$max measurement was protocol dependent. They found that "fast" protocols (those with large work-rate increments per minute) and "slow" protocols (those with small work-rate increments per minute) caused underestimations of the true $\dot{V}O_2$max value, which was found using "intermediate-speed" protocols. Buchfuhrer et al. suggested that the fast protocols caused their subjects to terminate the GXT early because of insufficient muscle strength to accommodate the large work-rate increases during the final stages of the test. There are two likely reasons why Buchfuhrer et al. found low $\dot{V}O_2$max values for the slow protocols. First, these protocols, which lasted an average of 18 min for

cycle ergometry and 26 min for treadmill exercise, would be expected to result in a significant increase in core temperature. This increase, in turn, would result in a redistribution of the cardiac output so that less blood (and therefore less O_2) would be going to the exercising musculature and more blood would be going to the cutaneous circulation in an effort to dissipate heat. Less blood flow (and therefore less O_2 delivery) to the working muscles at maximal work rates would explain the lower $\dot{V}O_2$max values found for the slow protocols. A second plausible explanation for this finding is subject motivation. The slow protocols are particularly exhausting, requiring high motivation on the part of the subject to deal with the high levels of lactate and heat associated with heavy, prolonged exercise. Buchfuhrer et al. found the highest $\dot{V}O_2$max values with GXT protocols that lasted 8 to 12 min.

Using the results of Buchfuhrer et al., GXT protocols should be designed to cause the test to end somewhere between 8 and 12 min. An example will demonstrate how the increment size can be found. Consider a subject with a predicted $\dot{V}O_2$max of 3,000 ml · min^{-1} for a cycle ergometer GXT. According to Wasserman and Whipp (11), the relationship between $\dot{V}O_2$ in milliliters per minute (ml · min^{-1}) and work rate (WR) in watts (W) for cycle ergometry is given by the following linear regression equation:

$$\dot{V}O_2 = 10 \text{ ml} \cdot \text{min}^{-1} \cdot \text{W}^{-1}(\text{WR}) + 500 \text{ ml} \cdot \text{min}^{-1}$$

Solving for the work rate that would result in a $\dot{V}O_2$ of 3,000 ml · min^{-1} yields 250 W. The increment size per minute that would produce a test duration of 8 min is 31 W (250 W/8 min). For a test duration of 12 min, the increment size per minute would be 21 W (250 W/12 min). A prudent choice of the increment size per minute would be 25 W, which would produce a test duration of approximately 10 min.

The most widely used cycle ergometer GXT protocols have a warm-up period of approximately 4 min. The work rate during the warm-up period is typically unloaded cycling or a light work rate such as 15 W. Immediately after the 4-min warm-up, the work rate is incremented by x W each minute until the subject reaches his or her limit of tolerance; x is the increment size that is predicted to produce a test duration somewhere between 8 and 12 min from the time the work-rate increments begin. These cycle ergometer protocols can be used to test the entire spectrum of subjects, from elite athletes to patients with cardiopulmonary disease. Only the increment size needs to be adjusted. Regarding the pedal frequency during cycle ergometry GXT, Hermansen and Saltin (12) found that 60 rpm gave higher $\dot{V}O_2$max values than did 50, 70, or 80 rpm. Hence, it is suggested that the pedal frequency for cycle ergometry GXT be 60 rpm.

Of the treadmill GXT protocols, the Balke walking test (13) has been widely used. The protocol calls for a constant speed of 3.4 mph throughout the test. The grade is 0% for the first 2 min. The grade is then raised to 2% and increased 1% per minute thereafter until the subject reaches his or her limit of tolerance. For low-fit subjects, this protocol elicits valid $\dot{V}O_2$max values. However, for fitter subjects, the test duration is very long. Also, these subjects are required to walk at grades above 20% during the last few minutes of the test and complain of severe local discomfort in the lower back and calf muscles, which may limit their ability to achieve maximal work rates. McArdle, Katch, and Pechar (7) compared $\dot{V}O_2$max values measured using the Balke walking treadmill test to those measured using running treadmill tests in reasonably fit male subjects. They found that the Balke walking test yielded $\dot{V}O_2$max values that were approximately 5% lower than those obtained on the running tests. The Balke test could be modified to use a faster walking speed, which would likely result in increased $\dot{V}O_2$max values for fitter subjects.

A typical running treadmill protocol is that of Maksud and Coutts (14). It begins with the subject running at 6 mph on the level (0% grade) for 2 min. Thereafter, the grade is increased by 2.5% each 2 min; the speed is constant throughout the test.

Each of the protocols previously described is continuous. Some GXT protocols are discontinuous. An example is the treadmill test of Mitchell, Sproule, and Chapman (15). The test begins with the subject walking at 3 mph for 10 min at a 10% grade. Then the subject rests for 10 min. Next, the subject runs for 2.5 min at 6 mph up a 2.5% grade. After another 10-min rest period, the subject runs for 2.5 min at 6 mph up a 5.0% grade. This procedure (rest, 2.5% grade increase) is continued until the subject reaches his or her limit of tolerance.

The $\dot{V}O_2$max obtained using a continuous protocol is the same as that obtained using a discontinuous protocol. McArdle, Katch, and Pechar (7) compared the continuous Maksud and Coutts treadmill protocol to the discontinuous Mitchell, Sproule, and Chapman treadmill protocol in 15 college-aged males. The mean $\dot{V}O_2$max values for the continuous and discontinuous protocols were very similar, 4.109 and 4.145 L · min^{-1}, respectively. What differed markedly was the test duration: 12.3 min for the continuous test and 67.3 min for the discontinuous test. Both the subjects and the investigators preferred the continuous test for its shorter duration.

Three clinical treadmill protocols designed by cardiologists to test patients with heart disease are popular. Figure 2.3 shows the protocols of Naughton, Ellestad, and Bruce.

CRITERIA FOR ACHIEVEMENT OF $\dot{V}O_2$max

The most widely accepted criterion for the achievement of $\dot{V}O_2$max during GXT is a plateau in $\dot{V}O_2$ as the work rate continues to increase. However, typically less than 50% of subjects tested actually demonstrate a plateau. Cumming and Borysyk (16) administered GXT to 65 men aged 40 to 65 years. Only 43% of these men met the plateau requirement. Freedson et al. (17) found that fewer than 40% of 301 adults undergoing GXT demonstrated a plateau. Cumming and Friesen (18), Cunningham et al. (19), and Åstrand (20) found that fewer than 50% of young boys who underwent GXT actually demonstrated a plateau. Indeed, as Noakes (21) recently pointed out, even the original investigators who developed the plateau criterion failed to find a true plateau in $\dot{V}O_2$ as the work rate continued to increase.

There are three other criteria often used to defend the achievement of $\dot{V}O_2$max: (a) blood lactate concentration in the first 5 min of recovery > 8 mmol · L^{-1}, (b) respiratory exchange ratio at test termination > 1.00, and (c) heart rate at test termination > 85% of age-predicted maximum. The third criterion is the least rigorous because of the well-known large variation in maximal heart rate at any given age.

It has been suggested that if a subject fails to demonstrate a plateau in $\dot{V}O_2$ as the work rate continues to increase, he or she then reached a $\dot{V}O_2$peak, not a $\dot{V}O_2$max. However, given the current controversy concerning the plateau criterion for achievement of $\dot{V}O_2$max, many investigators readily accept that the subject has achieved $\dot{V}O_2$max if he or she meets any of the four previously listed criteria.

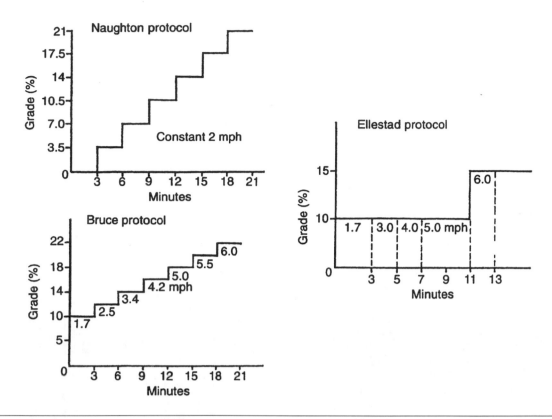

Figure 2.3 Three commonly used treadmill protocols for patients with heart disease.
From *American College of Sports Medicine: Guidelines for Exercise Testing and Prescription*, 3rd ed. (p. 20), 1986, Philadelphia: Lea & Febiger. Copyright 1986 by Lea & Febiger. Adapted by permission.

For patients, especially those with heart disease, a special term has been developed: *symptom-limited* $\dot{V}O_2max$. This is simply the highest $\dot{V}O_2$ measured before the patient had to stop exercising because of symptoms (e.g., severe angina).

NORMATIVE DATA

Many factors are known to influence $\dot{V}O_2max$. Bed rest causes it to go down, whereas endurance exercise training increases it (22). When $\dot{V}O_2max$ is expressed in terms of liters per minute, large people (those with increased height and/or weight) have higher values. Women have lower $\dot{V}O_2$-max values than do men. Old adults have lower $\dot{V}O_2max$ values than do young adults. These factors (extent of physical activity in leisure time, height, weight, gender, and age) can be used to predict $\dot{V}O_2max$ with some degree of confidence. Jones et al. (23) performed cycle ergometer GXTs on 50 male and 50 female subjects of various fitness levels who ranged in age from 15 to 71 years. From the data collected, they developed the following multiple linear regression equation:

$$\dot{V}O_2max \ (L \cdot min^{-1}) = 0.025 \ (Ht) -$$

$$0.023 \ (Age) - 0.542 \ (Gender) +$$

$$0.019 \ (Wt) + 0.15 \ (Lei) - 2.32 \ L \cdot min^{-1}$$

where *Ht* is standing height in centimeters, *Age* is in years, and *Wt* is body weight in kilograms. For male subjects, the gender code is 0. For female subjects, the gender code is 1. *Lei* is leisure time spent per week in physical activity. The four grades of leisure activity are as follows: Grade 1 for less than 1 hr/week, Grade 2 for 1 to 3 hr/week, Grade 3 for 3 to 6 hr/week, and Grade 4 for more than 6 hr/week. An example will illustrate how this equation can be used to predict $\dot{V}O_2max$. Assume a 44-year-old male subject is 183 cm tall, his weight is 70 kg, and he jogs 2.5 hr per week (hence, his leisure activity grade is 2). Plugging these numbers into the previous equation yields a predicted $\dot{V}O_2max$ of 2.87 L · min⁻¹. The multiple correlation coefficient for this equation is .892, and the standard error of estimate is 0.415 L · min⁻¹. This latter statistic can be used to compute the upper and lower 95% confidence limits of the predicted value. In the previous example, the predicted $\dot{V}O_2max$ value of 2.87 L · min⁻¹ would have lower and upper 95% confidence limits of 2.05 and 3.69 L · min⁻¹, respectively.

Åstrand and Rodahl (24) have tabulated the $\dot{V}O_2max$ values of many athletic groups (see Figure 2.4). Note that endurance athletes have the highest values. For one male cross-country skier, $\dot{V}O_2max$ was

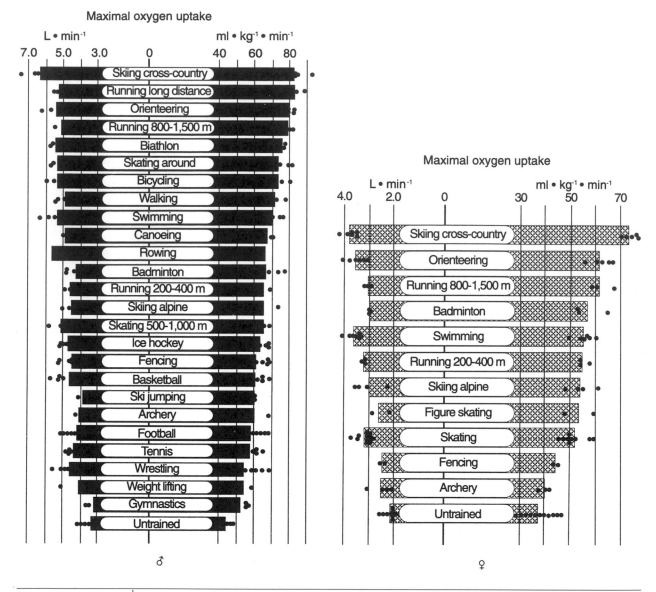

Figure 2.4 Maximal $\dot{V}O_2$ in L · min⁻¹ and ml · min⁻¹ · kg of body weight for male (left panel) and female Swedish national team athletes from different sports. Dots represent individual values that are higher than the mean value.
From *Textbook of Work Physiology* (pp. 414-415), 1986, New York: McGraw-Hill. Copyright 1986 by McGraw-Hill. Reprinted by permission.

measured at 7.4 L · min⁻¹ or 94 ml · min⁻¹ · kg⁻¹ body weight.

SUMMARY

Three systems are currently used to measure $\dot{V}O_2$max: the meteorological balloon/electronic gas analyzer system, the mixing chamber system, and the breath-by-breath system described in chapter 3. Each of these systems, when used properly, is capable of providing valid and reliable measurements of $\dot{V}O_2$max. Should readers desire additional information on this topic, I suggest that they read the excellent reviews of Thoden, Wilson, and MacDougall (25) and Holly (26).

REFERENCES

1. Whipp, B.J., Davis, J.A., Torres, F., & Wasserman, K. (1981). A test to determine the parameters of aerobic function during exercise. *Journal of Applied Physiology*, **50**, 217-221.
2. Wilmore, J.H., & Costill, D.L. (1974). Semiautomated systems approach to the assessment of oxygen uptake during exercise. *Journal of Applied Physiology*, **36**, 618-620.

3. Wilmore, J.H., Davis, J.A., & Norton, A.C. (1976). An automated system for assessing metabolic and respiratory function during exercise. *Journal of Applied Physiology*, **40**, 619-624.

4. Davis, J.A., & Lamarra, N. (1984). A turbine device for accurate volume measurement during exercise [Abstract]. *Aviation, Space, and Environmental Medicine*, **55**, 472.

5. Jones, N.L. (1984). Evaluation of a microprocessor-controlled exercise testing system. *Journal of Applied Physiology*, **57**, 1312-1318.

6. Fay, L., Londeree, B.R., LaFontaine, T.P., & Volek, M.R. (1989). Physiological parameters related to distance running performance in female athletes. *Medicine and Science in Sports and Exercise*, **21**, 319-324.

7. McArdle, W.D., Katch, F.I., & Pechar, G.S. (1973). Comparison of continuous and discontinuous treadmill and bicycle tests for max $\dot{V}O_2$. *Medicine and Science in Sports*, **5**, 156-160.

8. Davis, J.A., Vodak, P., Wilmore, J.H., Vodak, J., & Kurtz, P. (1976). Anaerobic threshold and maximal aerobic power for three modes of exercise. *Journal of Applied Physiology*, **41**, 544-550.

9. Davis, J.A., & Kasch, F.W. (1975). Aerobic and anaerobic differences between maximal running and cycling in middle-aged males. *Australian Journal of Sports Medicine*, **7**, 81-84.

10. Buchfuhrer, M.J., Hansen, J.E., Robinson, T.E., Sue, D.Y., Wasserman, K., & Whipp, B.J. (1983). Optimizing the exercise protocol for cardiopulmonary assessment. *Journal of Applied Physiology*, **55**, 558-564.

11. Wasserman, K., & Whipp, B.J. (1975). Exercise physiology in health and disease. *American Review of Respiratory Disease*, **112**, 219-249.

12. Hermansen, L., & Saltin, B. (1969). Oxygen uptake during maximal treadmill and bicycle exercise. *Journal of Applied Physiology*, **26**, 31-37.

13. *Guidelines for exercise testing and prescription* (3rd ed.). (1986). Philadelphia: Lea & Febiger.

14. Maksud, M.G., & Coutts, K.D. (1971). Comparison of a continuous and discontinuous graded treadmill test for maximal oxygen uptake. *Medicine and Science in Sports*, **3**, 63-65.

15. Mitchell, J.H., Sproule, B.J., & Chapman, C.B. (1958). The physiological meaning of the maximal oxygen uptake test. *Journal of Clinical Investigation*, **37**, 538-547.

16. Cumming, G.R., & Borysyk, L.M. (1972). Criteria for maximum oxygen uptake in men over 40 in a population survey. *Medicine and Science in Sports*, **14**, 18-22.

17. Freedson, P., Kline, G., Porcari, J., Hintermeister, R., McCarron, R., Ross, J., Ward, A., Gurry, M., & Rippe, J. (1986). Criteria for defining $\dot{V}O_2$max: A new approach to an old problem [Abstract]. *Medicine and Science in Sports and Exercise*, **18**, S36.

18. Cumming, G.R., & Friesen, W. (1967). Bicycle ergometer measurement of maximal oxygen uptake in children. *Canadian Journal of Physiology and Pharmacology*, **45**, 937-946.

19. Cunningham, D.A., Van Waterschoot, B.M., Paterson, D.H., Lefcoe, M., & Sangal, S.P. (1977). Reliability and reproducibility of maximal oxygen uptake measurement in children. *Medicine and Science in Sports*, **9**, 104-108.

20. Åstrand, P.-O. (1952). *Experimental studies of physical work capacity in relation to sex and age*. Copenhagen, Denmark: Munksgaard.

21. Noakes, T.D. (1988). Implications of exercise testing for prediction of athletic performance: A contemporary perspective. *Medicine and Science in Sports and Exercise*, **20**, 319-330.

22. Saltin, B., Blomquist, G., Mitchell, J.H., Johnson, R.L., Wildenthal, K., & Chapman, C.B. (1968). *Response to exercise after bed rest and after training*. New York: American Heart Association.

23. Jones, N.L., Makrides, L., Hitchcock, C., Chypchar, T., & McCartney, N. (1985). Normal standards for an incremental progressive cycle ergometer test. *American Review of Respiratory Disease*, **131**, 700-708.

24. Åstrand, P.-O., & Rodahl, K. (1986). *Textbook of work physiology* (3rd ed.). New York: McGraw-Hill.

25. Thoden, J.S., Wilson, B.A., & MacDougall, J.D. (1982). Testing aerobic power. In J.D. MacDougall, H.A. Wenger, & H.J. Green (Eds.), *Physiological testing of the elite athlete* (pp. 39-60). Ithaca, NY: Mouvement.

26. Holly, R.G. (1988). Measurement of the maximal rate of oxygen uptake. In S.N. Blair, P. Painter, R.R. Pate, L.K. Smith, and C.B. Taylor (Eds.), *Resource manual for guidelines for exercise testing and prescription* (pp. 171-177). Philadelphia: Lea & Febiger.

CHAPTER 3

Measurement of Pulmonary Gas Exchange

Norman Lamarra, PhD

University of California, Los Angeles

Brian Whipp, PhD, DSc

St. George's Hospital Medical School, London

Breath-by-breath measurement of pulmonary gas exchange (PGE) has become routine and essential for many investigations, from clinical diagnosis to scientific research. This chapter outlines the methods currently available for such measurement, and explores the (sometimes subtle) assumptions, implications, and error sources associated with each. The chapter progresses from discrete measurement of PGE through continuous measurement of nonsteady-state PGE, and contains a section on validation techniques. It ends with examples of state-of-the-art concepts, and the application of PGE measurement to exercise testing and evaluation. Some of the concepts are quite technical in nature, but unless they are understood adequately, erroneous interpretations might be drawn confidently from data that are (incorrectly) believed accurate, with potentially disastrous consequences.

The pattern of pulmonary gas exchange during muscular exercise in humans is currently being interpreted for determining the

- maximum O_2-uptake rate ($\mu \dot{V}O_2$),
- threshold of metabolic (lactic) acidosis ($\hat{\theta}_L$) (the estimator symbol [ˆ] is used when the variable or parameter under consideration is not directly measured, but estimated indirectly [39]),
- efficiency of muscular power generation (η),
- time constant for the O_2-uptake kinetics ($\tau \dot{V}O_2$),
- work-rate equivalent of the highest sustainable lactate ($\hat{\theta}_r$),
- partitions of the tolerable work-rate range representing different intensity domains, and
- optimal work rate, at least in theory, for use in endurance training.

It has also recently been developed as a means of

- discriminating among causes of exercise intolerance in patients with exertional dyspnea (shortness of breath),

- establishing categories of impairment in patients with cardiopulmonary (and other) diseases,
- assessing the efficacy of intervention programs aimed at improving systemic functioning in such patients, using both drug and rehabilitation strategies, and
- aiding in diagnosis of hitherto unsuspected disease.

The obvious importance of obtaining such information has led recently to more clinical exercise laboratories utilizing gas-exchange determinations. Laboratories also incorporate dynamic gas-exchange analysis into the array of assessment techniques they use to establish fitness profiles and develop training strategies for athletes.

The dogma that the interpretation cannot be better than the quality of the data themselves is rarely more applicable than in clinical exercise testing, where the consequences of misinterpretation based upon faulty data can be so dire. We shall therefore consider the fundamentals of determining the time course of pulmonary gas exchange (PGE) over prolonged time frames, then over the duration of a single breath, and finally even continuously within the breath.

BACKGROUND

An excellent review of the history behind the concepts discussed in this chapter may be found in the chapter by Perkins (33) in *Handbook of Physiology*. As described there, interest in the determination of gas exchange during exercise originated with the seminal work of Lavoisier (1, 34) in the 18th century. Contemporary exercise scientists also owe a great debt to the pioneering work of Geppert and Zuntz (2) in the later part of the 19th century, who established the fundamentals of pulmonary gas-exchange measurement, including correction for the disparity between inspired and expired volumes when the respiratory gas-exchange ratio ($R = \dot{V}CO_2/\dot{V}O_2$) does not equal unity (curiously, this is often termed the "Haldane" correction—see [3] for discussion). This correction is based upon the demonstration that the inspired N_2 fraction differs from the expired N_2 fraction if the inspiratory and expiratory tidal volumes are different, assuming no net nitrogen transport over the breath—a phenomenon that was first demonstrated by Lavoisier (1), using tedious but precise measurement techniques.

During the first half of this century, the development of reliable microtechniques for measuring respired gas concentrations by chemical extraction (such as the Haldane [4] or Scholander [5] methods) simplified the procedure somewhat, but these techniques were still extremely time consuming. Consequently, much information recently extracted by more sophisticated techniques was hidden from these early investigators. Today

it is routinely possible to measure respired gas concentrations with errors below 0.1% or even 0.01%, using instruments with response-time constants of a fraction of a second, incorporated into systems that automate the computation (and even allow immediate display) of the gas-exchange responses. However, certain fundamental facts of the determination must be understood *a fortiori* before such results can be taken for granted and interpretation attempted. With this in mind, the following sections outline the underlying methods available today for measurement of PGE and indicate the realm of applicability and the inherent assumptions associated with each.

DISCRETE MEASUREMENT OF PGE

Steady-State PGE

Discrete Measurement

The simplest useful measurement of ventilation and gas exchange is obtained by collecting the expirate of a subject believed to be in a steady state (e.g., at rest or in an equilibrium of moderate exercise). If only ventilation is required, the expirate may be collected directly into a spirometer (Tissot, rolling-seal, etc.) and the measurement requires only relatively simple transformation from the (ambient) collection conditions to either STPD (standard temperature and pressure, dry—i.e., 273 K and 760 Torr with no water vapor) or BTPS (body temperature and pressure, saturated—e.g., 310 K, ambient pressure, saturated). For example, suppose a subject in a steady state at rest exhales 20 L during a 3-min period through a two-way breathing valve directly into a calibrated spirometer; the (minute) ventilation $\dot{V}_E$ is

$$\dot{V}_E = \frac{20}{3} \cdot a \cdot b \cdot c \text{ L} \cdot \text{min}^{-1} \text{ STPD} \qquad (1)$$

where

$$a = (763 - 12)/763,$$
$$b = 273/(273 + 21), \text{ and}$$
$$c = 760/763.$$

Factor (a) removes the water vapor content from the saturated expirate at ambient temperature and pressure (12 Torr water vapor pressure here), giving dry ambient gas volume; factor (b) corrects this dry gas volume from collection temperature (21 °C here) to standard temperature (273 K); and factor (c) corrects the dry gas volume at standard temperature and ambient barometric pressure (763 Torr here) to standard pressure (760 Torr), finally producing the required STPD conditions. Typically, however, expiratory ventilation is expressed as BTPS, because the STPD value does not indicate what the subject's lungs were actually exhaling. The correction factor to convert the ventilation in Equation 1 from STPD to BTPS is

$$\dot{V}_E BTPS = \dot{V}_{\bar{E}} \; STPD \cdot a \cdot b \cdot c \qquad (2)$$

where

$$a = (273 + 37)/273,$$
$$b = 760/(760 - 47), \text{ and}$$
$$c = 763/760.$$

Factor (a) corrects temperature from 0 °C to 37 °C; factor (b) corrects water vapor content from dry to saturated at body temperature (47 Torr partial pressure); and factor (c) corrects pressure from standard to ambient (in this case, 763 Torr). Even such a simple calculation, however, requires several assumptions: for instance, that the two-way breathing valve, plumbing, and spirometer did not leak; that the expirate had actually settled to the ambient saturated conditions (21 °C) before the volume measurement was made; and that a whole number of breaths was collected. Some of these assumptions can be independently verified, and some may have very small influence on the calculation, but the cumulative effect of even small errors can be surprisingly large, particularly for gas exchange.

Continuing with this simple expirate collection method (6, 7), the subject's oxygen uptake ($\dot{V}O_2$) and carbon dioxide output ($\dot{V}CO_2$) can be calculated from the ventilation by obtaining a single measurement of the average mixed-expired concentration of O_2 and CO_2, respectively, and applying a further set of simplifying assumptions as follows. Such an average mixed-expired gas may be obtained either by collecting the expirate in an evacuated Douglas bag or by passing the expirate through a mixing chamber. The latter is a box (typically 3 to 8 L in volume) whose inlet and outlet are separated by a series of baffles to improve the homogeneity of the mixture (8). The concentrations of the mixed expirate can be measured via a mass-spectrometer or gas-analyzer sampling probe inserted near the outlet of the mixing chamber or of the collection bag. Assuming that the subject's gas stores were the same at the beginning and end of the collection period (i.e., the subject did not lose or retain significant quantities of N_2, and end-expiratory lung volume—EELV—was unchanged), then carbon dioxide output may be estimated by

$$\dot{V}CO_2 = \dot{V}_E \cdot dF_E CO_2 \; L \cdot min^{-1} \; STPD \qquad (3)$$

where ventilation is calculated STPD (e.g., Equation 1), and $dF_E CO_2$ is the difference between mixed-expired

and ambient air CO_2 dry fractional concentrations. A similar calculation for $\dot{V}O_2$ would appear as

$$\dot{V}O_2 = \dot{V}_E \cdot dF_E O_2 \; L \cdot min^{-1} \; STPD \qquad (4)$$

where $dF_E O_2$ is the difference between mixed-expired and ambient air dry O_2 fractions. However, as mentioned earlier, an implicit assumption in Equations 3 and 4 is that the gas-exchange ratio R is equal to 1. If this is so, then both equations will give identical values for $\dot{V}CO_2$ and $\dot{V}O_2$, and both will be accurate. If not, then Equation 4 is in error by an amount that may be large, depending on both the actual value of R and the ambient concentrations of O_2 and CO_2 (9). The error in $\dot{V}O_2$ is shown in Figure 3.1 for three inspirates (room air, a hypoxic, and a hyperoxic mixture) and is generalized by the equation

$$\% \text{ error in } \dot{V}O_2 = F_I O_2 \cdot (1 - 1/R) \cdot 100 \qquad (5)$$

where $F_I O_2$ is the fraction of O_2 in the inspirate. Equation 4 may be improved to take account of this effect by making further use of the assumption that there was no net N_2 transport during the collection period (i.e., that the subject inhaled and exhaled equal quantities of N_2), thus allowing mass balance to be applied as follows. The quantity of N_2 exhaled (and inhaled) is

$$Q_E N_2 = \dot{V}_E \cdot F_E N_2 \cdot T_c = Q_I N_2 \; L \; STPD \qquad (6)$$

where $F_E N_2$ is the average mixed-expired dry fraction of N_2 in the mixing chamber or bag, $\dot{V}_E$ is the average expired ventilation STPD, and the collection period was T_c minutes. Because the inspired air contains a fixed ratio of O_2 to N_2, $F_I O_2 / F_I N_2$, with a value normally about 0.265, the quantity of O_2 inhaled may be calculated as

$$Q_I O_2 = Q_I N_2 \cdot 0.265 = \dot{V}_E \cdot F_E N_2 \cdot 0.265 \cdot T_c \; L \; STPD$$
$$(7)$$

As in Equation 6, the quantity of O_2 exhaled is

$$Q_E O_2 = \dot{V}_E \cdot F_E O_2 \cdot T_c \; L \; STPD \qquad (8)$$

and combining Equations 7 and 8 gives oxygen uptake as

$$\dot{V}O_2 = (Q_I O_2 - Q_E O_2)/T_c = \dot{V}_E(F_E N_2 \cdot 0.265 - F_E O_2)$$
$$(9)$$

(If $F_E N_2$ is not directly measured, then $[1 - F_E CO_2 - F_E O_2]$ may be substituted.) Note that Equation 9 differs from Equation 4 only in the correction factor ($F_E N_2 / F_I N_2$) applied to the inspired O_2 fraction: If, as mentioned before, the gas-exchange ratio R = 1 and the subject's lung stores do not change, then $F_E N_2 = F_I N_2$, and Equation 9 reduces exactly to Equation 4. If dry gas concentrations are not directly obtainable (e.g., discrete gas analyzers are used rather than a mass spectrometer),

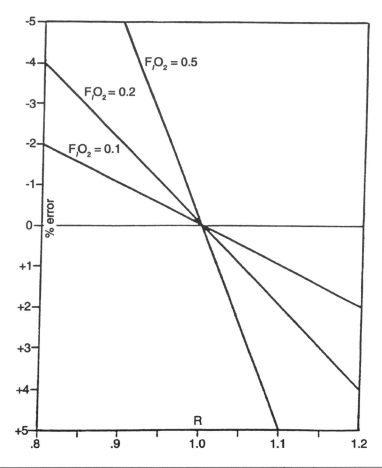

Figure 3.1   Error in $\dot{V}O_2$ calculated by Equation 4, when gas-exchange ratio R is not equal to unity. Error increases with F_IO_2.
From "Quantitative Relationships in Steady-State Gas Exchange" by A.B. Otis. In *Handbook of Physiology* (Vol. 1, pp. 681-698) by W.O. Fenn and H. Rahn (Eds.), 1964, Washington, DC: American Psychological Society. Copyright 1964 by the American Physiological Society. Reprinted by permission.

then the algorithm requires further modification, as discussed in Beaver, Wasserman, and Whipp (12). Other investigators have attempted to heat, cool, or dry the expirate in order to simplify these calculations, but the techniques are generally not suitable for the breath-by-breath analysis to be described later in this chapter, and will not be further discussed here. Further caution is required when considering inspirates different from room air: The above algorithms tend to become computationally unstable for values of F_IO_2 greater than about 0.8, and break down for 100% O_2 inspirate, therefore they may require modification to include measurement of both inspired and expired gases (10).

Continuous Measurement

The foregoing demonstrates that a single measurement of ventilation and gas exchange can be obtained by a straightforward though tedious method, but relies on certain key assumptions. To allow continuous measurement, the calculations may be automated by utilizing continuous sampling of both flow and concentration of the expirate. For example, if the expirate is passed through a flow- or volume-measurement device (such as a pneumotachograph, turbine, hot-wire, or ultrasonic flowmeter), then a microcomputer can be utilized to determine the length and volume of each breath, and thence the average ventilation. The gas concentrations in the mixing chamber can similarly be sampled and averaged by the computer, in order to estimate the average mixed-expired fractional concentrations. Equations 3 and 9 can then be applied to the measurements of $\dot{V}_E$ and mixed-expired concentrations—for example, by taking the average of the nearest whole number of breaths in each consecutive 30-s time interval. The results can be printed on-line while the computer continues to collect data or can be stored for later analysis. Several commercially available systems perform such computation and graphical display; they also automate the procedure of calibrating the transducers that measure flow and gas concentration. As can be seen from the simplicity of the equations, the required computational power is very small and is easily achieved by personal computers and even by programmable calculators (38).

The accuracy of the techniques we have described depends on the adequacy of the mixing, which in turn depends on the size of the mixing chamber relative to the tidal volume. If the tidal volume is high, then each breath will displace a large fraction of the mixed gas in the chamber, potentially making the gas concentration at the outlet change with each breath. If this occurs, then an accurate estimate of mixed-expired concentration can be obtained only by careful selection of the time period used for averaging the measured concentration. Clearly, the larger the volume of the mixing chamber (the larger the number of breaths averaged), the less important this consideration becomes, but on the other hand the longer will be the time taken to reach a steady state, and the more prominent will be the "slurring" of the response if it is actually changing, as we shall see in what follows.

Nonsteady-State PGE

The preceding discussion is based on the assumption that the subject is in a metabolic steady state. However, in awake daily life, a steady state is rarely achieved, and for the purposes of patient evaluation or research study it is often not particularly useful. Analysis of the nonsteady state, on the other hand, provides even more diagnostic information regarding the cardiorespiratory system's behavior, such as the responses to an abrupt change from one level of exercise to another. Accurate study of such responses, however, necessitates careful reevaluation of the assumptions outlined in Equations 1 through 9. A typical protocol requires a normal subject to remain at rest or to exercise for 6 min on a cycle ergometer with no load ("0" watts), after which the load is suddenly increased to 100 W (step change); the subject's heart rate, ventilation, and gas-exchange responses will adjust to the increased metabolic demand in an approximately exponential manner (13, 14, 15) as shown by the breath-by-breath response in Figure 3.2. Clearly, collecting the expirate in a spirometer would allow very few measurements to be made during the transition period, which lasts only 2 to 4 min. However, continuous measurements provided by the mixing chamber arrangement could be utilized to provide average values for $\dot{V}_E$, $\dot{V}CO_2$ and $\dot{V}O_2$ every 15 to 30 s, for example. Unfortunately, the accuracy of even such

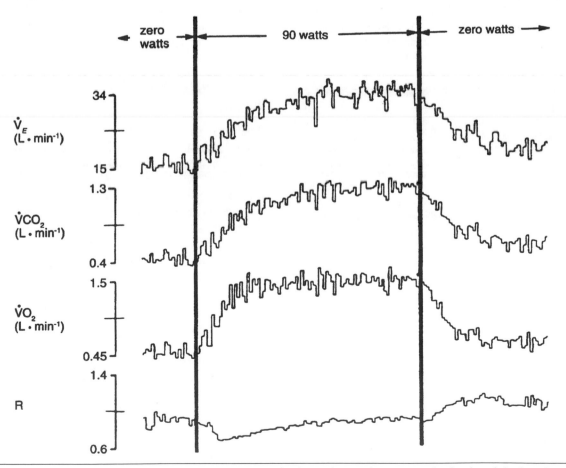

Figure 3.2 Pulmonary gas-exchange response pattern to a step change in exercise, measured using breath-by-breath computation.

"continuous" measurement becomes quite dependent (in the nonsteady state) on correct alignment of the gas-concentration measurements with the flow measurements (8), and quite large systematic errors are possible.

There are three approaches to improving the achievable measurement accuracy in these situations (i.e., for nonsteady-state PGE):

- Attempting to perform appropriate time alignment of the flow signal with the mixed-expired concentration signal
- Attempting to establish the time profile of the gas concentration signal at the "input" of the mixing chamber (i.e., the time course of the *subject's* mixed-expired concentration) from that measured at the "output," using system-analytic techniques (*deconvolution*, or modeling)
- Performing discrete analysis on each breath separately (breath-by-breath measurement)

The problem with the first approach is that, in the nonsteady state, the subject's mixed-expired concentration is typically changing, but the "inertia" of the mixing chamber causes the output values to be "slurred." A simplified view of this slurring has been proposed by several investigators, who note that a step change of mixed-expired concentration at the input to the mixing chamber produces an exponentially rising response at the output, with a time constant that depends on the size of the mixing chamber and the average flow rate through it. If the subject's mixed-expired concentration is changing more rapidly than this time constant, no simple technique will allow adequate reconstruction of the input from the output time course. However, when it changes slowly with respect to this time constant, a useful approximation to the desired input can be obtained by observing the output one time constant later. Because the value of this time constant depends linearly on the flow rate, it can be expressed in terms of an effective "volume shift" on the flow signal (8).

In many cases, this approach gives acceptable results, but in others there may still be systematic errors. This is because the output signal values might never reach those of the input signal, and when they do not, the desired input signal cannot be derived by using *any* time shift of the output. A simple example illustrates the problem: If the mixed-expired CO_2 concentration rises linearly, then begins to fall linearly—a profile characteristic of incremental exercise testing—then the output signal will rise linearly to follow the input, with a time lag proportional to the chamber's time constant; but it will never reach the peak value of the input, because it will level off and begin to fall before reaching the peak input value. In such cases, a simple time shift of the output signal clearly cannot accurately reconstruct the input signal.

There is an analytical solution to this problem: The input signal can be accurately reconstructed from the output by what has been termed "deconvolution"—solving the dynamic equations for the relationship between the output and input, that is, finding and inverting the transfer function of the mixing chamber (16). This requires the application of fairly sophisticated mathematics, but in principle it allows exact reconstruction of the input signal, hence removing systematic errors in situations like the one described. However, the approach requires an accurate (and tractable) model of the transfer function of the mixing chamber, and, to obtain this, several simplifying assumptions must be made (such as complete mixing of each breath into the chamber volume and displacement of the breath volume of this mixture out of the chamber).

If the goal of nonsteady-state analysis is to accurately characterize the dynamic behavior of the cardiorespiratory response, an alternative perspective suggests that separate analysis of each unit of gas exchange (viz., each breath) would provide a simpler and potentially more accurate approach. For breath-by-breath analysis, slurring becomes insignificant because the time period of a single typical breath is so short. Moreover, PGE calculation for each breath also provides the highest possible density of information for respiratory measurement in breathing animals such as humans.

Breath-by-Breath Measurement of PGE

When PGE is calculated separately for every breath, many of the simplifying assumptions we have suggested become unnecessary, but unfortunately an entirely new set must be considered for accurate measurement. This section considers the factors contributing to this accuracy when continuous measurements of flow (or volume) and gas concentration signals, such as those shown in Figure 3.3, are utilized to produce discrete breath-by-breath measurements such as the response to a step change in exercise level, as shown in Figure 3.2.

Alignment of Gas Concentration Signals

Earlier we considered the time alignment of gas concentration with flow signals for measurements at the output of a mixing chamber; for accurate breath-by-breath computation, the accuracy of such alignment becomes considerably more important (10, 17, 35). In Figure 3.3, the time course of inspiratory and expiratory flow is plotted for a single breath in Panels 1 and 2, together with the concentration signals shown in Panels 3 and 4. To obtain correct values for gas transport for a single breath, the intrabreath response of the gas analyzer must be considered in some detail, as follows.

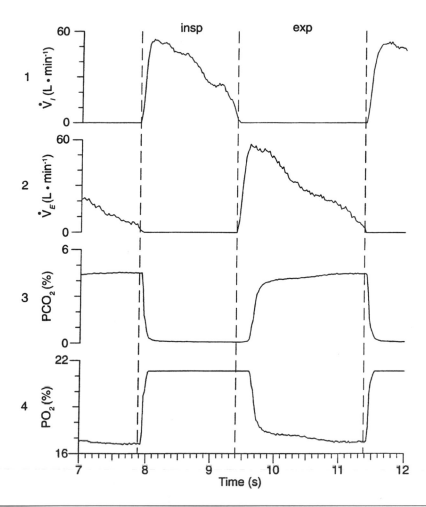

Figure 3.3 Single-breath pulmonary gas-exchange response of a subject at rest, showing, from top, inspiratory flow, expiratory flow, airway PCO_2, airway PO_2.

First, there is a time lag between the concentration signal and the flow signal, caused by two primary factors: the transit time of the gas from the sample probe (e.g., at the mouthpiece) to the analyzer, and the subsequent response time of the transducer and its associated electronics. To demonstrate these characteristics for a mass spectrometer, an experimental arrangement was used whereby an electrically operated (solenoid) valve switches either of two calibration gases, each at a separate input port, to the first of two output ports (in which the probe is placed). The second output port is arranged to allow the alternate gas to vent to room air, in order to prevent the pressure from rising in the outlets, while allowing high flow rates to ensure that the concentration at the probe tip changes sufficiently rapidly to be considered a step change when the electrical signal is applied.

The resultant concentration signal (measured at the output of the mass spectrometer) is shown in Figure 3.4, which is labeled to show the transit time (T_D) for CO_2 and O_2, and the half-time (τ') for the response to the step change in input. The former lag is easily

and accurately corrected by a simple time shift of the gas-concentration signal, but the latter requires more detailed consideration. If the response is monoexponential, with time constant τ, then, as discussed above, an acceptable approximation to the input signal can be derived from the output by utilizing an additional time shift equal to τ (which should be independent of both flow and mean concentration). However, if the transducer response is not first-order (e.g., is "sigmoidal" in shape, indicating higher-order transient dynamics), then a better approximation is obtained by estimating the time at which equal areas appear on each side of the response. If the response is symmetrical, then this time is equal to the half-time (i.e., the time taken to reach the midpoint of the step response). Note that T_D and τ' may both be different for each gas species, and may also depend on the gas mixture; for example, the mass spectrometer described exhibits an increase in T_D of 10 to 20 ms for both CO_2 and O_2 when the inspirate contains 80% O_2 rather than room air. This is due to the higher viscosity of O_2, which causes the

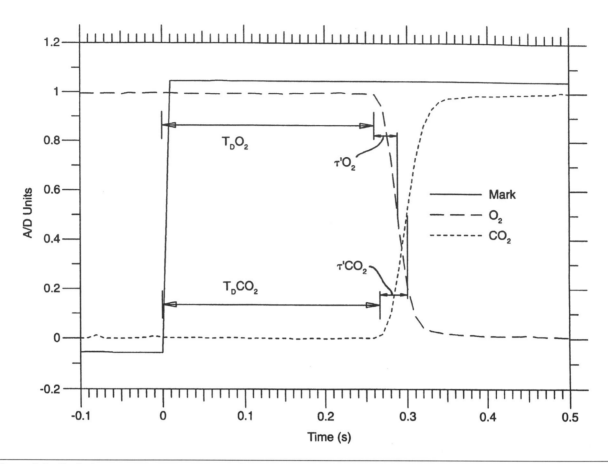

Figure 3.4 Typical mass-spectrometer response for CO_2 and O_2 from a step change in gas concentration produced by an electrically operated low-dead-space solenoid valve switched at time = 0.

velocity of the gas down the sampling catheter to be reduced.

Once a total "effective lag time" (e.g., $T_D + \tau'$) of the concentration signal to a step response has been obtained, the flow signal must be delayed by this amount in order to align it to the concentration signal at the probe tip. Figure 3.3 shows the result after performing such alignment, and the flow and concentration signals thus represent those at the mouth. Notice, however, that there remains an additional apparent delay in the concentration signals just after the start of both inspiration and expiration. These delays do not need further time-delay compensation, and represent the time taken to wash out the "proximal" and "distal" series dead-space volumes, respectively: The former volume is approximately that of the airways and breathing apparatus up to the probe tip, and the latter is that of the breathing apparatus from the probe tip to the outside air (e.g., the remainder of the breathing valve).

The actual quantity of each gas species passing the probe tip during expiration ($V_E CO_2$), and inspiration ($V_I CO_2$) can now be calculated by integrating the product of instantaneous flow with instantaneous (aligned) gas concentration, performing the integration over the appropriate (expiratory or inspiratory) phase of the breath; for instance:

$$V_E CO_2 = \int_{exp} [\dot{V}_E(t) \cdot F_E CO_2(t)] \cdot dt \ \text{L STPD} \quad (10)$$

where $F_E CO_2(t)$ is the dry fraction of CO_2 in the expirate at time t, and $\dot{V}_E$ is the ventilation STPD.

The lowest panel of Figure 3.5 illustrates the results of applying Equation 10 to Panels 2 and 3 of Figure 3.3; the quantity $V_E CO_2$ is the end-expiratory value of this curve, and is marked with an asterisk in the figure.

At this point it is instructive to consider this integral more carefully—it is that quantity of CO_2 exhaled past the mass-spectrometer probe (e.g., at the mouth); but this is not necessarily equal to that escaping from the body into the atmosphere, because some is reinspired on the next inspiration (viz., that stored in the distal dead space). Accurate calculation of CO_2 uptake (i.e., "net" PGE) requires that this inspired quantity be subtracted from that given in the previously mentioned integral. A simple expedient is to assume that the volume of the distal dead space is equal to that of the breathing valve, and that at end expiration it is filled

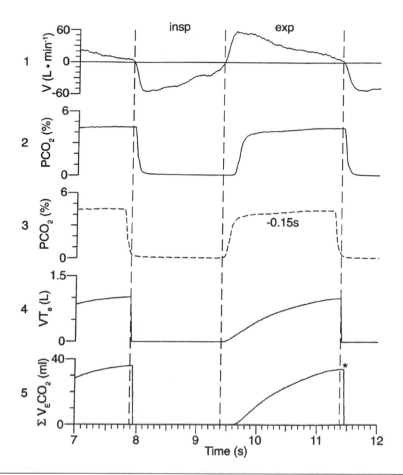

Figure 3.5   Single-breath pulmonary gas-exchange response of a subject at rest, showing further details of PGE computation (see also Figure 3.2).

with gas at end-tidal concentration (12). For this simplification, the quantity to be subtracted becomes

$$V_ICO_2 = V_D \cdot F_{ET}CO_2 \quad L \text{ STPD} \qquad (11)$$

Similar considerations apply for O_2, and these have been termed "breathing-valve" corrections.

It is also instructive to consider what is represented by a further time shift of the gas concentration signal so that the step response is aligned to the start of expiration as shown in the third panel of Figure 3.5. The integral in Equation 10 for this case could then be considered to be an estimate of the quantity of CO_2 evolved from the *alveolus*—that is, the amount crossing the "stationary interface," which is the boundary between convective airflow and diffusion-dominated flow. Of course, this quantity also does not equal the desired CO_2 output, because now the CO_2 stored in *both* the proximal *and* the distal dead spaces will be reinspired on the next breath. As before, if this inspired amount could be calculated and subtracted from the expiratory integral, the result would be the amount that escapes from the

body (and should be equal to that obtained at the mouth in the earlier calculation).

Figure 3.6 quantifies the effect of misalignment error in the gas-concentration signal on the volume calculated by Equation 10. This allows determination of error bounds on the achievable accuracy of the breath-by-breath gas exchange or, conversely, allows specification of the accuracy to which the concentration signal must be known at the probe tip, in order to achieve the required accuracy in gas-exchange computation. Note that the correct result (at time error = 0) does *not* occur at the peak of the curve for either CO_2 or O_2; this emphasizes the impossibility of deriving the correct time shift without measuring it independently (e.g., as shown in Figure 3.4 above) to an accuracy of 10 to 20 ms or better.

In contrast to these considerations, the mixing chamber system described earlier requires knowledge of this alignment only to the order of a few seconds, because the mixing chamber contains a gas mixture that already closely represents mixed-expired gas. Unfortunately, this value cannot be calculated from the time course of F_ECO_2 at the mouth without correct flow weighting. In

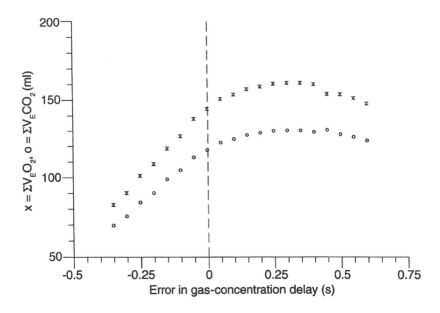

Figure 3.6   Effect of error in estimation of effective gas-concentration delay on calculation of pulmonary gas exchange from Equation 10. Note that the correct value (dashed line) does not occur at the peak of the curve.

other words, V_ECO_2 does *not* equal the product of the tidal volume ($\int \dot{V}_E(t) \cdot dt$) and the time-averaged CO_2 concentration ($\int F_ECO_2(t) \cdot dt$) except fortuitously. Rather, it is given by the integral of the product of these variables ($\int \dot{V}_E(t) \cdot F_ECO_2(t) \cdot dt$), where all integrals are taken over the expiratory phase.

Water Vapor Content

During exhalation, the water vapor content of expirate increases from ambient room air (about 1.5% content for 50% relative humidity) to saturated at end expiration (about 4.5% content for expirate saturated at 32 °C leaving the mouth [18]). Because it is difficult (and relatively expensive) to measure instantaneous water vapor content continuously throughout the breath, simplifying assumptions are usually made. A simple expedient is to consider the water vapor content to be ambient (e.g., 1.5%) as long as the expiratory CO_2 fraction is below some threshold, and saturated (e.g., 4.5%) when above it; a reasonable value for such a threshold is $F_ECO_2 = 0.02$.

Transducer Linearity

When a mass spectrometer is used, gas-concentration measurements are likely to be quite linear over the physiological range, but this might not be true for other types of gas analyzer (e.g., oxygen cell, infrared capnometer), either in the steady state or during a transient. Similarly, flow meter accuracy may depend systematically on flow rate (even on the profile within a breath). Furthermore, both flow and concentration signals may exhibit dynamic distortions caused by the transducer's own dynamic characteristics, thus making accuracy dependent on (possibly nonlinear) dynamic equations. In practice, simplifying assumptions can often reduce such known types of systematic errors to acceptably low values. However, the cumulative effect of such errors (even those remaining after simple correction) can be significant in certain cases, such as for certain experimental protocols, breathing patterns, or combinations of transducers.

Computational Errors

Because the most prevalent form of inexpensive computation today is the digital microcomputer, the (usually analog) transducer signals must be sampled by an analog-to-digital converter (A/D) and processed as a sequence of discrete quantized samples. It requires some sophistication to optimally process such samples and minimize cumulation of the errors mentioned earlier. Fortunately, such sophistication is usually limited not by the available microcomputers or languages, but rather by the programmer's knowledge of the transducers' characteristics and their interrelated dynamics. At the minimum, however, the sampling rate of the A/D should be twice the frequency of the most rapidly changing transducer output (e.g., that measuring flow). Rates of 50 to 150 Hz are typically adequate.

VALIDATION OF PGE MEASUREMENTS

As we have described in some detail, many factors contribute to the final accuracy of PGE measurements.

After each known factor has been independently addressed and its error contribution has been corrected to an acceptable (and known) level, the combined system must be validated to ensure that the unknown errors (and the residual after correcting the known ones) do not conspire to produce unacceptable results.

For example, the steady-state error of a system calculating breath-by-breath results can be evaluated by accumulating the results for a specific set of N breaths while simultaneously collecting the same breaths in an evacuated Douglas bag. The computed true CO_2 (TCO_2) for the set is given by

$$TCO_2 = \sum_i^N (\dot{V}CO_2/f)_i / N_{TOT} \qquad (12)$$

where

$$V_{TOT} = \sum_i^N (\dot{V}_E/f)_i \qquad (13)$$

and if f_i is the breathing frequency of breath i. The value of TCO_2 obtained from the balloon is

$$(TCO_2)_{bag} = F_ECO_2 - F_ICO_2 \qquad (14)$$

where F_ICO_2 is the inspired concentration of CO_2 (e.g., for room air, $F_ICO_2 = .0007$). Comparison of the two values of TCO_2 gives an estimate of the overall system error in the steady state. Similar considerations apply for O_2 in this and the following examples.

Next, the same balloon may be emptied into a calibrated spirometer to measure its volume (which is likely to be at ATPS conditions), and this volume can be converted to STPD (see the first section of this paper) for comparison with the computed value given by Equation 13, assuming that $\dot{V}_E$ is also computed STPD. Errors of less than 5% in both comparisons (TCO_2 and $\dot{V}_E$) are achievable and probably acceptable for many purposes, but extreme care is required to significantly reduce this error magnitude.

Assuming that acceptable errors are achieved for a particular steady state, the system's accuracy should next be determined for a series of steady-state responses ranging from rest to maximal exercise, and for a variety of subjects, because certain systematic errors can be dependent on breathing pattern. In this way, the range of applicability of a given system will be known, as will the aproximate repeatability of the measurements. A system that produces less than 5% error in TCO_2 and $\dot{V}_E$ over the range of metabolic rates represented by O_2 uptake in the range 0.25 to 5.0 L · min^{-1} (i.e., from rest to athlete maximum $\dot{V}O_2$) is unlikely to be achievable without rigorous attention to the above considerations and highly practiced experimental technique for balloon collection and measurement.

Regarding the nonsteady state, this collection and comparison can be performed systematically over the nonsteady-state domain of interest. For example, the set of breaths collected could be cued to represent the first 2 min of exercise after a step change in work rate. Again, average values of computed TCO_2 and $\dot{V}_E$ can be compared with bag measurements, and repeated for a variety of step increments (in both directions) and a variety of subjects. Validation of the system should always be performed for the specific protocols required for a particular investigation or clinical test, and should be repeated periodically (e.g., weekly or monthly) to ensure that unnoticed problems have not arisen in the interim.

Finally, some discussion of the concept of physical calibrators (i.e., those that can simulate aspects of breathing) is appropriate. It is possible to validate many aspects of a system's performance to a high degree of accuracy and repeatability using a calibrated variable-speed pump and calibrated gas mixtures (40). Briefly, the accuracy of ventilation measurements can be determined by calculating the average stroke volume computed by the system and comparing it with that of the pump (determined by collecting the pump expirate directly into a spirometer). Repeating the procedure for a range of pump frequencies enables the linearity of the system's ventilation measurement to be determined over the flow range of interest, though at the higher frequencies direct collection may produce erroneous measurements due to spirometer inertia. Caution is required in interpreting such results, because such physical calibrators can exhibit systematic differences from human breathing, and hence can produce unexpected (though perhaps correct and useful) results. For example, suppose a system is calibrated using a 3-L hand syringe, and during calibration the computer algorithm corrects for the known ambient temperature, pressure, and water vapor content of the gas. Next, an experiment is performed in which the subject is actually the same syringe, and for which the breaths are collected while the computer calculates the usual respiratory variables. It is likely that, for this mode, the computer algorithms are assuming that the expirate is at 32 °C, saturated, because the system is not likely to be directly measuring either temperature or saturation intrabreath. The computed ventilation will thus be incorrectly scaled and may require further correction to the appropriate conditions before their absolute accuracy can be determined.

Figure 3.7 shows the result of such a study performed using a turbine flow meter and an electrically operated syringe pump of nominal 1.5-L stroke, whose cycle time is varied electronically from 5 to 60 breaths per minute. The average calculated volume of inspiration and expiration is plotted against breathing frequency, and shows that the relative error is below 0.1% for

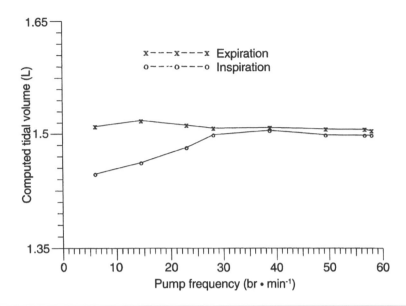

Figure 3.7 Error in computation of average stroke volume of a syringe pump versus the pump frequency. Note that error is 0.1% to 0.3% over a range of ventilation spanning rest to heavy exercise.

expiration, and below 0.3% for inspiration, over the range of flows from 7.5 to 90 L · min⁻¹. It is important to realize, however, that even such excellent results are not sufficient to guarantee accuracy for a human subject, because the (sinusoidal) flow profile of the pump is quite dissimilar to the abrupt flow transients typical of human breathing. Conversely, if a given system cannot produce stable and accurate output even for such a simple validation experiment, then it is unlikely to be usable for real testing.

The same pump arrangement can be further modified to investigate the system's response to simulated breathing, by introducing a steady stream of test gas into the expiratory path of the pump before the gas is sampled by the analyzer probe. It is possible in this way to produce cyclic profiles of CO_2 and O_2 that look remarkably similar to human breathing patterns, and the reproducibility and flexibility of such a device makes it particularly suitable for system evaluation (40). However, even further caution is required in interpreting the results of such studies, because several assumptions embedded in the computer algorithms may be violated by the simulated breathing. It may be possible to correct the computed values to reflect such known errors in the assumptions (e.g., by entering the expiratory temperature to be ambient rather than 32 °C). Comparison of the computed and measured values for $\dot{V}CO_2$ and $\dot{V}O_2$ may thus require deep understanding of the algorithms being tested. If these calculations can be manipulated correctly, or an accurate nomograph constructed, then it is possible to achieve high accuracy and repeatability. For example, computed $\dot{V}CO_2$ can be compared with the independently measured flow rate of CO_2 out of the

test gas tank, to determine whether the computer is correctly calculating the critical cross-product integrals (Equation 11), hence estimating the system's absolute accuracy. Considerations for O_2 can be even more complicated, but they will not be addressed further here.

Given all this, it is prudent to consider carefully the claimed attention given to error analysis and reduction by commercial vendors of PGE measurement equipment. Unfortunately, at present there is no accepted way of independently evaluating such critical combinations of devices against standard validation tests, and, as we have seen, it is not sufficient to guarantee the accuracy of every isolated component. It is thus possible only to estimate the total system accuracy, and then only for specified protocols and for a specific range of subject responses for which validation can be performed. *Caveat emptor!*

FURTHER ADVANCES IN BREATH-BY-BREATH MEASUREMENT OF PGE

As we have mentioned, breath-by-breath measurement of PGE provides the highest density of information for respiratory variables; however, work in the 1980s attempted to address two interesting and fruitful areas: estimation of ''alveolar'' gas exchange and study of intrabreath gas exchange.

''Alveolar'' Gas Exchange

As was described earlier, measurement of average PGE at the mouth should reflect that at the alveolus. However, this relies on the major assumption that there is no change in the lung gas stores from one breath to the next. Such an assumption obviously can be violated by almost every breath (but must be true, at least asymptotically, over the longer term for the steady state). There are thus random variations observable in the computed values of PGE for each breath (19). Such random variations have been termed "noise," and several investigators have attempted to reduce the magnitude of such noise by various computational techniques, each of which, however, depends on further assumptions. Changes in lung stores can produce large changes in CO_2 output and O_2 uptake at the mouth (10, 11, 20, 21), so it was reasoned that estimation of the changes in lung stores from breath to breath would allow more accurate estimation of the transport between alveolus and capillary, particularly for situations in which the EELV (end-expiratory lung volume) can change rapidly, such as the onset of muscular exercise from prior rest (41). This can create major errors in the interpretation of the gas-exchange ratio R: Imagine that the inspiratory and expiratory volumes of O_2 and CO_2 are each accurately measured, but that no concern is given to the change in EELV. Then, as measured at the mouth, $\dot{V}CO_2 = (V_ECO_2 - V_ICO_2)$ will be an *overestimate* of the alveolar exchange when EELV *decreases* (i.e., some "extra" CO_2 will be evolved from the lung gas stores). But because this process also vents *more* O_2 into the atmosphere, $\dot{V}O_2 = (V_IO_2 - V_EO_2)$ will decrease and *underestimate* the alveolar O_2 exchange. R will consequently be markedly high with respect to the actual alveolar gas exchange. Conversely, it will be markedly low when EELV increases between breaths. Interestingly, this effect is not seen when only expired quantities are measured, because one must assume what happened during inspiration from the expiratory measurements; this assumption, though erroneous, yields a close approximation to the actual alveolar R, as discussed by Ward, Lamarra, and Whipp (37)—but not, of course, for $\dot{V}CO_2$ or $\dot{V}O_2$ separately.

On the other hand, with further analysis it is possible to estimate closely the *actual* change in lung gas stores for each breath, and thence determine appropriate alveolar gas-exchange values for $\dot{V}CO_2$, $\dot{V}O_2$, and hence R. To address this, Wessel at al. (36) used measurement of inspired gas flow and concentration to estimate the net transport of each gas (including N_2) for each breath, and calculated net change in lung volume from the quantity $\dot{V}N_2 = (V_IN_2 - V_EN_2)$ by assuming no N_2 exchange at the alveolus. The lung was thus modeled as a mixing chamber of "fixed" initial end-expiratory volume to which the inspirate was added and from which the expirate was subtracted. This technique was further refined by Beaver, Lamarra, and Wasserman (10) to include estimates for changes in end-expiratory

lung gas concentrations as well as EELV between breaths. Swanson and Sherrill (21) further assumed that the "fixed" initial EELV could be chosen optimally to minimize the breath-to-breath fluctuations, the optimal value being interpreted as an "effective" lung volume. Because O_2 and CO_2 can be treated independently, an effective lung volume was computed separately for each gas, rather than assuming that this volume should be chosen to equal the subject's measured end-expiratory lung volume (10, 11, 35) (even if this value does not minimize the fluctuations). Because fluctuations might in fact occur at the alveolus (e.g., as a consequence of pulse-to-pulse variations in pulmonary blood flow), it is not necessarily imperative or correct to adopt the minimization strategy. However, all of the mentioned algorithms can demonstrate significant reduction in the observed breath-to-breath fluctuation when compared to expiratory-only methods, and the degree of improvement is itself relatively insensitive to the actual assumed value of lung volume.

Intrabreath Gas Exchange

Even more recently, renewed interest has been generated in the study of the pattern of gas exchange within the breath (22, 23, 24, 25), in the hope of achieving better understanding of the underlying (continuous) process of gas transport and its determinants in health and disease. Two such areas of interest are

- estimating the series "dead space" (23, 25)—this approximates the anatomical dead space, but in reality reflects the volume to the "stationary interface," and
- observing the time profile of the gas-exchange ratio, R (22, 24, 25).

The series dead space was computed by Cumming (23) on isolated breaths, and further investigated by Lamarra, Whipp, and Ward (26) and Whipp et al. (25) to allow measurement breath by breath, thence allowing on-line estimation of true mean alveolar PCO_2 from the equation

$$P_ACO_2 = 863 \cdot \dot{V}CO_2/\dot{V}_A \text{ Torr} \qquad (15)$$

where $\dot{V}_A = \dot{V}_E \cdot (1 - V_D/V_T)$, V_D is the series dead space, and V_T is the tidal volume. Comparisons of calculated values for P_ACO_2 with direct measurements of arterial PCO_2 (P_aCO_2) show a small but systematic difference for normal subjects performing moderate exercise (this difference being compatible with expected differences in alveolar-to-arterial CO_2 concentration). The technique thus provides a useful *noninvasive* and continuous estimator of P_aCO_2 at the minor expense of modest additional computation.

The intrabreath time profile of the gas-exchange ratio is also of considerable interest for determining whether simple indices of cardiorespiratory pathology may be obtained, as well as for its contribution to the understanding of the basic physiology of the underlying gas-transport dynamics. Detailed discussion of this topic is, however, outside the scope of this chapter.

APPLICATION TO EXERCISE TESTING AND EVALUATION

An important advantage of breath-by-breath analysis of pulmonary gas exchange during exercise is the improved precision in discriminating the indices of aerobic function—namely, maximum $\dot{V}O_2$ ($\mu\dot{V}O_2$), lactate threshold for $\dot{V}O_2$ ($\theta_L\dot{V}O_2$), work efficiency (η), and time constant for O_2 uptake ($\tau\dot{V}O_2$). For example, $\mu\dot{V}O_2$ determined from discrete collections of expired gases can provide only the mean value over the sampling interval. And as this is commonly 1 min or so, the average might not accurately represent the highest value obtained during the exercise—which is the object of the assessment. Furthermore, an investigator requiring evidence of a plateau in $\dot{V}O_2$ to meet the criterion for achieving $\mu\dot{V}O_2$ would require a minimum of two samples (or 2 min exercise) at or near $\mu\dot{V}O_2$. A plateau lasting less than a minute is therefore likely to be missed entirely. On the other hand, by using breath-by-breath analysis, whenever a plateau actually occurs it is observable, regardless of its duration.

Similarly, estimation of the lactate threshold in $\dot{V}O_2$ (28) needs interpolation of the sub- and suprathreshold pattern of response if the investigator uses discrete bag sampling. Naturally, the higher density of data afforded by breath-by-breath analysis provides the most accurate threshold discrimination.

High-density data acquisition is also crucial for interpreting the nonsteady-state phase of gas exchange, unless merely a general description (for example, of the O_2 deficit) is desired. The ability to characterize, or even demonstrate, the cardiodynamic phase (Phase 1) of pulmonary gas exchange (29) is precluded by the use of minute-by-minute sampling, as the phase lasts only some 20 s. Consequently, the measured response will not accurately reflect the underlying physiological pattern. However, with breath-by-breath analysis, Phase 1 can be characterized with respect to both its magnitude and its duration. The pattern is markedly altered in patients with cardiac disease (31) and may even be a discriminant in some cases, as shown in Figure 3.8. Furthermore, it can be dissected away from the analysis of the nonsteady-state phase, leaving Phase 2 (dominated by muscle extraction) for precise characterization and interpretation (see refs. 13 and 32 for discussion).

With respect to work efficiency η (i.e., the measured power generated divided by the incremental energy cost of that power generation), breath-to-breath analysis offers no advantages in rigor over the discrete bag-sampling technique. However, as it can be estimated from the same short-duration test that allowed τ, θ_L, and μ to be determined, some investigators are prepared to exchange a small potential error in η for the reduced time and patient stress required. This potential "error" results from the fact that the gas-exchange ratio R during a ramp or rapidly incrementing test is likely to underestimate the true tissue respiratory quotient (RQ) (due to discrepancies between $\tau\dot{V}O_2$ and $\tau\dot{V}CO_2$ at the mouth), but to date it has not been possible to determine a systematic difference.

The breath-to-breath fluctuations ("noise") mentioned earlier have been shown to be relatively uncorrelated from breath to breath (i.e., the direction and magnitude of the noise on one breath is not related to that on the previous one) and to possess a Gaussian distribution of values, that is, "white" Gaussian noise (19). This noise can be much more marked in some subjects than in others and is not devoid of physiological interest, because it contains information regarding pulmonary blood flow patterns; this, however, is also beyond the scope of the current chapter. On the other hand, it is usually in the investigator's interest to reduce or eliminate this noise in order to characterize more clearly the underlying response dynamics. This can be accomplished by averaging over each consecutive set of several breath samples in a single test, or by averaging the responses of several similar tests, cued to a common transition mark. Note, however, that the presence of the breath-to-breath noise imposes a degree of uncertainty in the estimation of the parameters of interest (such as $\tau\dot{V}O_2$), even when the noise is symmetrically distributed in a Gaussian manner. This is perhaps best illustrated by a simple exercise that is readily performed on a personal computer: A given exponential equation is established for $\dot{V}O_2$ (e.g., $\dot{V}O_2 = A + B[1 - \exp\{-t/\tau\}]$) with known values for τ, A, and B. Gaussian noise values with a given standard deviation are then added to the time samples, and the resulting noisy response is used for nonlinear estimation of τ (e.g., by finding the best-fit exponential). The estimation error ($\hat{\tau} - \tau$) can be quite different for each set of random noise values chosen, even if these have *precisely* the same standard deviation. In fact, this error itself will have a standard deviation that is related to that of the added noise (19). Unfortunately, some investigators have not given due consideration to this uncertainty when using parameter estimation (e.g., ref. 30) and cannot therefore rigorously justify conclusions regarding the effect on such an estimated parameter value of a particular intervention, such as training. Such an omission is akin

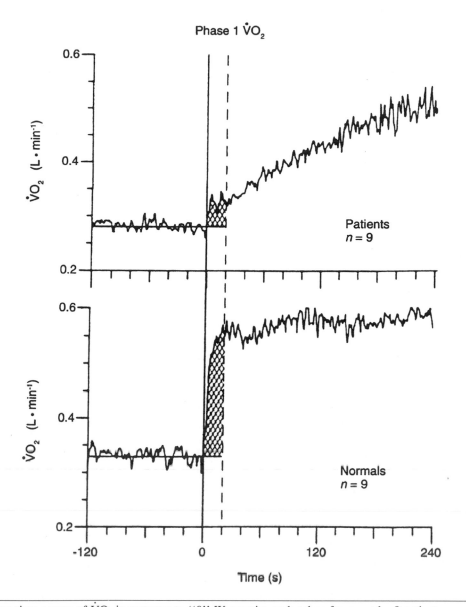

Phase 1 $\dot{V}O_2$

Patients
$n = 9$

Normals
$n = 9$

Figure 3.8 Mean time course of $\dot{V}O_2$ in response to "0" W exercise undertaken from rest by 9 patients. From "Dynamics of Oxygen Uptake During Exercise in Adults With Cyanotic Congenital Heart Disease" by K.E. Sietsema, D.M. Cooper, M.H. Rosove, J.K. Perloff, J.S. Child, M.M. Canobbio, B.J. Whipp, and K. Wasserman, 1986, *Circulation,* **73**, 1137-1140. Copyright 1986 by the American Heart Association. Reprinted by permission.

to neglecting to perform the well-known and required analysis when observing a different mean and standard deviation between two populations, which allows rigorous determination of whether such differences have sufficient significance for interpretation. These issues are discussed in ref. 39 with specific regard to interpretation of PGE response dynamics.

SUMMARY

Technological advances in both respired gas analysis and airflow determination, coupled with the recent saltation in affordable computer power, have brought high-resolution analysis of respiratory gas exchange within

the reach of most exercise physiology research laboratories. This allows the investigator to probe the non-steady-state phase, which is necessary for improved understanding of the physiological determinants—and fundamental limits—of exercise responses. The technical procedures, however, are fraught with potential errors that, unless recognized, can lead to high or unwarranted confidence in the interpretation of unwittingly erroneous data. In this chapter, we have attempted to describe the nature of such potential errors, and attempted thereby to assist the wary investigator to confidently choose breath-to-breath analysis if appropriate. This allows the benefits to be reaped from choosing the optimum sample density for each phase of investigation:

for example, data acquisition, processing and display, dynamic analysis, and physiological interpretation.

REFERENCES

1. Lavoisier, A.L. Alterations qu'eprouve l'air respire. In *Oeuvres de Lavoisier* (Vol. II, pp. 676-687). Paris: Imprimerie Imperiale.

2. Geppert, J., & Zuntz, N. (1988). Ueber die Regulation der Atmung. *Pflugers Archiv Fur Die Gesamte Physiologie Des Menschen Und Der Tiere*, **42**, 189-245.

3. Poole, D.C., & Whipp, B.J. (1988). Letter to the editor. *Medicine and Science in Sports and Exercise*, **20**, 420-421.

4. Haldane, J.S. (1912). *Methods of air analysis*. London: Griffin.

5. Scholander, P.F. (1947). Analyser for accurate estimations of respiratory gases in one-half cubic centimetre samples. *Journal of Biological Chemistry*, **167**, 235-250.

6. Consolazio, C.F., Johnson, R.E., & Pecora, L.J. (1963). *Physiologic measurements of metabolic functions*. New York: McGraw-Hill.

7. Wilmore, J.H., & Costill, D.L. (1974). Semiautomated systems approach to the assessment of oxygen uptake during exercise. *Journal of Applied Physiology*, **36**, 618-620.

8. Hughson, R.L., Kowalchuk, J.M., Prime, W.M., & Green, H.J. (1984). Open circuit gas exchange analysis in the nonsteady-state. *Canadian Journal of Applied Sport Sciences*, **5**, 15-18.

9. Otis, A.B. (1964). Quantitative relationships in steady-state gas exchange. In W.O. Fenn & H. Rahn (Eds.), *Handbook of physiology* (Vol. 1, pp. 681-698). Washington, DC: American Physiological Society.

10. Beaver, W.L., Lamarra, N., & Wasserman, K. (1981). Breath-by-breath measurement of true alveolar gas exchange. *Journal of Applied Physiology*, **51**, 1662-1675.

11. Auchincloss, J.H., Gilbert, R., & Baule, G.H. (1966). Effect of ventilation on oxygen transfer during early exercise. *Journal of Applied Physiology*, **21**, 810.

12. Beaver, W.L., Wasserman, K., & Whipp, B.J. (1973). On-line computer analysis and breath-by-breath graphical display of exercise function tests. *Journal of Applied Physiology*, **34**, 128-132.

13. Whipp, B.J., Ward, S.A., Lamarra, N., Davis, J.A., & Wasserman, K. (1982). Parameters of ventilatory and gas exchange dynamics during exercise. *Journal of Applied Physiology*, **52**, 1506-1513.

14. Linnarsson, D. (1974). Dynamics of pulmonary gas exchange and heart rate at start and end of exercise. *Acta Physiologica Scandinavica*, **415**(Suppl.), 1-68.

15. Hughson, R.L., Sherrill, D.L., & Swanson, G.D. (1988). Kinetics of $\dot{V}O_2$ with impulse and step exercise in humans. *Journal of Applied Physiology*, **64**, 451-459.

16. Helstrom, C.W. (1968). *Statistical theory of signal detection*. New York: Pergamon.

17. Noguchi, H., Ogushi, Y., Yoshiya, I., Itakura, N., & Yamabayashi, H. (1982). Breath-by-breath $\dot{V}CO_2$ and $\dot{V}O_2$ require compensation for transport delay and dynamic response. *Journal of Applied Physiology*, **52**, 79-84.

18. Green, I.D., & Nesarajah, M.S. (1968). Water-vapor pressure of end-tidal air of normals and chronic bronchitics. *Journal of Applied Physiology*, **24**(2), 229-231.

19. Lamarra, N., Whipp, B.J., Ward, S.A., & Wasserman, K. (1987). Breath-to-breath "noise" and parameter estimation of exercise gas-exchange kinetics. *Journal of Applied Physiology*, **62**, 2003-2012.

20. Pearce, D.H., & Milhorn, H.T., Jr. (1977). Dynamic and steady-state respiratory responses to bicycle exercise. *Journal of Applied Physiology*, **42**, 959-967.

21. Swanson, G.D., & Sherrill, D.L. (1983). A model of breath-to-breath gas exchange. In B.J. Whipp & D.M. Wiberg (Eds.), *Modelling and control of breathing*. New York: Elsevier.

22. West, J.B., Fowler, K.T., Hugh-Jones, P., & O'Donnell, T.V. (1957). Measurement of the ventilation-perfusion ratio inequality in the lung by the analysis of a single expirate. *Clinical Science*, **16**, 529-547.

23. Cumming, G. (1981). Gas mixing in disease. In J.G. Scadding & G. Cumming (Eds.), *Scientific foundations of medicine*. London: Heinemann.

24. Kim, T.S., Rahn, H., & Farhi, L.E. (1966). Estimation of true venous and arterial PCO_2 by gas analysis of a single breath. *Journal of Applied Physiology*, **21**, 1338-1344.

25. Whipp, B.J, Lamarra, N., Ward, S.A., Davis, J.A., & Wasserman, K. (1990). Estimating arterial PO_2 from flow-weighted and time-averaged alveolar PCO_2 during exercise. In G.D. Swanson & F.S. Grodins (Eds.), *Respiratory control: Modelling perspective* (pp. 155-164). New York: Plenum.

26. Lamarra, N., Whipp, B.J., & Ward, S.A. (1988). Physiological inferences from intra-breath measurement of pulmonary gas exchange. *Proceedings of the I.E.E.E. Symposium*, New Orleans.

27. Whipp, B.J., Davis, J.A., Torres, F., & Wasserman, K. (1981). A test to determine the parameters of aerobic function during exercise. *Journal of Applied Physiology*, **50**, 217-221.

28. Wasserman, K. (1987). Determinants and detection of anaerobic threshold and consequences of exercise above it. *Circulation*, **76**, VI-29–VI-39.

29. Krogh, A., & Lindhard, J. (1913). The regulation of respiration and circulation during the initial stages of muscular work. *Journal of Physiology* (London), **47**, 112-136.

30. Cerretelli, P., Shindell, D., Pendergast, D.P., Di Prampero, P.E., & Rennie, D.W. (1977). Oxygen uptake transients at the onset and offset of arm and leg work. *Respiration Physiology*, **30**, 81-87.

31. Sietsema, K.E., Cooper, D.M., Rosove, M.H., Perloff, J.K., Child, J.S., Canobbio, M.M., Whipp, B.J., & Wasserman, K. (1986). Dynamics of oxygen uptake during exercise in adults with cyanotic congenital heart disease. *Circulation*, **73**, 1137-1140.

32. Barstow, T.J., Lamarra, N., & Whipp, B.J. (1990). Modulation of muscle and pulmonary O_2 uptakes by circulatory dynamics during exercise. *Journal of Applied Physiology*, **68**, 979-989.

33. Perkins, J.F., Jr. (1964). Historical development of respiratory physiology. In W.O. Fenn & H. Rahn (Eds.), *Handbook of physiology* (Vol. 1, pp. 1-62). Washington, DC: American Physiological Society.

34. Seguin, A., & Lavoisier, A.L. (1789). Premier memoire sur la respiration des animaux. *Memoirs de l'Academie des Sciences*, **185**.

35. Yamamoto, Y., Takei, Y., Mokushi, K., Morita, K., Mutoh, Y., & Miyashita, M. (1987). Breath-by-breath measurement of alveolar gas exchange with a slow-response gas analyzer. *Medical and Biological Engineering and Computing*, **25**, 141-146.

36. Wessel, H.U., Stout, R.L., Bastanier, C.K., & Paul, M.H. (1979). Breath-by-breath variation of FRC: Effect on $\dot{V}O_2$ and $\dot{V}CO_2$ measured at the mouth. *Journal of Applied Physiology*, **46**, 1122-1126.

37. Ward, S.A., Lamarra, N., & Whipp, B.J. (1990). Gas-exchange inferences for the proportionality of the cardiopulmonary responses during phase 1 of exercise. In G.D. Swanson & F.S. Grodins (Eds.), *Respiratory control: Modelling perspective* (pp. 137-146). New York: Plenum.

38. Sue, D.Y., Hansen, J.E., Blais, M., & Wasserman, K. (1980). Measurement and analysis of gas exchange during exercise using a programmable calculator. *Journal of Applied Physiology*, **49**, 456-461.

39. Lamarra, N. (1990). Variables, constants, and parameters: Clarifying the system structure. *Medicine and Science in Sports and Exercise*, **22**(1), 88-95.

40. Huszczuk, A., Whipp, B.J., & Wasserman, K. (1990). Respiratory gas-exchange simulator for routine calibration in metabolic studies. *European Respiratory Journal*, **3**, 465-468

41. Ward, S.A., Davis, J.A., Weissman, M.L., Wasserman, K., & Whipp, B.J. (1979). Lung gas stores and the kinetics of gas exchange during exercise. *Physiologist*, **22**(4), 129.

CHAPTER 4

Indirect Methods for Estimation of Aerobic Power

Ann Ward, PhD

University of Wisconsin

Cara B. Ebbeling, MS
Lynn E. Ahlquist, PhD

Directed measurement of maximum oxygen uptake requires specialized expensive equipment, may place certain groups within the supposed normal population at risk, and is not always practical for either general health screening or when assessing large numbers. For these reasons, other indirect methods have been extensively used for the evaluation of cardiovascular fitness and/or prediction of maximal oxygen uptake. Such tests may be either of a maximal or submaximal nature, utilize a variety of different exercise modalities, and may be specific to different populations and age groups. A sampling of these tests is included in this chapter.

Direct measurement of oxygen consumption during a maximal exercise test provides the most accurate assessment of aerobic power. However, measuring maximum oxygen consumption ($\dot{V}O_2$max) requires sophisticated equipment and trained staff. Due to the expense, the time required, and the risks associated with maximal exercise, direct measurement of $\dot{V}O_2$max is not practical in many situations, such as fitness testing in health clubs or testing large populations.

Consequently, many indirect measures for assessing aerobic power have been developed. Some are based on performance on a maximal or submaximal test. Other protocols use the heart rate (HR) at submaximal work loads or provide an estimate of $\dot{V}O_2$max from multiple regression equations. Because of the specificity of testing and training, we have included

tests representative of each usual mode of testing. The tests are organized as maximal exercise tests, submaximal tests, and tests designed for children. We could not include every available test, so we have tried to choose the most accurate, representative, and commonly used tests. We have excluded tests that require sophisticated laboratory equipment, such as gas analyzers.

When one is choosing a test, the accuracy of the test and the population on which the test was developed should be considered. We have included this information for each test when available, as well as the test protocol. For tests where $\dot{V}O_2$max is estimated from multiple regression equations, we would like to clarify three terms. In this chapter, the *development population* is the subject population on which the regression equation was developed. *Cross-validation* is the evaluation of the accuracy of the equation on an independent sample with characteristics similar to those of the development population. *Validation* is the evaluation of the accuracy of the test on a population with characteristics different from those of the original development population.

Many of the tests provide an estimate of $\dot{V}O_2$max, whereas others categorize individuals. For tests that estimate $\dot{V}O_2$max, we recommend the standards established by the American Heart Association (Table 4.1) to place individuals into fitness categories (1). For other tests, we have provided normative data when available.

Table 4.1 Normal Values of Maximum Oxygen Uptake at Different Ages[a]

Age	Men	Women
20-29	43 (± 22)	36 (± 21)
	12 METs	10 METs
30-39	42 (± 22)	34 (± 21)
	12 METs	10 METs
40-49	40 (± 22)	32 (± 21)
	11 METs	9 METs
50-59	36 (± 22)	29 (± 22)
	10 METs	8 METs
60-69	33 (± 22)	27 (± 22)
	9 METs	8 METs
70-79	29 (± 22)	27 (± 22)
	8 METs	8 METs

Note. MET = metabolic equivalent; 1 MET = 3.5 ml · kg^{-1} · min^{-1} oxygen uptake.

[a](ml · kg^{-1} · min^{-1})

From Exercise standards: A statement for health professionals from the American Heart Association, *Circulation*, **82**, 2286-2322. Copyright 1990 by the American Heart Association. Reprinted with permission.

MAXIMAL TESTS

Maximum oxygen consumption can be estimated from performance on standardized protocols on the treadmill, cycle ergometer, or arm ergometer. The protocol chosen often depends on the equipment available, the population being tested, and the primary purpose of the test. A test that starts with a low work load has 1- to 3-min stages, and an increase of no more than 3 METs per stage is generally recommended (2, 3). The test should be no longer than 15 to 20 min to avoid boredom and loss of motivation.

When using a protocol to estimate $\dot{V}O_2$max from performance, it is important to follow the protocol precisely. For example, Ragg et al. (4) found that performance time on a graded exercise test with constant walking speed increased from 15 to 25 min when subjects were allowed to hold on to the handrail.

Maximal Treadmill Protocols

Bruce Protocol

The Bruce protocol (5) is the most frequently used diagnostic test for coronary heart disease and the best validated test for estimating $\dot{V}O_2$max from a maximal performance. This protocol starts at a low work level, allowing time for warm-up and cardiovascular adaptation. The increases in work load are relatively large compared to some protocols (3-4 METs per stage); thus, the test can be completed quickly.

Bruce, Kusumi, and Hosmer (5) developed predictive equations for $\dot{V}O_2$max from performance time on the Bruce protocol. Stepwise multiple regression analysis was used to develop population-specific predictive equations for $\dot{V}O_2$max for healthy adults, active men, sedentary men, and cardiac men ($N = 393$). Correlation coefficients ranged from $r = .86$ to $r = .92$.

Foster et al. (6) developed generalized equations for estimating $\dot{V}O_2$max from the Bruce protocol. The subjects were 230 men who underwent symptom-limited graded exercise testing using the Bruce protocol with concurrent measurement of $\dot{V}O_2$max. The sample, which included patients with angina, coronary bypass surgery patients, cardiac rehabilitation patients, healthy adults, and athletes, was divided into a development group ($n = 200$) and a cross-validation group ($n = 30$). A cubic equation using time was developed with a multiple correlation of $R = .977$ and *SEE* less than 3.5 ml · kg^{-1} · min^{-1}. Adding health status, activity level, interaction between health and activity, and age to the equation improved prediction accuracy slightly. However, because of the difficulty in identifying health status and activity level, the equation including only time is recommended for use. When the Foster et al. generalized equation was compared to the Bruce et al. population-specific equations, the average prediction error of the generalized equation was significantly less than the average prediction error for the population-specific equations (6).

Equipment

- Motor-driven treadmill
- Timer
- Electrocardiogram (ECG) (for diagnostic test) or HR monitor

Protocol

The Bruce protocol is summarized in Table 4.2.

Prediction Equations

Population-specific equations from Bruce, Kusumi, and Hosmer (5):

Table 4.2 The Bruce Treadmill Protocol

Stage	Duration (min)	Speed (mph)	Grade (%)
1	3	1.7	10
2	3	2.5	12
3	3	3.4	14
4	3	4.2	16
5	3	5.0	18
6	3	5.5	20
7	3	6.0	22

	r	n

1) Active men: 0.906   44

$$\dot{V}O_2max = 3.778 \text{ (time)} + 0.19$$

2) Sedentary men: 0.906   94

$$\dot{V}O_2max = 3.298 \text{ (time)} + 4.07$$

3) Cardiac patients: 0.865   97

$$\dot{V}O_2max = 2.327 \text{ (time)} + 9.48$$

4) Healthy adults: 0.920   295

$$\dot{V}O_2max = 6.70 - 2.82 \text{ (gender)} + 0.056 \text{ (time)}$$

Where:

$\dot{V}O_2max$ = maximal oxygen uptake (ml · kg^{-1} · min^{-1})
time = maximal treadmill performance in minutes for Equations 1 to 3 and seconds for Equation 4
gender = males = 1, females = 2

Generalized equations from Foster et al. (6):

	R	SEE

1) $\dot{V}O_2max = 14.76 - 1.38 \text{ (time)}$ .977   3.35
$+ 0.451 \text{ (time}^2)$
$- 0.12 \text{ (time}^3)$
2) $\dot{V}O_2max = 13.30 - 0.3 \text{ (time)}$ .979   3.19
$+ 0.297 \text{ (time}^2)$
$- 0.0077 \text{ (time}^3)$
$+ 4.2 \text{ (health)}$
3) $\dot{V}O_2max = 12.95 + 0.0062 \text{ (time)}$ .980   3.20
$+ 0.27 \text{ (time}^2)$
$- 0.0071 \text{ (time}^3)$
$+ 1.97 \text{ (health)}$
$- 0.83 \text{ (act)}$
$+ 3.07 \text{ (health} \times \text{act)}$
4) $\dot{V}O_2max = 15.98 + 0.176 \text{ (time)}$ .981   3.12
$+ 0.24 \text{ (time}^2)$
$- 0.006 \text{ (time}^3)$

$+ 1.33 \text{ (health)}$
$- 0.94 \text{ (act)}$
$+ 4.08 \text{ (health} \times \text{act)}$
$- 0.05 \text{ (age)}$

Where:

$\dot{V}O_2max$ = maximal oxygen uptake (ml · kg^{-1} · min^{-1})
time = maximal treadmill performance in minutes
health = 1 = healthy, 0 = known coronary artery disease
act = 1 = physically active, 0 = sedentary
age = age in years

Balke Protocol

The Balke protocol is characterized by a constant walking speed. In the original protocol developed by Balke and Ware (7), treadmill speed was set at 3.3 mph (90 m · min^{-1}), grade increased 1% every minute, and the test was terminated at a HR of 180 beats per minute (bpm). Balke and Ware measured oxygen consumption ($\dot{V}O_2$) on 500 subjects utilizing this protocol and developed the following linear equation to estimate $\dot{V}O_2$:

$$\dot{V}O_2 = \text{speed} \times [0.073 + (\% \text{ grade}/100)] \times 1.8$$

Where:

$\dot{V}O_2$ = oxygen consumption in ml · kg^{-1} · min^{-1}
speed = treadmill speed in m · min^{-1}
% grade = final treadmill grade in %
1.8 = the factor constituting the oxygen requirement in ml · min^{-1} for 1 kilogram-meter (kgm) of work

As investigators began using the Balke protocol, it was modified so that subjects walked to volitional exhaustion rather than stopping the test at a heart rate of 180 bpm. Froelicher and Lancaster (8) developed the following regression equation to estimate $\dot{V}O_2max$ from maximal performance time on this protocol using 1,025 healthy men 20 to 53 years old:

$$\dot{V}O_2max \text{ (ml · kg}^{-1} \cdot \text{min}^{-1}) = 11.12 + 1.51 \times \text{time (min)}$$
$$(r = 0.72, SEE = 4.26 \text{ ml · kg}^{-1} \cdot \text{min}^{-1})$$

The Balke protocol has been modified several times. Some modifications use 2%, 2.5%, or 5% increases in grade every 2 or 3 min instead of 1% increases every minute. Another modification incorporates an individualized, comfortable walking speed for subjects, based on their ability, rather than having all subjects walk at 3.3 mph. Because regression equations have not been developed for all of these modifications, investigators who use modified Balke protocols typically measure $\dot{V}O_2max$ or estimate it from the speed and grade of the treadmill at maximal exercise using the American

College of Sports Medicine (ACSM) energy cost equation for walking (2). However, the ACSM equation overestimates $\dot{V}O_2$max because it was designed to estimate $\dot{V}O_2$ during submaximal steady-state aerobic exercise.

Maximal Cycle Ergometer Protocols

The cycle ergometer is frequently used for maximal testing because it is relatively inexpensive compared to a treadmill, can be portable, requires little space, and provides for stable ECG and blood pressure monitoring. Results for $\dot{V}O_2$max on cycle ergometer tests are generally lower than for treadmill tests, due to involvement of a smaller muscle mass. The following protocol is recommended by ACSM (2).

Equipment

- Mechanically or electronically braked cycle ergometer
- Timer
- ECG or HR monitor (optional)
- Metronome

Protocol

1. Adjust seat height and handlebars to fit the subject.
2. Pedal speed should be constant—usually 50 or 60 rpm.
3. Begin the test by having the subject pedal at a low resistance for a 2-min warm-up.
4. Increase external work by 150 to 300 kgm every 2 or 3 min until the subject can no longer maintain pedal speed. The magnitude of the increase in work depends on the body mass and fitness of the subject.
5. When the test is completed, decrease the resistance and have the subject continue pedaling for 3 to 5 min to prevent venous pooling.

Calculations

$\dot{V}O_2$max can be estimated from performance on the test using the ACSM equation for the energy cost of stationary cycling (2):

$$\dot{V}O_2 \text{ (ml} \cdot \text{min}^{-1}) = \text{kgm} \cdot \text{min}^{-1} \times 2 \text{ ml} \cdot \text{kgm}^{-1} + [3.5 \text{ ml} \cdot \text{kg}^{-1} \cdot \text{min}^{-1} \times \text{body mass (kg)}]$$

The mechanical power in kilogram-meters per minute (kgm $\cdot$ min^{-1}) is determined by the product of the weight applied (kg or kp), the distance this weight travels per revolution (m $\cdot$ rev^{-1}), and the number of revolutions per minute (rev $\cdot$ min^{-1})—or kgm $\cdot$ min^{-1} = (kg) × (m $\cdot$ rev^{-1}) × (rev $\cdot$ min^{-1}).

Maximum oxygen consumption can also be estimated from data presented in Table 4.3.

Maximal Arm Ergometry

Testing with an arm ergometer is useful in individuals who have lost the use of the legs or who have orthopedic or circulatory problems in the lower extremities that limit their ability to exercise on a cycle or treadmill. Arm $\dot{V}O_2$max is 20% to 30% less, and peak HR is 10 to 15 bpm lower, compared with leg ergometry. Arm ergometers are available commercially, and cycle ergometers can be modified for use with the arms (9).

Equipment

- Arm crank or cycle ergometer adapted for arm cranking
- Timer
- ECG or HR monitor (optional)
- Metronome

Protocol

1. The protocol for arm cranking is similar to that for leg ergometry (2). The arm ergometer should be

Table 4.3 Estimation of $\dot{V}O_2$max (ml $\cdot$ kg^{-1} $\cdot$ min^{-1}) From Cycle Ergometry

Body weight		Exercise rate (kgm · min⁻¹ and watts)						
kg	lb	300 / 50	450 / 75	600 / 100	750 / 125	900 / 150	1,050 / 175	1,200 / 200
50	110	18.0	24.0	30.0	36.0	42.0	48.0	54.0
60	132	15.0	20.0	25.0	30.0	35.0	40.0	45.0
70	154	12.9	17.1	21.4	25.7	30.0	34.3	38.6
80	176	11.3	15.0	18.8	22.5	26.3	30.0	33.8
90	198	10.0	13.3	16.7	20.0	23.3	26.7	30.0
100	220	9.0	12.0	15.0	18.0	21.0	24.0	27.0

Reprinted with permission from ACSM. (1986). *Guidelines for Exercise Testing and Prescription.* (3rd edition). Philadelphia: Lea & Febiger.

positioned so that the subject can arm-crank seated upright with the feet flat on the floor. The midpoint of the cycle sprocket should be positioned shoulder-high for each subject. The seat should also be positioned so that during arm cranking the arms are fully extended at maximal reach to facilitate maximal efficiency.

2. Follow the same protocol as for leg ergometry, except set the initial work load at 75 to 150 kgm and increase work output by 75- to 150-kgm increments. The test is terminated when the subject can no longer maintain the crank rate.

Calculations

$\dot{V}O_2$max can be estimated from the mechanical power using the following ACSM equation (2):

$$\dot{V}O_2 \ (ml \cdot min^{-1}) = kgm \cdot min^{-1} \times 3 \ ml \cdot kgm^{-1} + [3.5 \ ml \cdot kg^{-1} \cdot min^{-1} \times body \ mass \ (kg)]$$

Advantages and Disadvantages of Maximal Tests

Maximal protocols usually provide a better estimation of $\dot{V}O_2$max than do submaximal tests. However, maximal exercise presents a greater cardiovascular stress than submaximal exercise does, and therefore it is most ap-

propriate for young populations that have minimal incidence of heart disease and asymptomatic individuals who have been previously screened for heart disease risk. ACSM recommends that the test be supervised by a physician if it is being used to screen for the presence of coronary heart disease (2).

Treadmill walking and running offer the advantage of being activities that are more familiar to most adults than cycling or arm ergometry. The Bruce treadmill protocol can be performed relatively quickly and provides an accurate estimation of $\dot{V}O_2$max. The major disadvantages of this test are the large, abrupt changes in work load with each stage and awkward speeds. The Balke protocol has small increases in work load. The constant walking speed is more comfortable for the subject and decreases motion artifact that can interfere with monitoring blood pressure and the ECG. However, because of the small increases in work, this protocol may require more than 20 min in very fit subjects.

Similar values for directly measured $\dot{V}O_2$max can be achieved regardless of the treadmill protocol chosen. Pollock et al. (10) compared the results for $\dot{V}O_2$max from the Bruce, Balke, and Ellestad protocols, and a running protocol in 51 middle-aged men. As shown in Figure 4.1, the rate of increase in $\dot{V}O_2$ varied among the protocols, but there was little difference in $\dot{V}O_2$max. Comparable values were also observed at maximal exercise on each protocol for blood pressure, rating of perceived exertion, respiratory exchange ratio, and

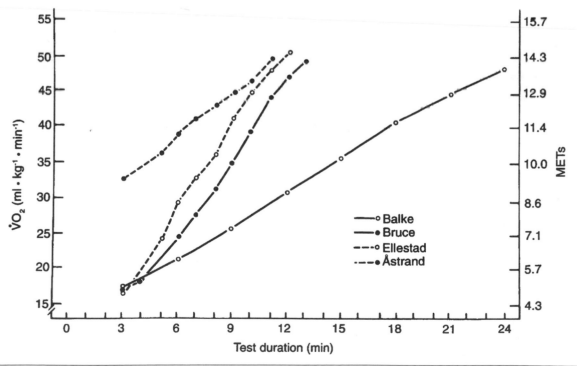

Figure 4.1 Rate of increase in oxygen consumption in four graded exercise protocols (10).
Reprinted with permission from Pollock, M.L., et al. (1976). A comparative analysis of four protocols for maximal treadmill stress testing. *American Heart Journal*, **92**, 36-46.

ventilation. Similar results have also been reported for women (11).

Cycle and arm ergometers are more portable and less expensive than treadmills; however, most Americans are not accustomed to these activities and experience local muscle fatigue before reaching their maximal capacity. There is less motion artifact with cycle ergometer tests so blood pressure and ECG are easier to obtain. Arm ergometer tests are useful in individuals who have lost the use of their legs or have orthopedic or circulatory limitations to exercise; however, blood pressure and ECG are difficult to assess with these.

SUBMAXIMAL AND FIELD TESTS

Submaximal or field tests may be more practical for estimating or categorizing aerobic capacity in many situations, such as when testing individuals over age 40, when testing large populations, or when time or equipment is limited.

Running and Walking Tests

Running and walking tests often are based on the time required to go a given distance (600 yd, 1.5 mi, 2 mi) or the total distance covered in a given time (9, 12, or 15 min). In addition, multiple regression equations based on track or treadmill running or walking have been developed to estimate $\dot{V}O_2$max.

12-Minute Field Performance Test

Balke (12) developed a field performance test using a 15-min run to assess the aerobic fitness of military personnel. The average energy cost, or oxygen consumption, for the test was calculated using time and distance measurements. Balke found that calculated values approximated $\dot{V}O_2$max (ml · kg^{-1} · min^{-1}).

Cooper (13, 14, 15) later shortened the test to 12 min and introduced the 1.5-mi run as an alternative to the 12-min run. He reported a correlation of $r = .90$ between 12-min run/walk distance and $\dot{V}O_2$max in 115 males aged 17 to 52 years. However, using different populations, other researchers have found correlations as low as $r = .30$ between run/walk scores and $\dot{V}O_2$max (16, 17). The highly significant correlation coefficient reported by Cooper may be explained by the wide age and fitness ranges of subjects in his sample.

Equipment

- Measured track or course
- Timer

Protocol

1. The concept of pacing should be explained to the subject.
2. Instruct the subject to cover the longest possible distance in 12 min (or to run 1.5 mi as fast as possible). Walking is permitted, but it is preferable to run.
3. When the test is completed, the subject should continue to walk slowly for 3 to 5 min to prevent venous pooling. Record the total distance covered in 12 min or the time required to run 1.5 mi.

Calculations

Cooper derived the following regression equation to describe the relationship between distance and $\dot{V}O_2$max:

$$\text{run/walk distance (miles)} = 0.3138 + 0.0278 \times \dot{V}O_2 \text{ (ml} \cdot \text{kg}^{-1} \cdot \text{min}^{-1})$$

This equation can be reorganized to estimate $\dot{V}O_2$max from the 12-min run:

$$\dot{V}O_2\text{max (ml} \cdot \text{kg}^{-1} \cdot \text{min}^{-1}) = 35.97 \text{ (miles)} - 11.29$$

For example, if a woman runs 1.2 mi in 12 min, her estimated $\dot{V}O_2$max would be 31.9 ml · kg^{-1} · min^{-1}.

$$\dot{V}O_2\text{max (ml} \cdot \text{kg}^{-1} \cdot \text{min}^{-1}) = 35.97 \text{ (1.2 mi)} - 11.29 = 31.9$$

One-Mile Walk Test

Kline et al. (18) tested 343 adults aged 30 to 69 years. Maximal oxygen consumption was measured directly during a graded treadmill test to volitional exhaustion using a modified Balke protocol. In addition, each subject performed a minimum of two 1-mi walk tests on a measured track on separate days.

Subjects were randomly assigned to a development group ($n = 174$) or a cross-validation group ($n = 169$). A multiple regression equation was generated to estimate $\dot{V}O_2$max using data from the development group, and the accuracy of the equation was assessed using data from the cross-validation group. Cross-validation analysis yielded a correlation of $r = .88$ between observed and estimated $\dot{V}O_2$max. When the equation subsequently was validated on 20- to 29-year-olds (19), 70- to 79-year-olds (20), and overweight women (21), correlations between observed and estimated $\dot{V}O_2$max ranged from $r = .78$ to $r = .88$.

The accuracy of the equation also has been assessed using a 1-mi treadmill walk as an alternative to a track walk (22). A correlation of $r = .91$ between observed and estimated $\dot{V}O_2$max was found when exercise HR at the end of the treadmill walk was used in the equation.

Equipment

- Measured track or course (or treadmill)
- Timer
- HR monitor (optional)

Protocol

1. Instruct the subject to walk 1 mi as fast as possible without running.
2. Record average HR for the last 2 complete min of the walk. If a HR monitor is not available, the subject must measure his or her 15-s pulse rate and record HR in beats per minute immediately upon completion of the test.
3. Record elapsed time to complete the walk to the nearest second.
4. When the test is completed, the subject should continue to walk slowly for 3 to 5 min to prevent venous pooling.

Calculations

Estimated $\dot{V}O_2max$

$$(ml \cdot kg^{-1} \cdot min^{-1}) = 132.85 - 0.077 \times \text{body weight (lb)} - 0.39 \times \text{age (y)} + 6.32 \times \text{gender (0 = F; 1 = M)} - 3.26 \times \text{elapsed time (min)} - 0.16 \times \text{HR (bpm)}$$

For example, estimated $\dot{V}O_2max$ can be calculated as follows for a 46-year-old female who weighs 155 lb and walks 1 mi in 15 min and 20 s (15.33 min), with a pulse rate of 36 beats/15 s (144 bpm) at the end of the walk:

Estimated $\dot{V}O_2max$

$$(ml \cdot kg^{-1} \cdot min^{-1}) = 132.85 - (0.077 \times 155) - (0.39 \times 46) + (6.32 \times 0) - (3.26 \times 15.33) - (0.16 \times 144)$$
$$= 132.85 - 11.94 - 17.94 - 49.98 - 23.04$$
$$= 29.95$$

Since the regression equation estimates $\dot{V}O_2max$ in milliliters per kilogram per minute ($ml \cdot kg^{-1} \cdot min^{-1}$), the standards established by the American Heart Association (Table 4.1) can be used to categorize individual fitness levels.

Single-Stage Submaximal Treadmill Walking Test

A single-stage submaximal treadmill test was developed to estimate $\dot{V}O_2max$ ($ml \cdot kg^{-1} \cdot min^{-1}$) (23). Subjects (67 men, 72 women) from 20 to 59 years walked at a constant speed (2.0-4.5 mph) at 5% grade for 4 min and then performed a $\dot{V}O_2max$ test. Maximal oxygen consumption was measured directly, and HR was assessed using a HR monitor. Multiple regression analysis was used to develop a model for estimating $\dot{V}O_2max$ from the 4-min stage at 5% grade in a development group ($n = 117$). To assess the accuracy of the model in a cross-validation group ($n = 22$), an estimated $\dot{V}O_2max$ value was obtained using the model. The correlation between observed and estimated $\dot{V}O_2max$ was $r = .96$ for the cross-validation group. For 90.9% of the subjects in the cross-validation group, residual scores (observed $\dot{V}O_2max$ – estimated $\dot{V}O_2max$) were within the range of ± 5 $ml \cdot kg^{-1} \cdot min^{-1}$.

Equipment

- Motor-driven treadmill
- Timer
- HR monitor (optional)

Protocol

1. Explain proper treadmill walking techniques to the subject, and allow the subject to practice walking at 0% grade until she or he is at ease on the treadmill.
2. A brisk, but comfortable, pace ranging from 2.0 to 4.5 mph should be established during a 2- to 4-min warm-up at 0% grade immediately prior to the test.
3. The subject then should walk for 4 min at 5% grade at the established individualized walking speed.
4. Measure HR at the end of the test using a HR monitor or by counting the pulse rate.
5. When the test is completed, the subject should continue to walk slowly for 3 to 5 min to prevent venous pooling.

Calculations

Estimated $\dot{V}O_2max$

$$(ml \cdot kg^{-1} \cdot min^{-1}) = 15.1 + 21.8 \times \text{speed (mph)} - 0.327 \times \text{HR (bpm)} - 0.263 \times \text{speed} \times \text{age (y)} + 0.00504 \times \text{HR} \times \text{age} + 5.98 \times \text{gender (0 = F; 1 = M)}.$$

For example, estimated $\dot{V}O_2max$ can be calculated as follows for a 34-year-old male who weighs 170 lb, walks at 4.0 mph, and has a HR of 142 bpm at the end of the test:

Estimated $\dot{V}O_2max$

$$(ml \cdot kg^{-1} \cdot min^{-1}) = 15.1 + (21.8 \times 4.0) - (0.327 \times 142) - (0.263 \times 4.0 \times 34) + (0.00504 \times 142 \times 34) + (5.98 \times 1)$$
$$= 15.1 + 87.2 - 46.4 - 35.8 + 24.3 + 5.98$$
$$= 50.4$$

Because the regression equation estimates $\dot{V}O_2$max in milliliters per kilogram per minute ($ml \cdot kg^{-1} \cdot min^{-1}$), the standards established by the American Heart Association (Table 4.1) can be used to categorize individual fitness levels.

Submaximal Cycle Ergometry Tests

The most commonly used submaximal cycle ergometer tests are the single-stage test developed by Åstrand and Ryhming (24, 25) and a multistage test originally developed by Sjostrand (26). Both tests are based on the linear relationship between HR and $\dot{V}O_2$ and the assumption that a younger or more fit individual will have a lower submaximal steady-state HR at any given level of power output.

Åstrand-Ryhming Test

The original Åstrand-Ryhming nomogram (24) was developed on data from 58 subjects aged 18 to 30 years who performed submaximal tests on a cycle ergometer and maximal tests on either a cycle ergometer or a treadmill. The test is based on the observation that at 50% $\dot{V}O_2$max, males had an average HR of 128 bpm, and females, 138 bpm. At 70% $\dot{V}O_2$max, the average HRs were 154 and 164 bpm for males and females, respectively. Åstrand (27) later tested 144 additional subjects and modified the nomogram to include an age-correction factor, because maximal HR decreases with age.

Other authors have found correlations between measured $\dot{V}O_2$max and $\dot{V}O_2$max predicted from the Åstrand-Ryhming nomogram ranging from $r = .74$ to $r = .83$ (28, 29, 30, 31). Patton, Vogel, and Mello (32) found no correlation ($r = .58$) between measured and predicted $\dot{V}O_2$max in 12 women aged 18 to 33 years ($\bar{x} \pm SD = 24 \pm 2$ years). Teraslinna, Ismail, and MacLeod (33) demonstrated the importance of using the age-correction factor for older subjects. The correlation between measured and predicted $\dot{V}O_2$max increased from $r = .69$ to $r = .92$ when the age-correction factor was used for a group of 31 sedentary men aged 23 to 49 years ($\bar{x} \pm SD = 36 \pm 6$ years).

Legge and Bannister (34) have modified the nomogram. The new nomogram is based on the linear relationship between $\dot{V}O_2$ and the elevation in HR above that reached during zero-load pedaling at 90 rpm. The authors found that the correlation between measured $\dot{V}O_2$max and that predicted from the new nomogram ($r = .98$) was higher than the correlation between measured $\dot{V}O_2$max and predictions made from the original Åstrand-Ryhming nomogram ($r = .80$) in 14 males aged 20 to 29 years.

Equipment

- Mechanically or electronically braked cycle ergometer
- Timer
- HR monitor (optional)
- Metronome

Protocol

1. Adjust seat height and handlebars to fit the subject.
2. Set pedal speed at 50 rpm.
3. Set initial work loads at 150, 100, or 75 W for well-trained, moderately trained, and untrained subjects, respectively.
4. The work load should be maintained for 6 min. HR should be measured at the end of Minutes 5 and 6.
5. If the HRs for the 5th and 6th min do not differ by more than 5 bpm and if their mean value is between 130 and 170 bpm, the test should be terminated.
6. If the HR mean value is less than 130 bpm, the work load should be increased by 50 to 100 W, and the test continued another 6 min.
7. If the HRs at Minutes 5 and 6 differ by more than 5 bpm, the test should be continued until the HRs at two consecutive minutes do not differ by more than 5 bpm.
8. When the test is completed, decrease the resistance and have the subject continue pedaling for 3 to 5 min to prevent venous pooling.

Calculations

On Figure 4.2, draw a line between the work rate on the cycle ergometer test and the mean value for the HRs during the last 2 min of the test. The line will cross the estimated $\dot{V}O_2$ in liters per minute ($L \cdot min^{-1}$).

These estimates of $\dot{V}O_2$max are influenced by a person's maximal HR, which decreases with age. A correction factor from the table embedded in Figure 4.2 corrects the $\dot{V}O_2$max value when either the maximal HR or age is known. Multiply the $\dot{V}O_2$max value from the nomogram by the correction factor.

For example, the results of a cycle ergometer test for a 40-year-old man who worked at 200 W with a HR of 166 bpm is shown in Figure 4.2. A dashed line is drawn between the 200-W work rate and the HR value of 166 bpm. The estimated $\dot{V}O_2$max is 3.6 $L \cdot min^{-1}$. Because the man is 40 years old, this value is multiplied by the age-correction factor (0.83) for 40-year-olds. The resultant $\dot{V}O_2$max value for the 40-year-old man is 2.99 $L \cdot min^{-1}$.

A 25-year-old woman worked at 100 W with a HR of 156 bpm. Another dashed line is drawn between the 100-W work rate and her HR of 156 bpm. The estimated $\dot{V}O_2$max is 2.4 $L \cdot min^{-1}$. The age-correction factor for

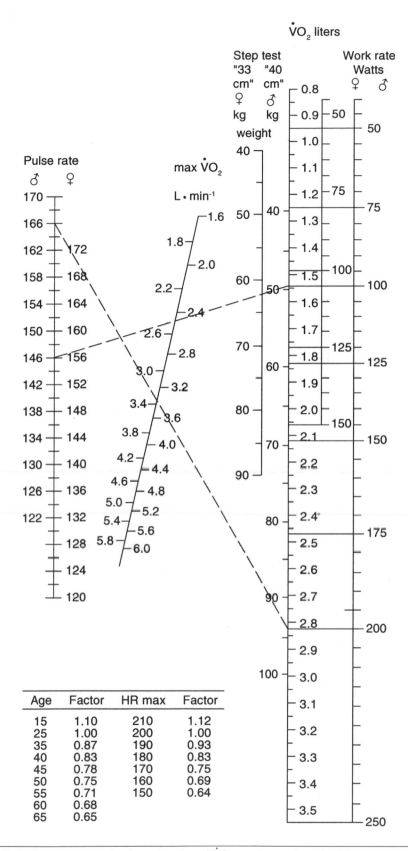

Age	Factor	HR max	Factor
15	1.10	210	1.12
25	1.00	200	1.00
35	0.87	190	0.93
40	0.83	180	0.83
45	0.78	170	0.75
50	0.75	160	0.69
55	0.71	150	0.64
60	0.68		
65	0.65		

Figure 4.2   Åstrand-Ryhming nomogram for the estimation of $\dot{V}O_2$max from submaximal heart rate values on either a cycle ergometer or a step test.

Reprinted with permission from Åstrand, P.O., and Rodahl, K. (1986). *Textbook of Work Physiology.* New York: McGraw-Hill Book Company.

a 25-year-old is 1.0, so her estimated $\dot{V}O_2$max is 2.4 L $\cdot$ min^{-1}.

YMCA Cycle Ergometer Test

The YMCA cycle ergometer test (35) uses the extrapolation method. Heart rate is measured at two or three 3-min submaximal work loads and extrapolated to the subject's estimated maximal HR (220 − age). The only precaution is that the HRs from two work loads must be in the linear portion of the HR/$\dot{V}O_2$ relationship.

Equipment
Same as Åstrand-Ryhming test

Protocol

1. Adjust seat height and handlebars to fit the subject.
2. Each stage lasts 3 min. HR is obtained during the last 30 s of each stage. The test is terminated when two work loads have been completed with HRs between 110 and 150 bpm.
3. The test begins at 25 W. After 3 min, HR is measured. The increase in work load is based on a branching protocol and is inversely related to HR (35).

Calculations

1. Plot HR against work (watts) on the graph illustrated in Figure 4.3.
2. Draw a line connecting the HRs and extrapolate to the subject's age-predicted maximum heart rate (maximum heart rate = 220 − age).
3. Drop a vertical line from the maximal HR to the x-axis. This point represents the estimated maximum work rate (watts). The corresponding estimated $\dot{V}O_2$max can be calculated from watts using the following equation (2):

$$\dot{V}O_2\text{max (ml} \cdot \text{min}^{-1}) = (\text{watts} \times 6 \text{ kpm/watt}) \times 2\text{ml/kpm} + 300$$

For example, a 40-year-old man completed three work loads. His HRs were 105, 120, and 150 bpm for the three stages. The three HRs are plotted against work rate (Figure 4.3). A line is drawn through the three points and extrapolated to 180 bpm (220 − 40 = 180). A vertical line is dropped to the baseline. The predicted maximum work load is 150 W. The $\dot{V}O_2$max corresponding to this work load is 2.1 L $\cdot$ min^{-1}.

Siconolfi Cycle Ergometer Test

Siconolfi, Cullinane, Carlton, and Thompson (36) developed and cross-validated a submaximal cycle ergometer test on 113 men and women aged 20 to 70 years. This test is a modification of the YMCA protocol that

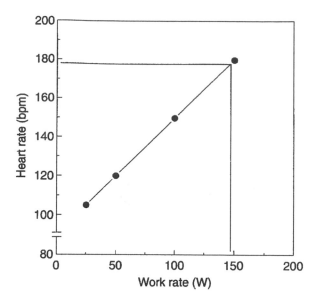

Figure 4.3   Sample graph for the extrapolation method of estimating maximum workrate and $\dot{V}O_2$max from heart rate responses to submaximal work rates.

uses the Åstrand-Ryhming nomogram. Regression equations were derived to estimate $\dot{V}O_2$max for men and women with multiple correlations of $R = .86$ and $R = .97$, respectively. Cross-validation yielded correlations of $r = .88$ and $r = .87$ for men and women, respectively, and no differences between measured and estimated $\dot{V}O_2$max.

Equipment
Same as Åstrand-Ryhming test

Protocol

1. Set initial work rate:
   Men under age 35: 300 kgm $\cdot$ min^{-1}
   Men over age 35 and all women: 150 kgm $\cdot$ min^{-1}
2. Increase work rate by the magnitude of the initial work rate every 2 min.
3. The test is terminated when a HR $\geq$ 70% of estimated maximal HR is reached.

Calculations
Find the estimated $\dot{V}O_2$max from the Åstrand-Ryhming nomogram as described under the Åstrand-Ryhming protocol. Use the following equations to calculate the age-corrected $\dot{V}O_2$max:
For males:

$$\dot{V}O_2\text{max (L} \cdot \text{min}^{-1}) = 0.348\ (x_1) - 0.035\ (x_2) + 3.011\ (r = .86,\ SEE = 0.359 \text{ L} \cdot \text{min}^{-1})$$

For females:

$$\dot{V}O_2max \ (L \cdot min^{-1}) = 0.302 \ (x_1) - 0.019 \ (x_2) + 1.593 \ (r = .97, \ SEE = 0.199 \ L \cdot min^{-1})$$

Where:

x_1 = $\dot{V}O_2max$ from Åstrand-Ryhming nomogram
x_2 = age in years

Submaximal Step Tests

Harvard Step Test

Brouha, Graybiel, and Heath (37) developed a simple single-stage step test on college-aged men at the Harvard Fatigue Laboratory. This test uses duration of exercise and recovery HR to determine an index of aerobic capacity.

$$Index = \frac{100 \times (duration \ of \ exercise \ in \ seconds)}{2 \times (sum \ of \ pulse \ counts \ in \ recovery)}$$

The sum of pulse counts is the number of heartbeats that occurred from 1 to 1.5, 2 to 2.5, and 3 to 3.5 min in recovery.

Based on his score the subject can be placed in one of the following classifications of aerobic capacity:

Index	Classification
> 90	Excellent
80-89	Good
65-79	High average
55-64	Low average
< 55	Poor

Equipment

- Platform 20 in. (50.8 cm) in height
- Metronome
- Timer

Protocol

1. Set the metronome at 120 bpm to elicit a stepping rate of 30 steps per minute.
2. Demonstrate the stepping cycle to the subject(s). A full cycle represents a 4-count beat: On Count 1, the subject places one foot on the step; on Count 2, the other leg is lifted onto the step and the subject straightens both the back and legs; on Count 3, the first foot is brought back down; followed by the second foot on Count 4.
3. The subject steps up and down on the platform at a rate of 30 steps per minute for a period of 5 min or until exhaustion. The subject is considered

exhausted when he or she cannot maintain the pace for 15 s.
4. At the end of the test, the subject immediately sits down. The duration of exercise is recorded.
5. Count the subject's pulse from 1 to 1.5, 2 to 2.5, and 3 to 3.5 min into recovery. The number of heartbeats during the three 30-s periods is recorded.

Calculations
For example, an individual stepped for 4 min, 12 s, with pulse counts of 78, 70, and 62 beats for the three recovery intervals. The calculated score is 60, which places the individual in the "low average" classification for fitness.

$$Index = \frac{100 \times (duration)}{2 \times (sum \ of \ pulses)} = \frac{100 \times (252)}{2 \times (210)} = 60$$

Queens College Step Test

McArdle et al. (38) developed a 3-min step test to evaluate aerobic fitness in 41 college-aged women. A 15-s HR was measured between 5 and 20 s of recovery. Test-retest reliability for recovery HR was $r = .92$. A correlation of $r = -.75$ was reported between recovery HR and $\dot{V}O_2max$ as determined directly using the Balke treadmill protocol. The regression equation for predicting $\dot{V}O_2max$ from recovery HR had a standard error of prediction of $\pm 2.9 \ ml \cdot kg^{-1} \cdot min^{-1}$.

Equipment

- Platform or step 16.25 in. (41.3 cm) in height (bleacher)
- Metronome or tape recorder and tape of prerecorded metronome rate of 88 bpm
- HR monitor (optional)
- Timer

Protocol

1. Set the metronome at 88 bpm to elicit a stepping rate of 22 steps per minute. Attach HR monitor if available.
2. Demonstrate the stepping cycle to the subject(s). A full cycle represents a 4-count beat as described for the Harvard step test.
3. The subject should practice for 15 s to adjust to the metronome cadence.
4. The subject performs the test by stepping for 3 min at a rate of 22 steps per minute.
5. After the test the subject remains standing. The pulse is counted for a 15-s period starting at 5 s into recovery (i.e., 5-20 s of recovery). Convert this value to beats per minute.

Calculations
The following equation was derived to estimate $\dot{V}O_2max$ from the recovery HR for women:

$\dot{V}O_2max$

$$(ml \cdot kg^{-1} \cdot min^{-1}) = 65.81 - [0.1847 \times$$
$$recovery\ HR\ (bpm)]$$

For example, if a woman has a 15-s recovery HR of 35 beats, her recovery HR is 4×35 beats, or 140 bpm.

$\dot{V}O_2max$

$$(ml \cdot kg^{-1} \cdot min^{-1}) = 65.81 - (0.1847 \times 140)$$
$$= 40\ ml \cdot kg^{-1} \cdot min^{-1}$$

Norms

Percentiles (39) based on data from 300 college-aged women are reported in Table 4.4.

McArdle, Katch, and Katch (40) reported a modification of this test to be used with college-aged men. The men performed a similar protocol except that they stepped at a rate of 24 steps per minute. The following regression equation was developed to estimate $\dot{V}O_2max$ for men from recovery HR:

$\dot{V}O_2max$

$$(ml \cdot kg^{-1} \cdot min^{-1}) = 111.33 - [0.42 \times$$
$$recovery\ HR\ (bpm)]$$

Siconolfi Step Test

Siconolfi, Garber, Laster, and Carleton (41) designed a multistage step test to assess aerobic fitness in the general population. This study included 48 healthy men and women aged 19 to 70 years. The subjects stepped for a maximum of three 3-min stages, or until their exercise HR for a stage exceeded 65% of age-predicted maximum. Exercise HR and submaximal $\dot{V}O_2$ estimated

Table 4.4 Percentile Norms for Recovery Heart Rate During the Queen's College Step Test

Percentile	Recovery heart rate (bpm)	Percentile	Recovery heart rate (bpm)
100	128	45	168
95	140	40	170
90	148	35	171
85	152	30	172
80	156	25	176
75	158	20	180
70	160	15	182
65	162	10	184
60	163	5	196
55	164	0	216
50	166		

Reprinted with permission from McArdle, W.D., Pechar, G.S., Katch, F.I., & Magel, J.R. (1973). Percentile norms for a valid step test in college women. *Research Quarterly*, **44**, 500.

using the ACSM equation for stepping (2) was recorded for the final stepping stage. Maximal oxygen consumption was estimated from the Åstrand-Ryhming nomogram, using the exercise HR and the estimated $\dot{V}O_2$ at the final stage. A correlation of $r = .92$ was reported between estimated $\dot{V}O_2max$ from this test and that measured directly using a cycle ergometer.

Equipment

- Platform or step 10 in. (25.4 cm) in height
- Metronome or tape recorder and tape of prerecorded metronome rates of 68, 104, and 136 bpm
- HR monitor
- Timer

Protocol

1. Attach HR monitor.
2. Set metronome rate at 68 bpm to elicit a stepping rate of 17 steps per minute (Stage 1). Demonstrate the stepping cycle to the subject(s) as described for the Harvard step test.
3. The subject performs Stage 1 by stepping up and down on the step for 3 min at a stepping rate of 17 steps per minute. Record the subject's HR in beats per minute during the last 30 s of this stage.
4. At the end of Stage 1, the subject sits for 1 min of recovery. If the recorded HR for Stage 1 is less than 65% of the subject's age-predicted maximum (220 − age), then the subject goes to Stage 2. If the HR is greater than 65% of the age-predicted maximum, the test is terminated.
5. For Stage 2, set the metronome rate at 104 bpm to elicit a stepping rate of 26 steps per minute. The subject steps for 3 min. Record heart rate (bpm) for the last 30 s of exercise.
6. At the completion of Stage 2, the subject sits for 1 min of recovery. If the Stage 2 HR is less than 65% of the age-predicted maximum, the subject will continue to Stage 3; else, the test is terminated.
7. For Stage 3, set the metronome at 136 bpm for a stepping rate of 34 steps per minute. The subject steps for 3 min at this rate. Record heart rate (bpm) for the last 30 s of exercise.

The protocol is summarized in Table 4.5:

Calculations

Values for $\dot{V}O_2$ estimated from the ACSM stepping equation (2) are 16.29, 24.91, and 33.53 $ml \cdot kg^{-1} \cdot min^{-1}$ for Stages 1, 2, and 3, respectively. The $\dot{V}O_2$ for the final completed stage is converted to liters per minute $(L \cdot min^{-1})$ by multiplying by body mass in kilograms and dividing by 1,000. The $\dot{V}O_2$ value in liters per minute and the HR during the final stage are used to find the subject's $\dot{V}O_2max$ on the Åstrand-Ryhming

Table 4.5   Siconolfi Step-Test Protocol

Stage	Stepping rate (steps/min)	Metronome rate (bpm)	Time (min)
1	17	68	3
Sitting recovery	—	—	1
2	26	104	3
Sitting recovery	—	—	1
3	34	136	3

Adapted with permission from Siconolfi, S.F., Garber, C.E., Lasater, T.M. & Carleton, R.A. (1985). A simple, valid step test for estimating maximal oxygen uptake in epidemiologic studies. *American Journal of Epidemiology*, **121**, 385.

nomogram (Figure 4.2). This value is then adjusted for age using the equations for males and females from the Siconolfi cycle ergometer test.

For example, a 20-year-old woman with a body mass of 55 kg had a recorded HR of 125 bpm at Stage 1 and 148 bpm at Stage 2. The woman advanced to Stage 2 because her HR for Stage 1 did not exceed 65% of her age-predicted maximum.

Age-predicted maximum HR = 220 − 20 = 200 bpm

$$65\% \text{ of age-predicted maximum HR}$$
$$= 200 \times 0.65 = 130 \text{ bpm}$$

$$\dot{V}O_2 \text{ at the final stage} = (24.91 \text{ ml} \cdot \text{kg}^{-1} \cdot \text{min}^{-1} \times$$
$$55 \text{ kg})/1{,}000$$
$$= 1.37 \text{ L} \cdot \text{min}^{-1}$$

Using the Åstrand-Ryhming nomogram, draw a straight line between the point that corresponds to 1.37 $\text{L} \cdot \text{min}^{-1}$ on the submaximal $\dot{V}O_2$ scale and the point that corresponds to 148 bpm on the heart rate scale. The line intercepts the $\dot{V}O_2$max scale at 2.4 $\text{L} \cdot \text{min}^{-1}$. The age-adjusted $\dot{V}O_2$max is calculated using the equations from the Siconolfi cycle ergometer test (36):

$$\dot{V}O_2\text{max (L} \cdot \text{min}^{-1}) = 0.302 \times (\text{nomogram } \dot{V}O_2\text{max})$$
$$- 0.019 \times (\text{age}) + 1.593$$
$$= 0.302 \times (2.4 \text{ L} \cdot \text{min}^{-1}) -$$
$$0.019 \times (20 \text{ yrs}) + 1.593$$
$$= 1.94$$

Advantages and Disadvantages of Submaximal Tests

Because most submaximal tests are based on the measurement of HR at one or more work loads, they have several limitations (28, 42). First, for any given rate of submaximal work, HR can vary independently of $\dot{V}O_2$ due to emotional state or degree of excitement. Heart rate can also vary with elapsed time after the previous meal, total circulating hemoglobin, degree of hydration, and ambient temperature (28).

Second, these tests are based on the assumption that HR is a linear function of $\dot{V}O_2$ throughout the range of work rates up to maximum. However, Maritz, Morrison, Peter, Strydom, and Wyndham (43) showed that HR reaches its maximum value at a slightly lower work rate than $\dot{V}O_2$. This asymptotic relationship between HR and $\dot{V}O_2$ causes a slight underestimation of $\dot{V}O_2$max.

Third, the variation in maximum HR with age is approximately 5% (42). Therefore, if the maximum HR is estimated at 200 bpm, it could actually be anywhere from 180 to 220 bpm. As a result, $\dot{V}O_2$max for an individual with a true maximum HR of 180 bpm will be overestimated. For an individual with a true maximum HR of 220 bpm, $\dot{V}O_2$max will be underestimated.

The 12-min run test and the 1-mi walk test involve activities that are familiar to most individuals, and many can be tested simultaneously. Because the 12-min run requires a near-maximal effort, the 1-mi walk test may be more appropriate for older, sedentary, or overweight individuals. On the other hand, the 1-mi walk test may underestimate $\dot{V}O_2$max in subjects with $\dot{V}O_2$max values greater than 55 ml · kg^{-1} · min^{-1}. The 1-mi walk test can also be administered on a treadmill. The single-stage treadmill test is time-efficient, requiring only 4 min to complete. Although the test was developed on both men and women who varied widely in age and fitness level, the test has not been validated in individuals over 60 years of age.

The submaximal cycle ergometer and step tests have the advantages of utilizing portable, inexpensive equipment. The major disadvantage of the cycle ergometer is that most Americans are unaccustomed to cycling. Consequently, $\dot{V}O_2$max can be underestimated by 5% to 25%, depending on the individual's level of conditioning (3).

The step tests can be administered to many people at the same time. However, the Harvard step test may be too strenuous for older, less fit individuals, and the 20-in. step height may cause local leg fatigue in shorter or heavier individuals. The Queen's College step test and Siconolfi step test avoid this limitation because they utilize a lower step. The Siconolfi test may be particularly useful for older or unfit subjects.

NONEXERCISE ESTIMATION OF $\dot{V}O_2$max

Researchers at the University of Houston have developed a method to estimate $\dot{V}O_2$peak that does not involve any form of exercise testing (44). Multiple regression equations were developed to estimate $\dot{V}O_2$peak (ml · kg^{-1} · min^{-1}) from age, physical activity status, and percent body fat or body mass index (BMI). The percent fat equation is slightly more accurate than the BMI equation. Physical activity is rated from the subject's exercise habits using the following code:

I. Does not participate regularly in programmed recreation sport or physical activity.
> 0 Avoids walking or exertion (e.g., always uses elevator, drives whenever possible instead of walking).
> 1 Walks for pleasure, routinely uses stairs, occasionally exercises sufficiently to cause heavy breathing or perspiration.

II. Participates regularly in recreation or work requiring modest physical activity, such as golf, horseback riding, calisthenics, gymnastics, table tennis, bowling, weight lifting, or yard work:
> 2 10 to 60 minutes per week.
> 3 Over one hour per week.

III. Participates regularly in heavy physical exercise (such as running or jogging, swimming, cycling, rowing, skipping rope, running in place) or engages in vigorous aerobic type activity (such as tennis, basketball, or handball).
> 4 Runs less than one mile per week or spends less than 30 minutes per week in comparable physical activity.
> 5 Runs 1 to 5 miles per week or spends 30 to 60 minutes per week in comparable physical activity.
> 6 Runs 5 to 10 miles per week or spends 1 to 3 hours per week in comparable physical activity.
> 7 Runs over 10 miles per week or spends over 3 hours per week in comparable physical activity.

The physical activity rating (PA-R) is used in the following equations to estimate $\dot{V}O_2$peak in ml · kg^{-1} · min^{-1}:

% Fat model ($R = .81$, $SEE = 5.35$ ml · kg^{-1} · min^{-1})
$$\dot{V}O_2\text{peak} = 50.513 + 1.589 \,(\text{PA-R}) - 0.289 \,(\text{age}) - 0.552 \,(\% \text{ fat}) + 5.863 \,(F = 0, M = 1)$$

BMI model ($R = .783$, $SEE = 5.70$ ml · kg^{-1} · min^{-1})
$$\dot{V}O_2\text{peak} = 56.363 + 1.921 \,(\text{PA-R}) - 0.381 \,(\text{age}) - 0.754 \,(\text{BMI}) + 10.987 \,(F = 0, M = 1)$$

For example, the estimated $\dot{V}O_2$peak for a 35-year-old man with 15% body fat and a physical activity rating of 6 would be

$$\dot{V}O_2\text{peak} = 50.513 + 1.589 \,(6) - 0.289 \,(35) - 0.552 \,(15) + 5.863 \,(1)$$
$$= 47.5 \text{ ml} \cdot \text{kg}^{-1} \cdot \text{min}^{-1}$$

The estimated $\dot{V}O_2$peak using the BMI model for a 35-year-old woman who is 65 in. tall, weighs 130 lb, and has an activity rating of 6 would be

$$\dot{V}O_2\text{peak} = 56.363 + 1.921 \,(6) - 0.381 \,(35) - 0.754 \,(59/1.65^2) + 10.987 \,(0)$$
$$= 38.2 \text{ ml} \cdot \text{kg}^{-1} \cdot \text{min}^{-1}$$

The nonexercise test is useful as an initial estimate of $\dot{V}O_2$max or for mass screening, because the required information can be collected through self-report. It appears to be accurate in subjects with $\dot{V}O_2$peak less than 55 ml · kg^{-1} · min^{-1}. It also has the advantage of not relying on heart rate as a predictor variable, so it might be useful in evaluating individuals taking medications that affect HR.

INDIRECT DETERMINATION OF AEROBIC POWER IN CHILDREN

Aerobic power in children has been determined indirectly using both maximal and submaximal protocols similar to those described for adults (45). Assessment of aerobic power in children, as in adults, is often based on performance measures or heart rates at submaximal work loads. Indices of aerobic power include endurance time on the treadmill, elapsed time to run a given distance, and physical working capacity at a heart rate of 170 bpm.

Bruce Treadmill Test

Cumming, Everatt, and Hastman (46) assessed treadmill endurance time in 53 girls and 24 boys using the Bruce protocol (Table 4.2). In addition, $\dot{V}O_2$ was measured directly during the test. Correlations between endurance time and $\dot{V}O_2$max were $r = .88$ for the girls and $r = .85$ for the boys. To assess reliability of the Bruce test in children, an additional 20 subjects aged 7 to 13 years performed the test on 2 separate days. The correlation between endurance times for the two trials was $r = .94$.

Oxygen consumption obtained from 38 subjects during the last minute of each of the first three stages varied with age, and the youngest children were the least efficient. Because many factors other than aerobic capacity may contribute to endurance time in children, Cumming et al. (46) did not estimate $\dot{V}O_2$max. However, percentile charts for treadmill endurance time using the Bruce protocol were constructed based on data obtained from 327 children and youth aged 4 to 18 years who were diagnosed as having an innocent heart murmur (Table 4.6).

Table 4.6 Bruce Treadmill Test Endurance Times (min) in Clinic Children With an Innocent Murmur

Age group		n	Percentiles					M	SD
			10	25	50	75	90		
Boys	4-5	40	8.1	9.0	10.0	12.0	13.3	10.4	1.9
	6-7	28	9.7	10.0	12.0	12.3	13.5	11.8	1.6
	8-9	30	9.6	10.5	12.4	13.7	16.2	12.6	2.3
	10-12	31	9.9	12.0	12.5	14.0	15.4	12.7	1.9
	13-15	26	11.2	13.0	14.3	16.0	16.1	14.1	1.7
	16-18	12	11.3	12.1	13.8	14.5	15.8	13.5	1.4
Girls	4-5	36	7.0	8.0	9.0	11.2	12.3	9.5	1.8
	6-7	34	9.5	9.6	11.4	13.0	13.0	11.2	1.5
	8-9	26	9.9	10.5	11.0	13.0	14.2	11.8	1.6
	10-12	28	10.5	11.3	12.0	13.0	14.6	12.3	1.4
	13-15	24	9.4	10.0	11.5	12.0	13.0	11.1	1.3
	16-18	12	8.1	10.0	10.5	12.0	12.4	10.7	1.4

Reprinted with permission from Cumming, G.R., Everatt, D., & Hastman, L. (1978). Bruce treadmill test in children: Normal values in a clinic population. *The American Journal of Cardiology*, **41**, 69-75.

Equipment

- Motor-driven treadmill
- Timer
- Equipment for monitoring HR

Protocol

1. Prepare to monitor HR throughout the test.
2. Explain proper treadmill walking techniques to the subject, and allow the subject to practice walking at 0% grade until she or he is at ease on the treadmill. A technician should stand beside or behind the child during the warm-up period and throughout the test.
3. Explain to the child that he or she must stay on the treadmill until totally exhausted and unable to continue walking or running. It is important that the child understand precisely what she or he is asked to do.
4. During the test, the child should not hold on to the handrails.
5. The speed and grade of the treadmill should increase every 3 min as outlined by Bruce, Kusumi, and Hosmer (5) (Table 4.2). Verbal encouragement should be given to the subject throughout the test. The child should continue to volitional exhaustion.
6. Record elapsed time at the end of the test.
7. Upon completion of the test, the child should continue to walk slowly for at least 3 to 5 min.

Calculations

Elapsed time should be expressed in 1/10ths of a minute for comparison to percentile charts.

For example, if a 14-year-old boy completed 14 min and 20 s (14.3 min) of the Bruce protocol, he would fall

at the 50th percentile compared to the data of Cumming, Everatt, and Hastman (46) (Table 4.6).

One-Mile Run/Walk Test

Several fitness test batteries have incorporated a 1-mi run/walk test as a measure of aerobic capacity, or cardiovascular endurance (46, 47, 48, 49). Cureton, Boileau, Lohman, and Misner (51) obtained a validity coefficient of $r = -.66$ between $\dot{V}O_2max$ obtained during a treadmill test and 1-mi run/walk time for 196 boys and girls aged 7 to 12 years. In another study, Krahenbuhl, Pangrazi, Petersen, Burkett, and Schneider (52) reported test-retest reliability coefficients of $r = .82$ to $r = .92$ for schoolchildren in Grades 1 through 3.

Traditionally, interpretation of test scores has been based on normative data, so that a child's performance on the test is interpreted relative to the scores of children in a reference group. Recently, the use of criterion-referenced standards for 1-mi run/walk time have been incorporated in several test batteries (47, 48, 50, 53, 54). Using the reference-standard approach, performance evaluation is based on scores associated with desirable levels of $\dot{V}O_2max$, the criterion for aerobic power. If run/walk performance is equal to or better than the standard, it is concluded that the child has an acceptable level of aerobic power.

Cureton and Warren (53) provide a detailed description of the derivation of Fitnessgram criterion-referenced standards for 1-mi run/walk time. Values for $\dot{V}O_2max$ of 42 ml · kg^{-1} · min^{-1} for males and 35 ml · kg^{-1} · min^{-1} for females were adopted as the criteria for adolescents aged 17 years or older. Because age has little effect on $\dot{V}O_2max$ expressed relative to body mass for boys aged 5 to 17 years, a $\dot{V}O_2$max criterion of 42 ml · kg^{-1} · min^{-1} was used for boys of all ages. However, the $\dot{V}O_2$max criterion was increased to 40 ml · kg^{-1} · min^{-1} for girls aged 5 to 9 years to account for lower average levels of body fat compared to older girls, and the criterion was decreased by 1 ml · kg^{-1} · min^{-1} per year to 35 ml · kg^{-1} · min^{-1} for girls aged 14 to 17 years. The $\dot{V}O_2$max criterion was multiplied by the average percentage of $\dot{V}O_2$max (80%-85% for children aged 5 to 9 years; 90%-100% for children aged 10 to 17 years) assumed to be utilized during the test. Finally, the average running speed needed to elicit the percentage of $\dot{V}O_2$max assumed to be utilized was calculated and converted to a reference standard for 1-mi run/walk time.

Equipment

- Measured track or course
- Timer

Protocol

1. The concept of pacing should be explained to the child. If possible, the child should be given an opportunity to practice before the day of the test.
2. Instruct the child to try to run the entire distance. If the child cannot complete the mile by running, walking is permitted.
3. Elapsed time is recorded at the end of the test.
4. When the test is completed, the subject should cool down by walking for 3 to 5 min.

Reference Standards

Reference standards proposed by Fitnessgram and AAHPERD are presented in Table 4.7. At the present

Table 4.7   Criterion-Referenced Standards Proposed by Fitnessgram and AAHPERD for 1-Mi Run/Walk Time (Minutes:Seconds)

Age	Boys		Girls	
	Fitnessgram	AAHPERD	Fitnessgram	AAHPERD
5	16:00	13:00	17:00	14:00
6	15:00	12:00	16:00	13:00
7	14:00	11:00	15:00	12:00
8	13:00	10:00	14:00	11:30
9	12:00	10:00	13:00	11:00
10	11:00	9:30	12:00	11:00
11	11:00	9:00	12:00	11:00
12	10:00	9:00	12:00	11:00
13	9:30	8:00	11:30	10:30
14	8:30	7:45	10:30	10:30
15	8:30	7:30	10:30	10:30
16	8:30	7:30	10:30	10:30
17	8:30	7:30	10:30	10:30

Data are from Fitnessgram (48) and AAHPERD (47).

time, a single set of standards has not been adopted by both groups, and the Fitnessgram standards are lower than the AAHPERD standards. For example, if a 7-year-old girl completes a mile in 14:21, her score would be considered acceptable by Fitnessgram standards but unacceptable by AAHPERD standards.

Physical Working Capacity at a Heart Rate of 170 (PWC$_{170}$)

In 1948, Wahlund (55) first presented the concept of estimating physical working capacity at a pulse rate of 170 bpm using increasing work loads on a cycle ergometer. Since that time, several protocols have been used to assess physical working capacity, or mechanical power, at a HR of 170 bpm in children (45). Franz, Wiewel, and Mellerowicz (56) reported a correlation coefficient of $r = .87$ between $\dot{V}O_2$max and PWC$_{170}$ in boys aged 1.42 ± 0.9 years. However, Petzl, Haber, Schuster, Popow, and Haschke (57) noted correlations between $\dot{V}O_2$max and PWC$_{170}$ expressed relative to body mass ranging from $r = .12$ for 10-year-old boys to $r = .67$ for 14-year-old boys. The latter authors suggested that although the PWC$_{170}$ test is valid for children aged 11 years or older, it perhaps should not be used as an indicator of $\dot{V}O_2$max for children aged 10 years or younger.

Equipment

- Cycle ergometer (Mechanically braked ergometers may be used, but electronically braked ergometers are preferred because power output is not dependent on pedal frequency. When a mechanically braked ergometer is used, a revolution counter is recommended, because most children have difficulty pedaling at a constant rate.) Pediatric ergometers should be used, or adult models should be modified in size (58)
- Metronome (if using a mechanically braked cycle ergometer)
- HR monitor

Protocol

1. Pedal rate must be explained to the child, especially when a mechanically braked cycle ergometer is used for testing. Pedal rates of approximately 60 rpm are recommended when using a mechanically braked ergometer.
2. Allow adequate warm-up time for the child to become accustomed to riding the cycle ergometer. Most children require at least 5 min of practice.
3. Several submaximal continuous cycling protocols are available for determining PWC$_{170}$ (45). The McMaster protocol is presented in Table 4.8.

Table 4.8   The McMaster Cycling Protocol

Body height (cm)	Initial load (watts)	Increments (watts)	Duration of each load (min)
< 119.9	12.5	12.5	2
120-139.9	12.5	25.0	2
140-159.9	25.0	25.0	2
> 160.0	25.0	25.0 (females) 50.0 (males)	2

Reprinted with permission from Bar-Or, O. (1983). *Pediatric Sports Medicine for the Practitioner: Physiologic Principles of Clinical Applications.* New York: Springer-Verlag.

4. The stage at which a HR of 170 bpm is reached should be completed even if the heart rate exceeds 170 bpm.
5. Upon completion of the test, the child should continue to pedal slowly for approximately 3 to 5 min.

Calculations

Three, or more, HR measurements are plotted against mechanical power (Figure 4.4). To decrease measurement error, one of the HRs should be within 160 to 180 bpm. The power output corresponding to a HR of 170 bpm is PWC_{170}.

For example, data for two subjects are plotted in Figure 4.4. Values for PWC_{170} for Subjects 1 and 2 are 1.51 and 2.16 W · kg^{-1}, respectively. If Subject 2 is a 12-year-old girl, she would be placed in the 90th percentile, based on the data collected in our laboratory on 458 boys and girls aged 6 to 13 years (Table 4.9).

Advantages and Disadvantages of Tests for Children

The Bruce treadmill protocol, commonly used to assess maximal exercise capacity in adults, also is suited for testing youth. The low initial loads allow for adequate warm-up time for most children. Treadmill endurance time is highly correlated to $\dot{V}O_2$max.

Little equipment is needed to administer the 1-mi run/walk test, and many children can be tested simultaneously. Thus, this test has been included in several fitness test batteries used in schools. Factors that affect performance on the 1-mi run/walk test include experience, motor efficiency, environmental conditions, and motivation. The theory underlying use of criterion-referenced standards to interpret scores on the 1-mi run/walk test is sound, but the standards must be validated on a large sample of children. Experts in the field of exercise science and physical education must come to a consensus on a single set of reference standards.

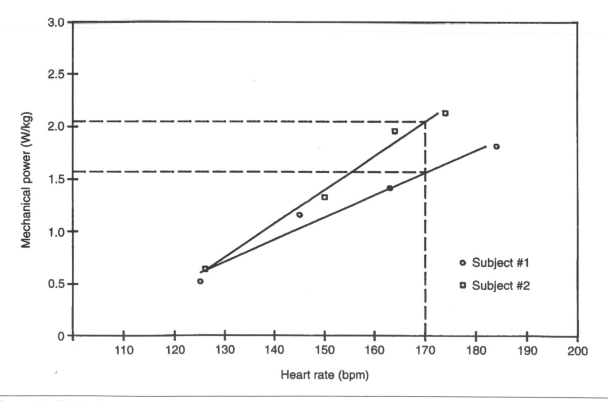

Figure 4.4   Calculation of PWC_{170} for two subjects.

Table 4.9   PWC$_{170}$ in Boys and Girls Ages 6 to 13 Years

Age group		n	| Percentiles 10	25	50	75	90	M	SD
Boys	6-7	45	1.29	1.48	1.85	2.17	2.56	1.87	0.51
	8-9	64	1.39	1.67	1.99	2.31	2.59	2.01	0.43
	10-11	53	1.34	1.73	2.12	2.32	2.69	2.05	0.48
	12-13	59	1.40	1.76	2.15	2.36	2.70	2.12	0.50
Girls	6-7	54	1.13	1.42	1.72	2.03	2.16	1.70	0.41
	8-9	65	1.30	1.48	1.69	2.02	2.19	1.74	0.38
	10-11	64	1.15	1.37	1.54	1.94	2.20	1.64	0.39
	12-13	54	1.18	1.50	1.73	1.96	2.21	1.74	0.41

Heart rate is used as a single independent variable to determine PWC$_{170}$. Although HR at any given work load may reflect the physical working capacity of an individual, there are limitations associated with using HR as a single independent variable. Heart rate can vary apart from fitness level and is often related to emotional state, environmental stresses, or elapsed time after a previous meal. Many children are not accustomed to cycling and may be overly excited or nervous at the start of the test, resulting in elevation in HR. PWC$_{170}$ may not be valid for assessing the fitness of an individual child under the age of 11 years. However, PWC$_{170}$ can provide useful information in population studies (45).

REFERENCES

1. American Heart Association. (1990). Exercise standards: A statement for health professionals from the American Heart Association. *Circulation*, **82**, 2286-2322.
2. American College of Sports Medicine. (1991). *Guidelines for exercise testing and prescription* (4th ed.). Philadelphia: Lea & Febiger.
3. Pollock, M.L., & Wilmore, J.H. (1990). *Exercise in health and disease: Evaluation and prescription for prevention and rehabilitation* (2nd ed.). Philadelphia: W.B. Saunders.
4. Ragg, K.E., Murray, T.F., Karbonit, L.M., & Jump, D.A. (1980). Errors in predicting functional capacity from a treadmill exercise stress test. *American Heart Journal*, **100**, 581-583.
5. Bruce, R.A., Kusumi, F., & Hosmer, D. (1973). Maximal oxygen intake and nomographic assessment of functional aerobic impairment in cardiovascular disease. *American Heart Journal*, **85**, 545-562.
6. Foster, C., Jackson, A.S., Pollock, M.L., Taylor, M.M., Hare, J., Sennett, S.M., Rod, J.L., Sarwar, M., & Schmidt, D.H. (1984). Generalized equations for predicting functional capacity from treadmill performance. *American Heart Journal*, **107**, 1229-1234.
7. Balke, B., & Ware, R. (1959). An experimental study of Air Force personnel. *U.S. Armed Forces Medical Journal*, **10**, 675-688.
8. Froelicher, V.F., & Lancaster, M.C. (1974). The prediction of maximal oxygen consumption from a continuous exercise treadmill protocol. *American Heart Journal*, **87**, 445-450.
9. Franklin, B.A. (1985). Exercise testing, training and arm ergometry. *Sports Medicine*, **2**, 100-199.
10. Pollock, M.L., Bohannon, R.L., Cooper, K.H., Ayres, J.J., Ward, A., White, S.R., & Linnerud, A.C. (1976). A comparative analysis of four protocols for maximal treadmill stress testing. *American Heart Journal*, **92**, 39-46.
11. Pollock, M.L., Foster, C., Schmidt, D., Hellman, C., Linnerud, A.C., & Ward, A. (1982). Comparative analysis of physiologic responses to three different maximal graded exercise test protocols in healthy women. *American Heart Journal*, **103**, 363-373.
12. Balke, B. (1963). A simple field test for the assessment of physical fitness. *Civil Aeromedical Research Institute Report*, **63**(6), 1-8.
13. Cooper, K.H. (1968). A means of assessing maximal oxygen intake. *Journal of the American Medical Association*, **203**, 135-138.
14. Cooper, K.H. (1970). *The new aerobics*. New York: Bantam.
15. Cooper, K.H. (1977). *The aerobics way*. New York: Bantam.
16. Safrit, M.J., Costa, M.G., Hooper, L.M., Patterson, P., & Ehlert, S.A. (1988). The validity generalization of distance run tests. *Canadian Journal of Sport Sciences*, **13**, 188-196.
17. Jessup, G.T., Tolson, H., & Terry, J.W. (1974). Prediction of maximal oxygen intake from the Åstrand-Ryhming test, 12-minute run, and anthropometric variables using stepwise multiple regression.

American Journal of Physical Medicine, **53**, 200-207.

18. Kline, G.M., Porcari, J.P., Hintermeister, R., Freedson, P.S., Ward, A., McCarron, R.F., Ross, J., & Rippe, J.M. (1987). Estimation of V̇O₂max from a one-mile track walk, gender, age, and body weight. *Medicine and Science in Sports and Exercise*, **19**, 253-259.

19. Coleman, R.J., Wilkie, S., Viscio, L., O'Hanley, S., Porcari, J., Kline, G., Keller, B., Hsieh, S., Freedson, P.S., & Rippe, J. (1987). Validation of 1-mile walk test for estimating V̇O₂max in 20-29 year olds. *Medicine and Science in Sports and Exercise*, **19**, S29.

20. O'Hanley, S., Ward, A., Zwiren, L., McCarron, R., Ross, J., & Rippe, J.M. (1987). Validation of a one-mile walk test in 70-79 year olds. *Medicine and Science in Sports and Exercise*, **19**, S28.

21. Ward, A., Wilkie, S., O'Hanley, S., Trask, C., Kallmes, D., Kleinerman, J., Crawford, B., Freedson, P., & Rippe, J. (1987). Estimation of V̇O₂max in overweight females. *Medicine and Science in Sports and Exercise*, **19**, S29.

22. Widrick, J.J., Ward, A., Ebbeling, C., & Rippe, J.M. (1992). Treadmill validation of an over-ground walking test to predict maximal oxygen consumption. *European Journal of Applied Physiology*, **64**, 304-308.

23. Ebbeling, C.B., Ward, A., Puleo, E.M., Widrick, J., & Rippe, J.M. (1991). Development of a single-stage submaximal treadmill walking test. *Medicine and Science in Sports and Exercise*, **23**, 966-973.

24. Åstrand, P.-O., & Ryhming, I. (1954). A nomogram for calculation of aerobic capacity (physical fitness) from pulse rate during submaximal work. *Journal of Applied Physiology*, **7**, 218-221.

25. Åstrand, P.O., & Rodahl, K. (1986). *Textbook of work physiology*. New York: McGraw-Hill.

26. Sjostrand, T. (1947). Changes in the respiratory organs of workmen at an oil smelting works. *Acta Medica Scandinavica*, **196**, 687-699.

27. Åstrand, I. (1960). Aerobic work capacity in men and women with special reference to age. *Acta Physiologica Scandinavica*, **49**(Suppl. 169), 1-92.

28. Rowell, L.B., Taylor, H.L., & Wang, Y. (1964). Limitations to prediction of maximal oxygen intake. *Journal of Sports Medicine*, **19**, 919-927.

29. Glassford, R.G., Baycroft, G.H.Y., Sedgwick, A.W., & MacNab, R.B.J. (1965). Comparison of maximal oxygen uptake values determined by predicted and actual methods. *Journal of Applied Physiology*, **20**, 509-514.

30. DeVries, H.A., & Klafs, C.E. (1965). Prediction of maximal oxygen uptake from submaximal tests. *Journal of Sports Medicine*, **5**, 207-214.

31. Davies, C.T.M. (1968). Limitations to the prediction of maximum oxygen uptake from cardiac frequency measurements. *Journal of Applied Physiology*, **24**, 700-706.

32. Patton, J.F., Vogel, J.A., & Mello, R.P. (1982). Evaluation of a maximal predictive cycle ergometer test of aerobic power. *European Journal of Applied Physiology*, **49**, 131-140.

33. Teraslinna, P., Ismail, A.H., & MacLeod, D.F. (1966). Nomogram by Åstrand and Ryhming as a predictor of maximum oxygen intake. *Journal of Applied Physiology*, **21**, 513-515.

34. Legge, B.J., & Banister, E.W. (1986). The Åstrand-Ryhming nomogram revisited. *Journal of Applied Physiology*, **61**, 1203-1209.

35. Golding, L.A., Meyers, C.R., & Sinning, W.E. (1989). *Y's way to physical fitness: The complete guide to fitness testing and instruction* (3rd ed.). Champaign, IL: Human Kinetics.

36. Siconolfi, S.F., Cullinane, E.M., Carleton, R.A., & Thompson, P.D. (1982). Assessing V̇O₂max in epidemiologic studies: Modification of the Åstrand-Ryhming test. *Medicine and Science in Sports and Exercise*, **14**, 335-338.

37. Brouha, L., Graybiel, A., & Heath, C.W. (1943). The step test: A simple method of measuring physical fitness for hard muscular work in adult man. *Revue Canadienne de Biologie*, **2**, 86-92.

38. McArdle, W.D., Katch, F.I., Pechar, G.S., Jacobson, L., & Ruck, S. (1972). Reliability and interrelationships between maximal oxygen intake, physical work capacity and step-test scores in college women. *Medicine and Science in Sports*, **4**, 182-186.

39. McArdle, W.D., Pechar, G.S., Katch, F.I., & Magel, J.R. (1973). Percentile norms for a valid step test in college women. *Research Quarterly*, **44**, 498-500.

40. McArdle, W.D., Katch, F.I., & Katch, V.L. (1986). *Exercise physiology: Energy, nutrition and human performance* (2nd ed.). Philadelphia: Lea & Febiger.

41. Siconolfi, S.F., Garber, C.E., Laster, T.M., & Carleton, R.A. (1985). A simple, valid step test for estimating maximal oxygen uptake in epidemiologic studies. *American Journal of Epidemiology*, **121**, 382-390.

42. Wyndham, C.H. (1967). Submaximal tests for estimating maximum oxygen intake. *Canadian Medical Association Journal*, **96**, 736-742.

43. Maritz, J.S., Morrison, J.F., Peter, J., Strydom, N.B., & Wyndham, C.H. (1961). A practical method of estimating an individual's maximal oxygen intake. *Ergonomics*, **4**, 97-122.

44. Jackson, A.S., Blair, S.N., Mahar, M.T., Wier, L.T., Ross, M., & Stuteville, J.E. (1990). Prediction of

functional aerobic capacity without exercise testing. *Medicine and Science in Sports and Exercise*, **22**, 863-870.

45. Bar-Or, O. (1983). *Pediatric sports medicine for the practitioner: From the physiologic principles to clinical applications*. New York: Springer-Verlag.

46. Cumming, G.R., Everatt, D., & Hastman, L. (1978). Bruce treadmill test in children: Normal values in a clinic population. *The American Journal of Cardiology*, **41**, 69-75.

47. American Alliance for Health, Physical Education, Recreation and Dance. (1988). *The AAHPERD physical best program*. Reston, VA: AAHPERD.

48. Institute for Aerobics Research. (1987). *Fitnessgram user's manual*. Dallas: Author.

49. Franks, B.D. (1989). *YMCA youth fitness test manual*. Champaign, IL: Human Kinetics.

50. Safrit, M.J. (1990). The validity and reliability of fitness tests for children: A review. *Pediatric Exercise Science*, **2**, 9-28.

51. Cureton, K.J., Boileau, R.A., Lohman, T.G., & Misner, J.E. (1977). Determinants of distance running performance in children: Analysis of a path model. *Research Quarterly*, **48**, 270-279.

52. Krahenbuhl, G.S., Pangrazi, R.P., Petersen, G.W., Burkett, L.N., & Schneider, M.J. (1978). Field testing of cardiorespiratory fitness in primary school children. *Medicine and Science in Sports*, **10**, 208-213.

53. Cureton, K.J., & Warren, G.L. (1990). Criterion-referenced standards for youth health-related fitness tests: A tutorial. *Research Quarterly for Exercise and Sport*, **61**, 7-19.

54. Blair, S.N., Clark, D.G., Cureton, K.J., & Powell, K.E. (1989). Exercise and fitness in childhood: Implications for a lifetime of health. In G.V. Gisolfi & D.R. Lamb (Eds.), *Perspectives in exercise science and sports: Youth, exercise, and sport* (pp. 401-430). Indianapolis: Benchmark Press.

55. Wahlund, H. (1948). Determination of the physical working capacity. *Acta Medica Scandinavica*, **132**(Suppl. 215).

56. Franz, I.-W., Wiewel, D., & Mellerowicz, H. (1984). Comparative measurements of $\dot{V}O_2max$ and PWC_{170} in schoolchildren. In H. Lollgen & H. Mellerowicz (Eds.), *Progress in ergometry: Quality control and test criteria* (pp. 247-250). New York: Springer-Verlag.

57. Petzl, D.H., Haber, P., Schuster, E., Popow, C., & Haschke, F. (1988). Reliability of estimation of maximum performance capacity on the basis of submaximum ergometric stress tests in children 10-14 years old. *European Journal of Pediatrics*, **147**, 174-178.

58. Klimt, F., & Voigt, G.B. (1971). Investigations on the standardization of ergometry in children. *Acta Pediatrica Scandinavica*, **60**(Suppl. 217), 35-36.

CHAPTER 5

Blood Lactate and Respiratory Measurement of the Capacity for Sustained Exercise

Carl Foster, PhD
Matthew Schrager, MS
Milwaukee Heart Institute

Ann C. Snyder, PhD
University of Wisconsin—Milwaukee

Estimates of the ability to perform prolonged exercise are usually made on the basis of changes in the pattern of pulmonary ventilation or of blood lactate accumulation during incremental exercise. However, there are so many different approaches using various markers that understanding what is really being measured is very difficult. In this chapter we attempt to compare the various approaches to estimating prolonged exercise capacity, and present a scheme for understanding how to use and interpret the various techniques.

HISTORICAL CONTEXT

The observation of abrupt increases in blood lactate concentration during incremental exercise is not new (3, 12, 88), nor is the observation of an apparently inappropriately increased ventilation at the same work load that elicits blood lactate accumulation. As early as the mid-1920s, Hill (48) suggested that the increase in blood lactate was attributable to an inadequacy of oxygen delivery to the working muscles, the beginnings of anaerobic metabolism.

In the 1960s, Wasserman and McIlroy (117) and Hollmann (49, 50) independently described the concept of anaerobic threshold (tissue hypoxia leading to anaerobic metabolism) and the concept of noninvasive detection by measurement of respiratory metabolism. Since the early 1980s the central concepts of the anaerobic threshold hypothesis have been both vigorously challenged and defended. These arguments are well summarized in the point/counterpoint papers of Brooks (8) and Davis (19). We will not fully review the topic, but it seems possible to agree that blood (and, for that matter, muscle) lactate accumulation can be attributed to disparities in the rate of lactate production and removal, whether or not lactate production is related to an O_2 deficiency (anaerobic conditions) in the muscle. The more important of the causes of lactate accumulation is probably a failure in blood lactate removal as blood flow to the renal and splanchnic lactate removal sites decreases with increasing exercise intensity (26, 76). Further, although several specific conditions have been shown to uncouple the accumulation of blood lactate and the disproportionate hyperpnea of exercise, the mechanistic link between the buffering of lactate by bicarbonate leading to an increased need to ventilate to maintain P_aCO_2 within normal limits is attractive as a general principle.

The accumulation of lactate in the blood and the appearance of excess ventilation both appear to be related to the capacity to perform prolonged exercise. During steady-state exercise at intensities equal to or greater than those that during incremental exercise would be associated with increased lactate and/or disproportionate ventilation, there is a progressive accumulation of blood lactate, progressively increasing ventilation, and a relatively short time to exhaustion. Thus, the anaerobic threshold is related in some way to the maximal exercise intensity consistent with a steady state of blood lactate concentration, the maximal lactate steady state.

RELATIONSHIP OF BLOOD AND MUSCLE LACTATE

Blood lactate may be thought of as a shadow of muscle lactate. Figure 5.1 compares muscle and blood lactate from literature studies. In practical terms, blood lactate is always less than the associated muscle lactate. The

magnitude of difference between muscle and blood depends upon the circumstances of measurement. The studies indicated by filled symbols represent either peak postexercise blood lactate values compared to end exercise muscle lactate values or simultaneous muscle and blood lactate values obtained during long (> 5 min) exercise stages. The best-fit line representing these studies is the dotted line. The data from Jacobs (56), shown by the solid line, represent simultaneous muscle and blood lactate values after 4-min stages. The data (dashed line) from Green (44) represent simultaneous muscle and blood lactate values during rapidly incremented exercise (1-min stages).

Blood lactate depends upon the presence of a net positive gradient for lactate between muscle and blood and is tempered by dilution in the body water, removal in the lactate sinks, and the temporal lag before lactate produced in the muscle appears in the blood. The rate of release of lactate from muscle to blood is only partially concentration-dependent and is maximal in the range of 4 mmol · kg^{-1} wet weight of muscle. Thus, with high muscle lactate concentrations there may be a substantial time lag before lactate equilibrates with the blood (60). A variety of studies have provided direct comparisons between muscle (vastus lateralis) and blood lactate during cycle ergometer exercise. In the case where peak postexercise lactate is measured (40, 41, 62, 65, 66, 120), or with simultaneous sampling after relatively long (approx. 5 min) exercise stages (98), there appears to be a reasonably consistent, although not 1:1, relationship between muscle and blood lactate. In the case of shorter exercise stages

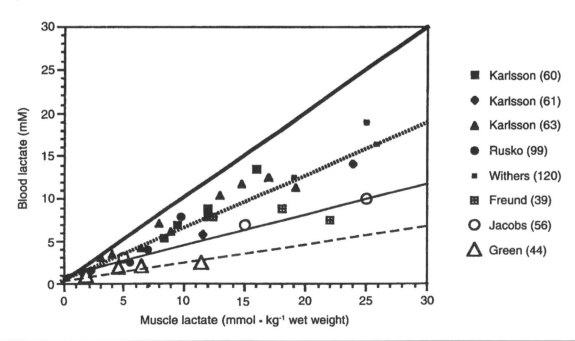

Figure 5.1 Comparison of blood and muscle lactate from literature studies.

(< 4 min) there appears to be a progressive underestimation of the degree of muscular lactic acidosis by simultaneously measured blood lactate values (57). With rapidly incremented exercise tests, the difference between simultaneous muscle and blood lactate concentrations may be rather large (44). Tesch, Daniels, and Sharp (114) have pointed out that inconsistencies in the magnitude of gradient between muscle and blood can be resolved by noting the magnitude of increase in blood lactate 1 min following cessation of exercise, which is not unlike the taking of serial samples to ascertain the peak blood lactate concentration. This problem is addressed conceptually with the individual anaerobic threshold technique of Stegmann, Kindermann, and Schnabel (110).

The evolution kinetics of blood lactate after exercise have been discussed in terms of a two-compartment model by Freund et al. (38-41). Their data suggest that, with relatively brief periods of exercise (approx. 3 min), blood lactate may be expected to increase during the first moments of recovery. With longer exercise stages (approx. 6 min) there may be little or no postexercise increase in blood lactate.

Thus, to some degree blood lactate is an effective shadow of intramuscular conditions and can reflect the degree of lactic acidosis present in the muscle. This relationship is dependent upon the length of the exercise stages and the behavior of blood lactate following exercise. Keep these concepts in mind as we discuss the various invasive and noninvasive approaches to measuring anaerobic threshold.

PRACTICAL SIGNIFICANCE OF THE ANAEROBIC THRESHOLD

Given the controversy that has surrounded the term *anaerobic threshold* (and its clones), why should we be interested in measuring it? There are three practical reasons for this interest. $\dot{V}O_2$max increases with the onset of training in previously sedentary individuals but is comparatively insensitive to the substantial and prolonged training undertaken by athletes (18, 34). The percent of $\dot{V}O_2$max that can be sustained for prolonged exercise, which is conceptually equivalent to anaerobic threshold, increases with training beyond the point where $\dot{V}O_2$max fails to increase (21, 25, 42, 50, 53, 58, 65, 74, 91, 92, 100, 105, 112, 113, 118).

Secondly, anaerobic threshold is highly related to performance in a variety of endurance activities. In many cases the relationship is better than that between $\dot{V}O_2$max and performance (1, 9, 14, 15, 16, 30, 31, 45, 54, 55, 56, 57, 58, 61, 68, 69, 70, 72, 85, 86, 90, 99, 103, 106, 111, 119). Thus anaerobic threshold may

represent a superior index of endurance capacity compared to the traditional "gold standard" $\dot{V}O_2$max.

Thirdly, anaerobic threshold may allow a more relevant index of exercise intensity by which to provide guidelines for exercise training (13, 31, 46, 49, 50, 58, 67, 71, 84, 86, 101, 105, 109, 118, 125). Many physiologists and coaches feel that the greatest intensity compatible with a steady state for blood lactate might represent some practical upper-limit intensity for exercise training, in that the rate of aerobic metabolism is high but the negative consequences of disturbed acid-base status are absent. Clearly, at exercise intensities greater than the anaerobic threshold, the total volume of training is likely to be limited. Accordingly, training at about the intensity associated with the anaerobic threshold may optimize the intensity–duration relationship. Several authors have suggested that performance may stagnate if training is conducted too frequently at intensities associated with elevated blood lactate concentrations, although direct evidence for this is lacking (3, 46, 75, 105).

LABORATORY APPROACHES TO MEASUREMENT

One of the greatest problems in dealing with the blood lactate and ventilatory markers of limits to the capacity to do prolonged exercise, often loosely referred to as "anaerobic threshold," is deciding exactly what we mean by the use of any given term. Analogous to the four blind men describing an elephant—one thinks the elephant is like a fire hose, one like a large leaf on a giant tree, one like a tree trunk, and one like a malodorous cave—each marker is measuring something that isn't part of a smooth transition from rest to maximal exercise, something that has to do with the ability to sustain exercise. What is being measured?

Definitions

Even among texts in English (which do not include many important works in this area), a plethora of terminology is used to refer to discontinuities in blood lactate or ventilation during incremental exercise and to the presence or absence of steady-state conditions during constant-load exercise. These terms include *optimal ventilatory efficiency* (49, 50), *lactate threshold* (54), *anaerobic threshold* (116, 117), *respiratory compensation threshold* (117), *aerobic-anaerobic threshold* (67), *onset of blood lactate accumulation* (58), *onset of plasma lactate accumulation* (30), *individual anaerobic threshold* (110), *heart rate deflection* (14), and *aerobic threshold* and *anaerobic threshold* (107). Doubtless we have left out some important terms, but clearly this is a complicated topic.

Skinner and McLellan (107) and Kinderman (67) have independently suggested that there are at least two apparent points of discontinuity in the blood lactate/ventilatory response to incremental exercise that may serve as general concepts for many of the terms used by other authors. The first of these is associated with the first sustained increase in blood lactate above resting values and with the first discontinuity in ventilation represented by an increase in $\dot{V}_E$ relative to $\dot{V}O_2$. Given the biological "noise" in relation to blood lactate concentrations, this point is often consistent with a blood lactate concentration of about 2.0 to 2.5 mM. In the nomenclature of Skinner-McLellan-Kinderman this point is the *aerobic threshold*. The second of the discontinuities is represented by a very rapid increase in blood lactate concentration and an increase in ventilation relative to both $\dot{V}O_2$ and $\dot{V}CO_2$. It is also associated with a blood lactate concentration of about 4.0 mM. In the nomenclature of Skinner-McLellan-Kinderman this point is the *anaerobic threshold*. While acknowledging arguments concerning the use of the term *anaerobic* and the problems of whether a true threshold exists, we will use these two terms throughout the remainder of this chapter.

Fixed Blood Lactate Concentration

As a strategy for obviating the problems of biological noise associated with detecting the inflection of blood lactate, fixed blood lactate concentrations of about 2.0

mM and 4.0 mM are often used to detect the aerobic and anaerobic thresholds, respectively. In practice we have found 2.5 mM to be a more convenient marker of the aerobic threshold, because it is usually above the considerable biological noise evident at low exercise intensities. Figure 5.2 shows a schematic computation of aerobic and anaerobic threshold from fixed blood lactate concentrations during incremental exercise with 4-min stages. Aerobic threshold (AerT) is defined as the power output associated with a blood lactate concentration of 2.5 mM (some authors prefer 2.0 mM). The anaerobic threshold (AnT) is defined as the power output associated with a blood lactate concentration of 4.0 mM. In this example, because 4-min stages are used, AnT is equivalent to the onset of blood lactate accumulation (OBLA) described by Jacobs (57). Although rapidly incremented exercise stages may be used (44, 116), longer exercise stages of greater than 3 min are often used (46, 49, 50, 58, 67, 103-106, 109, 110, 118, 119). The actual work load or oxygen uptake associated with fixed blood lactate concentrations is determined by interpolation from visual plots of power output, velocity, or $\dot{V}O_2$ versus blood lactate. Simple curve-fitting programs available for most personal computers can help standardize interpolation.

Heck (46) has discussed the importance of stage duration and intrastage interval relative to measurement of the anaerobic threshold. With longer stages (6 min vs. 3 min) anaerobic threshold moves to lower values for velocity (e.g. $\dot{V}O_2$). With longer (90 s vs. 30 s) breaks between stages in discontinuous protocols, such as the interruption of running required to

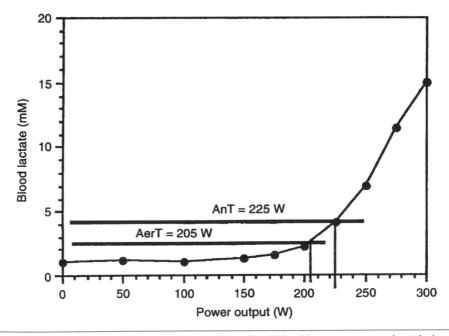

Figure 5.2 Computation of aerobic and anaerobic threshold from fixed blood lactate concentrations during incremental exercise with 4-min stages. (AerT = 2.5 mM, AnT = 4.0 mM).

allow sampling, anaerobic threshold moves to higher values. In view of the data of Freund et al. (38-41, 98), Rusko et al. (98), and Yoshida (125), 4 min represents a practical minimum stage duration for the determination of aerobic and anaerobic thresholds. The data of Tesch, Daniels, and Sharp (115) demonstrating an inconsistent relationship between blood and muscle lactate with 4-min stages as well as the muscle versus blood lactate data presented in Figure 5.1 support this concept, as does the data of Foxdal et al. (127).

Farrell et al. (30) and others (17, 45) have used very long (10 min) stage durations to define the onset of plasma lactate accumulation, which is conceptually equivalent to the aerobic threshold. Several investigators have used comparatively long stage durations to define the anaerobic threshold, particularly in field settings (31, 46, 127).

The decision regarding stage duration, number of stages, and interval between stages is probably mostly a matter of convenience and logistics within the laboratory. Certainly longer stages are to be preferred over shorter stages, and breaks between stages should be as brief as possible. We have shown the technique to be fairly robust, such that the differences in stage durations caused by using fixed-distance increments during field testing do not systematically affect the calculated value for either aerobic or anaerobic threshold (35).

Ventilatory Markers

Wasserman et al. (116, 117) and Hollman et al. (49, 50) independently noted that $\dot{V}_E$ increased disproportionately during exercise at about the same time as blood lactate began to increase (aerobic threshold). Wasserman et al. suggested the mechanistic link of the buffering of lactate by bicarbonate leading to excess $\dot{V}CO_2$ and, accordingly, disproportionate $\dot{V}_E$ in relation to $\dot{V}O_2$. Given that the increase in lactate is matched by a near 1:1 decrease in bicarbonate, P_aCO_2 is maintained at near resting levels, and pH is maintained, the period immediately following the aerobic threshold is characterized by a period of isocapnic buffering. At a somewhat greater exercise intensity bicarbonate is no longer able to defend the pH in the face of increasing blood lactate concentration. $\dot{V}_E$ increases again, this time out of proportion to both $\dot{V}O_2$ and $\dot{V}CO_2$, leading to a decrease in P_aCO_2. This has been termed the "respiratory compensation threshold" (116) and within the Skinner-McLellan-Kindermann nomenclature is the anaerobic threshold.

Ventilatory markers are usually easier to detect with fairly rapidly incremented protocols, the respiratory compensation threshold being particularly difficult to detect during slowly incremented exercise. Various detection strategies have been recommended, varying in their complexity in relation to the technical capabilities of the laboratory producing them. The simplest approach has been to plot $\dot{V}_E$ as a function of either power output or, more commonly, $\dot{V}O_2$. The initial nonlinear increase in $\dot{V}_E$, at about 50% $\dot{V}O_2$max, represents the aerobic threshold in the Skinner-McLellan-Kindermann nomenclature. If a second discontinuity is evident, usually at about 85% $\dot{V}O_2$max, it represents the anaerobic threshold. Wasserman et al. (116) and others (4, 5) have recommended using breath-by-breath measurements to increase the precision of detection. However, for comparatively crude measurements, like $\dot{V}_E$, samples integrated over convenient time intervals of 10 to 60 s can be just as useful in laboratories not equipped to make breath-by-breath measurements. The ventilatory equivalents for oxygen ($\dot{V}_E/\dot{V}O_2$) and for carbon dioxide ($\dot{V}_E/\dot{V}CO_2$) have been widely used as markers of aerobic threshold, on the premise that at the aerobic threshold $\dot{V}_E/\dot{V}O_2$ will increase while $\dot{V}_E/\dot{V}CO_2$ will remain constant, because the excess $\dot{V}_E$ is largely attributable to an excess $\dot{V}CO_2$ (22, 23, 24, 49, 77, 116, 121, 122). The subsequent nonlinear increase in $\dot{V}_E/\dot{V}CO_2$ can be used as a marker of the anaerobic threshold (10, 43, 52). Beaver, Wasserman, and Whipp (4) have suggested that simple plots of $\dot{V}CO_2$ versus $\dot{V}O_2$ and $\dot{V}_E$ versus $\dot{V}CO_2$ can also serve as useful markers of the aerobic and anaerobic thresholds, respectively. Changes in the concentrations of O_2 or CO_2 in the mixed-expired—or, better, end-tidal—gas may also be convenient markers of aerobic and anaerobic threshold. In our experience, given the impressive graphic capabilities of most computerized gas-exchange systems, it is best to plot several variables to establish candidates for aerobic and anaerobic threshold and depend upon agreement between two or more indices to arrive at the best answer (Figure 5.3).

Several authors, most notably Wasserman's group (116), have suggested collecting about 2 min of resting data and 2 min of unloaded exercise before beginning the incrementation of the protocol. Once incrementation begins, the rate of increase should be fairly rapid, with many small steps rather than fewer large steps. In the ideal world, an essentially infinite number of infinitely small steps could be taken (ramping). Ideally, the subject should be fatigued within 8 to 12 min after incrementation begins. This protocol seems to enhance the period of isocapnic buffering between aerobic and anaerobic thresholds and make detection of both points easier. With this technique, it is important to recognize that the aerobic and anaerobic thresholds will be expressed in terms of $\dot{V}O_2$ rather than velocity or power output as is common with fixed blood lactate concentration protocols. If the intent of measuring aerobic and anaerobic thresholds is to enhance the exercise prescription, then the $\dot{V}O_2$ will have to be translated into velocity and/or power output.

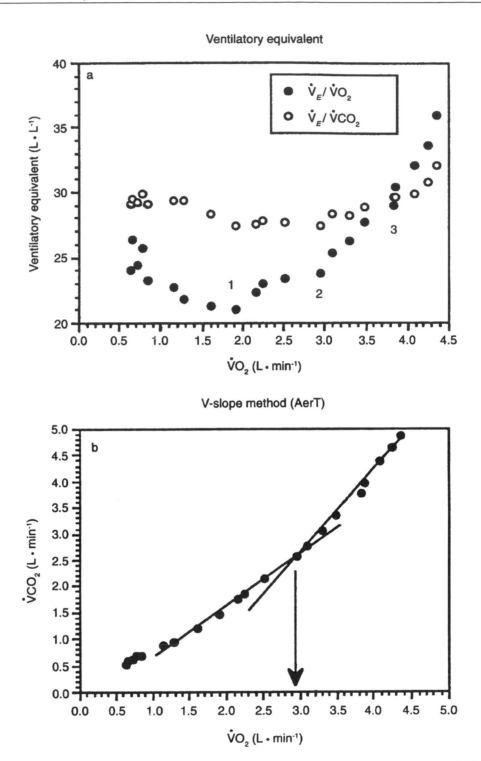

Figure 5.3 The aerobic (AerT) and anaerobic thresholds (AnT) may be computed from respiratory responses during an incremental exercise test on the cycle ergometer with the power output incremented in a ramp fashion with a slope of 40 Watts · min⁻¹. Candidates for AerT (1, 2; top) are identified at a $\dot{V}O_2$ of 1.95 and 2.90 liters · min⁻¹ from changes in the $\dot{V}_E/\dot{V}O_2$. A candidate for AnT (3) is identified from changes in the $\dot{V}_E/\dot{V}CO_2$ at a $\dot{V}O_2$ of 3.70 liters · min⁻¹. Using the V-slope technique of Beaver et al. (ref 5) plots of $\dot{V}CO_2$ versus $\dot{V}O_2$ (bottom) and $\dot{V}_E$ versus $\dot{V}O_2$ (next page, top) are made. By fitting straight lines through the lower and upper segments of the data points (in this case 30s data collection increments), the point of intersection (indicated by arrows) may be taken as a candidate for AerT. In both figures the intersection is a $\dot{V}O_2$ of 2.90 liters · min⁻¹, in agreement with candidate #2 from

Ventilation (AerT)

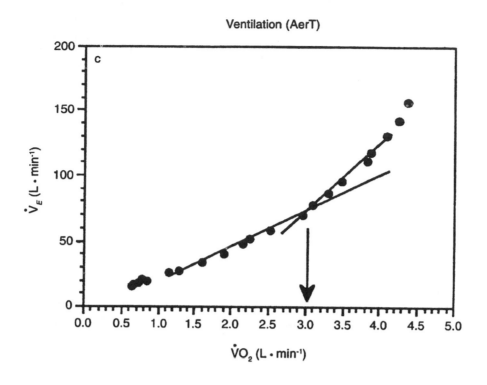

V-slope method (AnT)

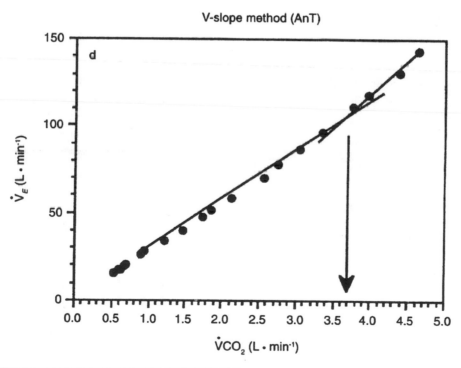

Figure 5.3 *(continued)*

the $\dot{V}_E/\dot{V}O_2$ data. Accordingly, AerT is defined. By plotting $\dot{V}_E$ versus $\dot{V}CO_2$ (bottom) and drawing lines through the upper and lower segments of the data points, we have another method for defining AnT. In this case (indicated by the arrow), the $\dot{V}CO_2$ is 3.70 liters · min^{-1}. We note from the $\dot{V}CO_2$ versus $\dot{V}O_2$ plot (previous page, bottom) that a $\dot{V}CO_2$ of 3.70 liters · min^{-1} corresponds to a $\dot{V}O_2$ of 3.70 liters · min^{-1}, which is in agreement with the $\dot{V}_E/\dot{V}CO_2$ data from the figure (previous page, top). Accordingly, AnT is defined. The numerical correspondence of $\dot{V}O_2$ and $\dot{V}CO_2$ at AnT in this example is coincidential and has no special relevance.

Individual Anaerobic Threshold

Stegmann, Kindermann, and Schnabel (110) have noted that steady-state blood lactate concentrations vary widely across individuals. On this basis, as well as based on arguments founded on the diffusion of lactate from muscle to blood, they have proposed the concept of individual anaerobic threshold. The individual anaerobic threshold is defined in terms of blood lactate responses both during and following exercise (Figure 5.4). Kindermann et al. (67) have suggested that the individual anaerobic threshold may be significantly better than a fixed blood lactate concentration in defining the maximal lactate steady state. The concept of the individual anaerobic threshold has been supported in data from other laboratories (78, 79). Coen et al. (13) have demonstrated the value of using the velocity associated with the individual anaerobic threshold in designing training programs for athletes.

Typically, stage durations for individual anaerobic threshold tests are at the short end of the continuum (3-4 min) compared to those used in fixed blood lactate concentration tests (3-10 min).

Blood lactate is sampled during a brief pause at the end of each stage, or without pause if cycle ergometry is used. Blood is also sampled during the first several minutes of recovery. A plot of blood lactate versus test time is made, and separate curves plotted for the exercise and recovery portions of the test. The time during recovery where the blood lactate concentration equals that at the end of the exercise portion of the test is used as an anchor for fitting

a tangent to the lactate curve during exercise. The velocity (power output) and blood lactate associated with the time-versus-blood-lactate and tangent curves represents the individual anaerobic threshold.

Figure 5.4 presents a schematic computation of the individual anaerobic threshold according to Stegmann, Kindermann, and Schnabel (110) from blood lactate responses during and following an incremental exercise test with stages of 50 W every 3 min. The exercise blood lactate response curve (AB) is fitted using either a second- or third-order polynomial. The recovery blood lactate curve (CD) is fitted using a third-order polynomial. The correspondence between peak exercise blood lactate and the same blood lactate during recovery is noted (EF). A tangent is fit between F and the exercise blood lactate response. The point of contact of the tangent (G) represents the individual anaerobic threshold. The blood lactate concentration at the individual anaerobic threshold is noted (GH), 3.8 mM in this example. The time during the test at which the individual anaerobic threshold occurred is GI. In this example the individual anaerobic threshold occurred at 18 min, which represents a power output of 300 W.

The individual anaerobic threshold is somewhat dependent upon the degree to which the test is truly maximal (79), the nature and intensity of activity during the recovery period (83), and the duration of exercise stages. In general, however, it is a remarkably robust measurement. The exercise intensity and blood lactate concentration associated with the individual anaerobic threshold are usually intermediate between the aerobic and anaerobic

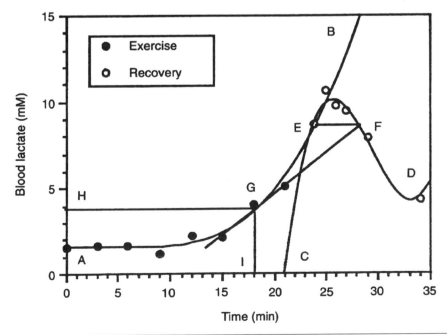

Figure 5.4   Schematic computation of the individual anaerobic threshold according to Stegmann, Kindermann, and Schnabel (110).

thresholds. The absolute blood lactate concentration at the individual anaerobic threshold is highly individual. Beyond intrinsic individual patterns, highly trained individuals often have lower concentrations (2-3 mM), and less fit individuals have higher concentrations (4-7 mM), of blood lactate (109, 110).

In most settings, the individual anaerobic threshold is a good measure of the capacity for sustained exercise, the maximal steady state. Whether or not it is substantially superior to the aerobic or anaerobic thresholds determined by fixed blood lactate concentrations or respiratory markers remains to be determined. The one direct comparison of the two methods, by Stegmann and Kindermann (109), suggested that the anaerobic threshold (4 mM lactate) significantly overestimated the sustainable exercise tolerance and that the individual anaerobic threshold provided a valid estimate of the maximal steady state. In fairness, however, anaerobic threshold was estimated using short (2 min) exercise stages, which tends to inflate the power output at anaerobic threshold.

Heart Rate Deflection

Conconi, Ferrari, Ziglio, Droghetti, and Codeca (14) have proposed that the linearity of the velocity–heart rate relationship is lost at fairly high velocities in well-trained runners. They further noted that the velocity at the deflection of heart rate (Vd) was associated with blood lactate accumulation. The Vd was well correlated with, and more or less equal to, the velocity in races of 1-hour duration. The Vd was also well correlated with (although certainly not equal to) velocity in 5,000 m and

marathon races. This technique is particularly appealing because it can be conducted in the field using the athletes' own sport idiom. Some authors have suggested that Vd can be used to control training in athletes (59). The Vd technique can also be used with athletes in other sports, such as swimming (11), canoeing, skiing, cycling, skating, rowing, and racewalking (28) (Figure 5.5). In activities like cycling and skating where resistance is provided primarily by air resistance, the Vd relationship is better appreciated by using velocity squared in the *x*-axis. For water sports (swimming, rowing), velocity cubed is the appropriate term on the *x*-axis. Figure 5.5 presents a schematic representation of the velocity of deflection (Vd) described by Conconi et al. (14), which probably represents the AnT (95). The heart rate at the end of successively faster 200-m stages is plotted. Straight-line relationships are noted during the early and late portions of the test. The intersection of the lines represents Vd, in this case 4.45 m · s^{-1}.

Others have failed to demonstrate the departure from linearity of the relationship between velocity (power output) and heart rate when fixed-duration stages are performed in the laboratory (37). Others have shown that Vd or power output at the heart rate deflection (Pd) is better related to the second ventilatory threshold (anaerobic threshold, in the Skinner-McLellan-Kindermann nomenclature) than to aerobic threshold (94). This same group has reported difficulty with the reproducibility of the technique, although Conconi et al. (14), Cellini et al. (11), and Droghetti et al. (28) report excellent reproducibility.

The mechanism that allows the Vd technique to work is probably the slowdown in oxygen uptake kinetics,

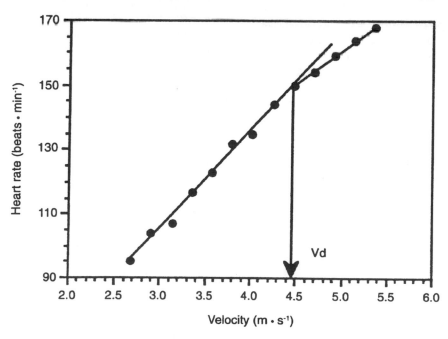

Figure 5.5 Schematic representation of the velocity of heart rate deflection (Vd) as described by Conconi et al. (14).

including heart rate, with increasing exercise intensity (116). This effect is accentuated with the field methods of Conconi et al. because they use stages of fixed distance and thus progressively shorter duration. The combination of slowed $\dot{V}O_2$ kinetics and progressively shorter stages acts to magnify the effect. In the original protocol, Conconi et al. recommend stages of 200 m. For well-conditioned athletes, capable of running at over 20 km/hour, the Vd may be observed during a stage that is only 36 s in duration.

Conconi has indicated (personal communication) that for the technique to work well, the subject must complete several stages at velocities well below Vd to allow for a well-developed velocity–heart rate relationship to be established. He has also suggested that devices such as pacing tapes or pacing lights to help control velocity may be useful. The primary limitation on obtaining good data seems to be the ability to make several measurements of heart rate with a large number of fairly evenly incremented stages in between. Strategies that facilitate this are likely to make the technique work better.

Percentage of Maximal Heart Rate

Several authors have examined heart rate responses associated with the aerobic threshold (9, 29, 82, 99), anaerobic threshold (67, 71, 94, 99, 109), individual anaerobic threshold (109), and maximal lactate steady state (108). Beyond the statement of Dwyer and Bybee (29) that heart rate, at whatever threshold one chooses, could be used to control subsequent training, there is little agreement about general heart rate guidelines. %HRmax after about 5 min of exercise varies from 66% to 95% HRmax at the aerobic threshold, to 85% to 91% HRmax at the individual anaerobic threshold or maximal lactate steady state, to 81% to 97% HRmax at the anaerobic threshold.

Presuming that an individually unique heart rate associated with the maximal lactate steady state can be identified, one still must account for cardiovascular drift. Heart rate can be expected to increase from 5 to 15 bpm over the course of a 30-min steady-state exercise bout when the work bout is performed in the range of intensities between the aerobic and anaerobic thresholds (46, 67, 71, 101, 108).

LABORATORY CONCERNS WITH AEROBIC AND ANAEROBIC THRESHOLDS

Sampling Technique

In the ideal world, arterial blood samples would be obtained to define variables related to blood lactate.

Because it is difficult to secure arterial blood, most investigators use either arterialized venous blood, capillary blood, or venous blood. Certainly some of the confusion surrounding variables related to blood lactate is due to the nature of blood sampling superimposed on other variables. The classical paper of Forster et al. (32) demonstrating that near-arterial blood concentrations for pH, lactate, and pCO_2, but not pO_2, could be obtained in arterialized venous blood (by hand warming) opened the possibility of systematically easier testing in many laboratories.

In general, venous blood sampling, without arterialization, results in lower blood lactate concentrations at any point in time compared to arterial blood (36, 96, 126). Capillary blood also usually underestimates arterial values somewhat (36).

Automated enzyme electrode systems are considered fairly reliable and to give only slightly different values than bench chemistry reference methods (63, 64), although important differences may exist (6, 7, 97).

Reproducibility

As might be expected, the groups with the most experience with the measurement of aerobic and anaerobic threshold report excellent reproducibility of blood (57, 58, 63, 64), respiratory (19, 116), and heart rate (14) methods of detection. Others (2, 47, 94) have reported problems with the reproducibility of various methods.

Nutritional Status

Several authors have demonstrated that blood lactate at any given exercise load is decreased in response to factors that might be expected to be associated with muscle glycogen depletion (27, 35, 51, 54, 57, 61, 73, 123). These findings are well within predictions, in that making lactate without its ultimate precursor, muscle glycogen, is virtually impossible. Some have suggested that the low blood lactate values found in athletes are as much a function of chronic muscle glycogen depletion as of a favorable ability to metabolize lactate. Certainly, the problem of relative glycogen depletion needs to be considered when evaluating exercise responses with blood lactate methods. Given that in athletes logistic requirements may make standardization of preevaluation diet and activity patterns difficult, we have proposed a strategy of using the maximal postexercise blood lactate concentration as a method of indexing submaximal blood lactate responses to the relative momentary nutritional status of the individual. Use of about 30% of the maximal blood lactate concentration in glycogen-depleted individuals predicts about the same power output as the power output at OBLA in rested athletes (35).

Others have noted that the ventilatory and blood lactate markers of aerobic and anaerobic threshold move in opposite directions in response to acute muscle glycogen depletion (51), although this uncoupling of ventilatory and blood lactate responses has not been observed in other laboratories (81). They have interpreted these observations as indicating that the discontinuity of $\dot{V}_E$ and blood lactate at the aerobic threshold are only coincidental and not related by any mechanistic link. Regardless of what these studies may say about the regulation of respiration by blood lactate, they reinforce the case for standardization of nutritional status prior to laboratory evaluations.

SUMMARY

Discontinuity in blood lactate accumulation and ventilation during exercise may be used as an index of endurance capacity and a guideline for exercise training. In general there are two main areas of discontinuity that seem to be present despite the substantial amount of methodological variation observed in the literature. These points of discontinuity—aerobic threshold and anaerobic threshold, in the nomenclature of Skinner-McLellan-Kindermann—are generally related to (for aerobic threshold) the first appearance of an elevated blood lactate concentration (up to a concentration of about 2.5 mM) and a disproportionate increase in $\dot{V}_E$ and $\dot{V}CO_2$ relative to $\dot{V}O_2$, and (for anaerobic threshold) the rapid accumulation of blood lactate (a concentration of about 4.0 mM is often used) and a disproportionate increase in $\dot{V}_E$ relative to $\dot{V}CO_2$. This point might also be associated with a negative deflection in the relationship between heart rate and work load. A unique exercise intensity, the individual anaerobic threshold as described by Stegmann and dependent upon blood lactate responses during both exercise and recovery, might be intermediate between the aerobic and anaerobic thresholds and, potentially, might be a better marker of sustainable exercise tolerance.

Markers related to blood lactate are often better appreciated with comparatively longer stage durations (> 4 min), whereas ventilatory markers are often better appreciated with fairly rapidly incremented stages. During the longer stage durations associated with blood lactate measurement, relevant thresholds may be related to work load (power output or velocity), whereas with the shorter stages used for respiratory measurement, relevant thresholds may be better related to $\dot{V}O_2$.

Various factors can act to modify the aerobic and anaerobic thresholds determined by either blood lactate or respiratory methods. In particular the short-term nutritional status of the individual may be important as well as the details of sampling of blood.

Our perspective suggests that much of the confusion relative to aerobic and anaerobic threshold might be related to the use of mix-and-match technology by various laboratories. For example, respiratory markers do not work particularly well with long exercise stages. If, in trying to combine blood lactate and respiratory markers, a lab uses stages that are too long, the respiratory markers are not going to be very revealing. A similar case is found with the use of short exercise stages for methods based on blood lactate. As a practical matter, unless one is doing studies trying to address unique methods, it seems to make sense to choose one of the well-established techniques and use it with minimal modification. Otherwise, it seems that one is likely to get the worst of each method, rather than the best result, by combining two or more methods for detecting aerobic and anaerobic threshold.

REFERENCES

1. Allen, W.K., Seals, D.R., Hurley, B.F., Ehsani, A.A., & Hagberg, J.M. (1985). Lactate threshold and distance running performance in young and older endurance athletes. *Journal of Applied Physiology*, **58**, 1281-1284.
2. Aunola, S., & Rusko, H. (1984). Reproducibility of aerobic and anaerobic thresholds in 20-50 year old men. *European Journal of Applied Physiology*, **53**, 260-266.
3. Bang, O. (1936). The lactate content of the blood during and after muscular exercise in man. *Skandivica Archives of Physiology Supplement*, **10**, 51-82.
4. Beaver, W.L., Wasserman, K., & Whipp, B.J. (1985). Improved detection of lactate threshold during exercise using a log-log transformation. *Journal of Applied Physiology*, **59**, 1936-1940.
5. Beaver, W.L., Wasserman, K., & Whipp, B.J. (1986). A new method for detecting the anaerobic threshold by gas exchange. *Journal of Applied Physiology*, **60**, 2020-2027.
6. Bishop, P.A., May, M., Smith, J.F., Kime, J. Mayo, J., & Murphy, M. (1992). Influence of blood handling techniques on lactic acid concentrations. *International Journal of Sports Medicine*, **13**, 56-59.
7. Bishop, P.A., Smith, J.F., Kime, J.C., Mayo, J.M., & Tin, Y.H. (1992). Comparison of a manual and an automated enzymatic technique for determining blood lactate concentrations. *International Journal of Sports Medicine*, **13**, 36-39.

8. Brooks, G.A. (1985). Anaerobic threshold: Review of the concept and directions for future research. *Medicine and Science in Sports and Exercise*, **17**, 22-31.

9. Bunc, V., Heller, J., Leso, J., Sprynarova, S., & Zdanowicz, S. (1987). Ventilatory threshold in various groups of highly trained athletes. *International Journal of Sports Medicine*, **8**, 275-280.

10. Caiozzo, V.J., Davis, J.A., Ellis, J.F., Azus, J.L., Vandagriff, R., Prietto, C.A., & McMaster, W.C. (1982). A comparison of gas exchange indices used to detect the anaerobic threshold. *Journal of Applied Physiology*, **53**, 1184-1189.

11. Cellini, M., Vitiello, P., Nagliati, A., Ziglio, P.G., Martinelli, S., Ballarin, E., & Conconi, F. (1986). Noninvasive determination of the anaerobic threshold in swimming. *International Journal of Sports Medicine*, **7**, 347-351.

12. Christansen, J., Douglas, C.G., & Haldand, J.S. (1914). The absorption and dissociation of carbon dioxide by human blood. *Journal of Physiology (London)*, **48**, 244-271.

13. Coen, B., Schwarz, L., Urhausen, A., & Kinderman, W. (1991). Control of training in middle and long distance running by means of the individual anaerobic threshold. *International Journal of Sports Medicine*, **12**, 519-524.

14. Conconi, F., Ferrari, M., Ziglio, P.G., Droghetti, P., & Codeca, L. (1982). Determination of the anaerobic threshold by a noninvasive field test in runners. *Journal of Applied Physiology*, **52**, 869-873.

15. Costill, D.L., Branam, G., Eddy, D., & Sparks, K. (1971). Determinants of marathon running success. *International Zeitschrift for Angewande Physiologie*, **29**, 249-254.

16. Costill, D.L., Thomason, H., & Roberts, E. (1973). Fractional utilization of the aerobic capacity during distance running. *Medicine and Science in Sports*, **5**, 248-252.

17. Coyle, E.F., Coggan, A.R., Hopper, M.K., & Walters, T.J. (1988). Determinants of endurance in well-trained cyclists. *Journal of Applied Physiology*, **64**, 2622-2630.

18. Daniels, J.T., Yarbrough, R.A., & Foster, C. (1978). Changes in V̇O₂max and running performance with training. *European Journal of Applied Physiology*, **39**, 249-254.

19. Davis, J.A. (1985). Anaerobic threshold: Review of the concept and directions for future research. *Medicine and Science in Sports and Exercise*, **17**, 6-18.

20. Davis, J.A., Caiozzo, V.J., Lamarra, N., Ellis, J.F., Vandagriff, R., Prietto, C.A., & McMaster, W.C. (1983). Does the gas exchange anaerobic threshold occur at a fixed blood lactate concentration of 2

or 4 mM. *International Journal of Sports Medicine*, **4**, 89-93.

21. Davis, J.A., Frank, M.H., Whipp, B.J., & Wasserman, K. (1979). Anaerobic threshold alterations caused by endurance training in middle aged men. *Journal of Applied Physiology*, **46**, 1039-1046.

22. Davis, J.A., Vodak, P., Wilmore, J.H., Vodak, J., & Kurtz, P. (1976). Anaerobic threshold and maximal aerobic power for three modes of exercise. *Journal of Applied Physiology*, **41**, 544-550.

23. Davis, J.A., Whipp, B.J., Lamarra, N., Huntsman, D.J., Frank, M.H., & Wasserman, K. (1982). Effect of ramp slope on determination of aerobic parameters from the ramp exercise test. *Medicine and Science in Sports and Exercise*, **14**, 339-344.

24. Davis, J.A., Whipp, B.J., & Wasserman, K. (1980). The relation of ventilation to metabolic rate during moderate exercise in man. *European Journal of Applied Physiology*, **44**, 97-108.

25. Denis, C., Fouquet, R., Poty, P., Geyssant, A., & Lacour, J.R. (1982). Effect of 40 weeks of endurance training on the anaerobic threshold. *International Journal of Sports Medicine*, **3**, 208-214.

26. Donovan, C.M., & Brooks, G.A., (1983). Endurance training affects lactate clearance, not lactate production. *American Journal of Physiology*, **244**, E83-E92.

27. Dotan, R., Rotstein, A., & Grodjinovsky, A. (1989). Effect of training load on OBLA determination. *International Journal of Sports Medicine*, **10**, 346-351.

28. Droghetti, P., Borsetto, C., Casoni, I., Cellini, M., Ferrari, M., Paolini, A.R., Ziglio, P.G., & Conconi, F. (1985). Noninvasive determination of the anaerobic threshold in canoeing, cross-country skiing, cycling, roller and ice skating, rowing and walking. *European Journal of Applied Physiology*, **53**, 299-303.

29. Dwyer, J., & Bybee, R. (1983). Heart rate indices of the anaerobic threshold. *Medicine and Science in Sports and Exercise*, **15**, 72-76.

30. Farrell, P.A., Wilmore, J.H., Coyle, E.F., Billing, J.E., & Costill, D.L. (1979). Plasma lactate accumulation and distance running performance. *Medicine and Science in Sports*, **11**, 338-344.

31. Fohrenbach, R., Mader, A., & Hollmann, W. (1987). Determination of endurance capacity and prediction of exercise intensities for training and competition in marathon runners. *International Journal of Sports Medicine*, **8**, 11-18.

32. Forster, H.V., Dempsey, J.A., Thomson, J., Vidruk, E., & DoPico, G.A., (1972). Estimation of arterial PO₂, PCO₂, pH and lactate from arterialized venous blood. *Journal of Applied Physiology*, **32**, 134-137.

33. Foster, C., Cohen, J., Donovan, K., Gastrau, P., Killian, P.J., Schrager, M., & Snyder, A. (1993). Fixed time versus fixed distance protocols for the blood lactate profile in athletes. *International Journal of Sports Medicine*, **14**, 264-268.

34. Foster, C., Pollock, M.L., Farrell, P.A., Maksud, M.G., Anholm, J.D., & Hare, J. (1982). Training responses of speed skaters during a competitive season. *Research Quarterly for Exercise and Sport*, **53**, 243-246.

35. Foster, C., Snyder, A.C., Thompson, N.N., & Kuettel, K. (1988). Normalization of the blood lactate profile in athletes. *International Journal of Sports Medicine*, **9**, 198-200.

36. Foxdal, P., Sjodin, A., Ostman, B., & Sjodin, B. (1991). The effect of different blood sampling sites and analyses on the relationship between exercise intensity and 4.0 mmol/l blood lactate concentration. *European Journal of Applied Physiology*, **63**, 52-54.

37. Francis, K.T., McClatchey, P.R., Sumsion, J.R., & Hansen, D.E. (1989). The relationship between anaerobic threshold and heart rate linearity during cycle ergometry. *European Journal of Applied Physiology*, **59**, 273-277.

38. Freund, H., Oyono-Euguelle, S., Heitz, A., Marbach, J., Ott, C., & Gartner, M. (1989). Effect of exercise duration on lactate kinetics after short muscular exercise. *European Journal of Applied Physiology*, **58**, 534-542.

39. Freund, H., Oyono-Euguelle, S., Heitz, A., Ott, C., Marbach, J., Gartner, M., & Pape, A. (1990). Comparative lactate kinetics after short and prolonged submaximal exercise. *International Journal of Sports Medicine*, **11**, 284-288.

40. Fruend, H., & Zouloumian, P., (1981). Lactate after exercise in man: Evolution kinetics in arterial blood. *European Journal of Applied Physiology*, **46**, 121-133.

41. Freund, H., Zouloumian, P. (1981). Lactate after exercise in man: Physiological observations and model predictions. *European Journal of Applied Physiology*, **46**, 161-176.

42. Gaesser, G.A., Poole, D.C., & Gardner, B.P. (1984). Dissociation between $\dot{V}O_2$max and ventilatory threshold responses to endurance training. *European Journal of Applied Physiology*, **53**, 242-247.

43. Gladden, L.B., Yates, J.W., Stremel, R.W., & Stamford, B.A. (1985). Gas exchange and lactate anaerobic thresholds: Inter- and intra-evaluator agreement. *Journal of Applied Physiology*, **58**, 2082-2089.

44. Green, H.J., Hughson, R.L., Orr, G.W., & Ranney, D.A. (1983). Anaerobic threshold, blood lactate and muscle metabolites in progressive exercise. *Journal of Applied Physiology*, **54**, 1032-1038.

45. Hagberg, J.M., & Coyle, E.F., (1983). Physiological determinants of endurance performance as studied in competitive racewalkers. *Medicine and Science in Sports and Exercise*, **15**, 287-289.

46. Heck, H., Mader, A., Hess, G., Mucke, S., Muller, R., & Hollmann, W. (1985). Justification of the 4 mmol/l lactate threshold. *International Journal of Sports Medicine*, **6**, 117-130.

47. Heitcamp, H.Ch., Holdt, M., & Scheib, M. (1991). The reproducibility of the 4 mmol/l lactate threshold in trained and untrained women. *International Journal of Sports Medicine*, **12**, 363-368.

48. Hill, A.V., Long, C.N.H., & Lupton, H. (1924). Muscular exercise, lactic acid and the supply and utilization of oxygen: Part VI. The oxygen debt at the end of exercise. *Proceedings of the Royal Society of London*, **97**, 127-137.

49. Hollmann, W. (1985). Historical remarks on the development of the aerobic-anaerobic threshold up to 1966. *International Journal of Sports Medicine*, **6**, 109-116.

50. Hollmann, W., Rost, R., Liesen, H., Dufaux, B., Heck, H., & Mader, A. (1981). Assessment of different forms of physical activity with respect to preventive and rehabilitative cardiology. *International Journal of Sports Medicine*, **2**, 67-80.

51. Hughes, E.F., Turner, S.C., & Brooks, G.A. (1982). Effects of glycogen depletion and pedaling speed on anaerobic threshold. *Journal of Applied Physiology*, **52**, 1598-1607.

52. Hughson, R.L., & Green, H.J. (1982). Blood acid-base and lactate relationships studied by ramp work tests. *Medicine and Science in Sports*, **14**, 297-302.

53. Hurley, B.F., Hagberg, J.M., Allen, W.K., Seals, D.R., Young, J.C., Cuddihee, R.W., & Holloszy, J.O. (1984). Effect of training on blood lactate levels during submaximal exercise. *Journal of Applied Physiology*, **56**, 1260-1264.

54. Ivy, J.L., Costill, D.L., van Handel, P.J., Essig, D.A., & Lower, R.W. (1981). Alteration in the lactate threshold with changes in substrate availability. *International Journal of Sports Medicine*, **2**, 139-142.

55. Iwaoka, K., Fuchi, T., Higuchi, M., & Kobayashi, S. (1988). Blood lactate accumulation during exercise in older endurance runners. *International Journal of Sports Medicine*, **9**, 253-256.

56. Iwaoka, K., Hatta, H., Atomi, Y. & Miyashita, M. (1988). Lactate, respiratory compensation thresholds and distance running performance in runners of both sexes. *International Journal of Sports Medicine*, **9**, 306-309.

57. Jacobs, I. (1981). Lactate, muscle glycogen and exercise performance in man. *Acta Physiologica Scandinavica*, (Suppl. 495), 1-35.

58. Jacobs, I. (1986). Blood lactate: Implications for training and sports performance. *Sports Medicine*, **3**, 10-25.

59. Janssen, P.G.J.M. (1989). *Training, lactate, pulse-rate*. Oulu, Finland: Polar Electro Oy.

60. Jorfeldt, L., Juhein-Dannfeldt, A., & Karlsson, J. (1978). Lactate release in relation to tissue lactate in human skeletal muscle during exercise. *Journal of Applied Physiology*, **44**, 350-352.

61. Karlsson, J. (1971). Lactate in working muscles after prolonged exercise. *Acta Physiologica Scandinavica*, **82**, 123-130.

62. Karlsson, J., Diamant, B., & Saltin, B. (1971). Muscle metabolites during submaximal and maximal exercise in man. *Scandinavian Journal of Clinical and Laboratory Investigation*, **26**, 385-394.

63. Karlsson, J., & Jacobs, I. (1982). Onset of blood lactate accumulation during muscular exercise as a threshold concept: Theoretical considerations. *International Journal of Sports Medicine*, **3**, 190-201.

64. Karlsson, J., Jacobs, I., Sjodin, B., Tesch, P., Kaiser, P., Sahl, O., & Karlberg, B. (1983). Semi-automatic blood lactate assay: Experiences from an exercise laboratory. *International Journal of Sports Medicine*, **4**, 52-55.

65. Karlsson, J., Nordesjo, L.O., Jorfeldt, L., & Saltin, B. (1972). Muscle lactate, ATP and CP levels during exercise after physical training in man. *Journal of Applied Physiology*, **33**, 199-203.

66. Karlsson, J., & Saltin, B. (1970). Lactate, ATP and CP in working muscles during exhaustive exercise in man. *Journal of Applied Physiology*, **29**, 598-602.

67. Kindermann, W., Simon, G., & Keul, J. (1979). The significance of the aerobic-anaerobic transition for the determination of work load intensities during endurance training. *European Journal of Applied Physiology*, **42**, 25-34.

68. Kumagai, S., Tanaka, K., Matsuura, Y., Matsuzaka, A., Hirakoba, K., & Asano, K. (1982). Relationships of the anaerobic threshold with the 5 km, 10 km and 10 mile races. *European Journal of Applied Physiology*, **49**, 13-23.

69. LaFontaine, T.P., Londeree, B.R., & Spath, W.K. (1981). The maximal steady state versus selected running events. *Medicine and Science in Sports and Exercise*, **13**, 190-192.

70. Lehmann, M., Berg, A., Kapp, R., Wessinghage, T., & Keul, J. (1983). Correlations between laboratory testing and distance running performance in marathoners of similar performance ability. *International Journal of Sports Medicine*, **4**, 226-230.

71. Ljunggren, G., Ceci, R., & Karlsson, J. (1987). Prolonged exercise at a constant load on a bicycle ergometer: Ratings of perceived exertion and leg aches and pain as well as measurements of blood lactate accumulation and heart rate. *International Journal of Sports Medicine*, **8**, 109-116.

72. Londeree, B.R., & Ames, S.A. (1975). Maximal steady state versus state of conditioning. *European Journal of Applied Physiology*, **34**, 269-278.

73. Maassen, N., & Busse, M.W. (1989). The relationship between lactic acid and work load: A measure for endurance capacity or an indicator of carbohydrate deficiency? *European Journal of Applied Physiology*, **58**, 728-737.

74. MacRae, H.S.H., Dennis, S.C., Bosch, A.N., & Noakes, T.D. (1992). Effects of training on lactate production and removal during progressive exercise in humans. *Journal of Applied Physiology*, **72**, 1649-1656.

75. Mader, A., & Heck, H. (1986). A theory of the metabolic origin of "anaerobic threshold." *International Journal of Sports Medicine*, **7**, 45-65.

76. Mazzeo, R.S., Brooks, G.A., Schoeller, D.A., & Budinger, T.F. (1986). Disposal of blood lactate in humans during rest and exercise. *Journal of Applied Physiology*, **60**, 232-242.

77. McLellan, T.M. (1985). Ventilatory and plasma lactate response with different exercise protocols: A comparison of methods. *International Journal of Sports Medicine*, **6**, 30-35.

78. McLellan, T.M., & Cheung, K.S.Y. (1992). A comparative evaluation of the individual anaerobic threshold and the critical power. *Medicine and Science in Sports and Exercise*, **24**, 543-550.

79. McLellan, T.M., Cheung, K.S.Y., & Jacobs, I. (1991). Incremental test protocol, recovery mode and the individual anaerobic threshold. *International Journal of Sports Medicine*, **12**, 190-195.

80. McLellan, T.M., & Gass, G.C. (1989). Metabolic and cardiorespiratory responses relative to the anaerobic threshold. *Medicine and Science in Sports and Exercise*, **21**, 191-198.

81. McLellan, T.M., & Gass, G.C. (1989). The relationship between the ventilation and lactate thresholds following normal, low and high carbohydrated diets. *European Journal of Applied Physiology*, **58**, 568-576.

82. McLellan, T.M., & Skinner, J.S. (1981). The use of the aerobic threshold as a basis for training. *Canadian Journal of Applied Sport Sciences*, **6**, 197-201.

83. McLellan, T.M., & Skinner, J.S. (1982). Blood lactate removal during active recovery related to

the aerobic threshold. *International Journal of Sports Medicine, 3,* 224-229.

84. Nagle, F., Robinhold, D., Howley, E., Daniels, J., Baptista, G., & Stoedefalke, K. (1970). Lactate accumulation during running at submaximal aerobic demands. *Medicine and Science in Sports, 2,* 182-186.

85. Nemoto, I., Iwaoka, I., Funato, K., Yoshioka, N., & Miyashita, M. (1988). Aerobic threshold, anaerobic threshold and maximal oxygen uptake of Japanese speed skaters. *International Journal of Sports Medicine, 9,* 433-437.

86. Olbrecht, J., Madsen, Ø., Mader, A., Liesen, A., & Hollmann, W. (1985). Relationship between swimming velocity and lactic concentration during continuous and intermittent training exercises. *International Journal of Sports Medicine, 6,* 74-77.

87. Orok, C.J., Hughson, R.L., Green, H.J., & Thompson, J.A. (1989). Blood lactate responses in incremental exercise as predictors of constant load performance. *European Journal of Applied Physiology, 59,* 262-267.

88. Owles, W.H. (1930). Alterations in the lactic acid content of the blood as a result of light exercise and associated changes in the CO_2 combining power of the blood and in the alveolar CO_2 pressure. *Journal of Physiology, 69,* 214-237.

89. Oyono-Euguelle, S., Gartner, M., Marbach, J., Heitz, A., Ott, C., & Fruend, H. (1989). Comparison of arterial and venous blood lactate kinetics after short exercise. *International Journal of Sports Medicine, 10,* 16-24.

90. Peronnet, F., Thibault, G., Rhodes, E.C., & McKenzie, D.C. (1987). Correlation between ventilatory threshold and endurance capability in marathon runners. *Medicine and Science in Sports and Exercise, 19,* 610-615.

91. Poole, D.C., & Gaesser, G.A. (1985). Response of ventilatory and lactate thresholds to continuous and interval training. *Journal of Applied Physiology, 58,* 1115-1121.

92. Poole, D.C., Ward, S.A., & Whipp, B.J. (1990). The effects of training on the metabolic and respiratory profile of high-intensity cycle ergometer exercise. *European Journal of Applied Physiology, 59,* 421-429.

93. Reybrouck, T., Ghesquiere, J., Cattaert, A., Fagard, R., & Amery, A. (1983). Ventilatory thresholds during short and long term exercise. *Journal of Applied Physiology, 55,* 1694-1700.

94. Ribeiro, J.P., Fielding, R.A., Hughes, V., Black, A., Bochese, M.A., & Knuttgen, H.G. (1985). Heart rate break point may coincide with the anaerobic but not the aerobic threshold. *International Journal of Sports Medicine, 6,* 220-224.

95. Rieu, M., Miladi, J., Ferry, A., & Duvallet, A. (1989). Blood lactate during submaximal exercises: Comparison between intermittent incremental exercises and isolated exercises. *European Journal of Applied Physiology, 59,* 73-79.

96. Robergs, R.A., Chwalbinska-Moneta, J., Mitchell, J.B., Pascoe, D.D., Houmard, J., & Costill, D.L. (1990). Blood lactate threshold differences between arterialized and venous blood. *International Journal of Sports Medicine, 11,* 446-451.

97. Rodriguez, F.A., Banquells, M., Pons, V., Drobnic, F., & Galilea, P.A. (1992). A comparative study of blood lactate analytic methods. *International Journal of Sports Medicine, 13,* 462-466.

98. Rusko, H., Luhdtanen, P., Rahkila, P., Viitasalo, J., Rehunen, S., & Harkonen, M. (1986). Muscle metabolism, blood lactate and oxygen uptake in steady state exercise at aerobic and anaerobic thresholds. *European Journal of Applied Physiology, 55,* 181-186.

99. Rusko, H., Rahkila, P., & Karvinen, E. (1980). Anaerobic threshold, skeletal muscle enzymes and fiber composition in young female cross country skiers. *Acta Physiologica Scandinavica, 108,* 263-268.

100. Saltin, B., Hartley, L.H., Kilbom, Å., & Åstrand, I. (1969). Physical training in sedentary middle aged and older men II: Oxygen uptake, heart rate and blood lactate concentration at submaximal and maximal exercise. *Scandinavian Journal of Clinical and Laboratory Investigation, 24,* 323-334.

101. Schnabel, A., Kindermann, W., Schmitt, W.M., Biro, G., & Stegmann, H. (1982). Hormonal and metabolic consequences of prolonged running at the individual anaerobic threshold. *International Journal of Sports Medicine, 3,* 163-168.

102. Simon, J., Young, J.L., Gutin, B., Blood, D.K., & Case, R.B. (1983). Lactate accumulation relative to the anaerobic and respiratory compensation thresholds. *Journal of Applied Physiology, 54,* 13-17.

103. Sjodin, B., & Jacobs, I. (1981). Onset of blood lactate accumulation and marathon running performance. *International Journal of Sports Medicine, 2,* 23-26.

104. Sjodin, B., Jacobs, I., & Karlsson, J. (1981). Onset of blood lactate accumulation and enzyme activities in m vastus lateralis in man. *International Journal of Sports Medicine, 2,* 166-170.

105. Sjodin, B., Jacobs, I., & Svedenhag, J. (1982). Changes in onset of blood lactate accumulation (OBLA) and muscle enzymes after training at OBLA. *European Journal of Applied Physiology, 49,* 45-57.

106. Sjodin, B., & Svedenhag, J. (1985). Applied physiology of marathon running. *Sports Medicine, 2,* 83-99.

107. Skinner, J.S., & McLellan, T.M. (1980). The transition from aerobic to anaerobic metabolism. *Research Quarterly for Exercise and Sport*, **51**, 234-248.

108. Snyder, A.C., Woulfe, T.J., Welsh, R., & Foster, C. (1994). A simplified approach to estimating the maximal lactate steady state. *International Journal of Sports Medicine*, **15**, 27-31.

109. Stegmann, H., & Kindermann, W. (1982). Comparison of prolonged exercise tests at the individual anaerobic threshold and the fixed anaerobic threshold of 4 mmol/l lactate. *International Journal of Sports Medicine*, **3**, 105-110.

110. Stegmann, H., Kindermann, W. & Schnabel, A. (1981). Lactate kinetics and individual anaerobic threshold. *International Journal of Sports Medicine*, **2**, 160-165.

111. Svedenhag, J., & Sjodin, B. (1984). Maximal and submaximal oxygen uptakes and blood lactate levels in elite male middle and long distance runners. *International Journal of Sports Medicine*, **5**, 255-261.

112. Svedenhag, J., & Sjodin, B. (1985). Physiological characteristics of elite male runners in and off season. *Canadian Journal of Applied Sport Sciences*, **10**, 127-133.

113. Tanaka, K., Watanabe, H., Konishi, Y., Mitsuzono, R., Sumida, S., Tanaka, S., Fukuda, T., & Makadomo, F. (1986). Longitudinal associations between anaerobic threshold and distance running performance. *European Journal of Applied Physiology*, **55**, 248-252.

114. Tesch, P.A., Daniels, W.L., & Sharp, D.S. (1982). Lactate accumulation in muscle and blood during submaximal exercise. *Acta Physiologica Scandinavica*, **114**, 441-446.

115. Tesch, P.A., Sharp, D.S., & Daniels, W.L. (1981). Influence of fiber type composition and capillary density on onset of blood lactate accumulation. *International Journal of Sports Medicine*, **2**, 252-255.

116. Wasserman, K., Hansen, J.E., Sue, D.Y., & Whipp, B.J. (1987). *Principles of exercise testing and interpretation*. Philadelphia: Lea & Febiger.

117. Wasserman, K., & McIlroy, M.B. (1964). Detecting the threshold of anaerobic metabolism. *American Journal of Cardiology*, **14**, 844-852.

118. Weltman, A., Seip, R.L., Snead, D., Weltman, J.Y., Haskvitz, E.M., Evans, W.S., Veldhuis, J.D., & Rogol, A.D. (1992). Exercise training at and above the lactate threshold in previously untrained women. *International Journal of Sports Medicine*, **13**, 257-263.

119. Weltman, A., Snead, D., Seip, R., Schurrer, R., Levine, S., Rutt, R., Reilly, T., Weltman, J., & Rogol, A. (1987). Prediction of lactate threshold and fixed blood lactate concentrations from 3200m running performance in male runners. *International Journal of Sports Medicine*, **8**, 401-406.

120. Withers, R.T., Sherman, W.M., Clark, D.G., Esselbach, P.C., Nolan, S.R., Mackay, M.H., & Brinkman, M. (1991). Muscle metabolism during 30, 60, and 90 s of maximal cycling on an air-braked ergometer. *European Journal of Applied Physiology*, **63**, 354-362.

121. Yamamoto, Y., Miyashita, M., Hughson, R.L., Tamura, S., Shinohara, M., & Mutoh, Y. (1991). The ventilatory threshold gives maximal lactate steady state. *European Journal of Applied Physiology*, **63**, 55-59.

122. Yeh, M.P., Gardner, R.M., Adams, T.S., Yanowitz, F.G., & Crapo, R.O. (1983). Anaerobic threshold: Problems of determination and validation. *Journal of Applied Physiology*, **55**, 1178-1186.

123. Yoshida, T. (1984). Effect of dietary modifications on lactate threshold and onset of blood lactate accumulation during incremental exercise. *European Journal of Applied Physiology*, **53**, 200-205.

124. Yoshida, T. (1984). Effect of exercise duration during incremental exercise on the determination of anaerobic threshold and the onset of blood lactate accumulation. *European Journal of Applied Physiology*, **53**, 196-199.

125. Yoshida, T., Suda, Y., & Takeuchi, N. (1982). Endurance training regimen based upon arterial blood lactate: Effects on anaerobic threshold. *European Journal of Applied Physiology*, **49**, 223-230.

126. Yoshida, T., Takeuchi, N., & Suda, Y. (1982). Arterial versus venous blood lactate increase in the forearm during incremental bicycle exercise. *European Journal of Applied Physiology*, **50**, 87-93.

127. Foxdal, P., Sjödin, B., Sjödin, A., & Östman, B. (1994). The validity and accuracy of blood lactate measurements for prediction of maximal endurance running capacity. *International Journal of Sports Medicine*, **15**, 89-95.

CHAPTER 6

Measurement of Anaerobic Power and Capacity

Carl Foster, PhD

Lisa L. Hector, MS

Kerry S. McDonald, PhD

Milwaukee Heart Institute

Ann C. Snyder, PhD

University of Wisconsin—Milwaukee

Because many sports activities and activities of daily living occur with rapid rest-to-exercise transitions and/or at high intensity, anaerobic energy expenditure is essential for human performance. This chapter describes several basic approaches to evaluating peak muscular power output, assumed to be primarily anaerobic. We also discuss some approaches to measuring anaerobic capacity, in particular the accumulated O_2 deficit which is the best of the newer approaches to measuring anaerobic capacity.

The maximum rate of muscle exercise attributable to aerobic metabolism is generally defined by maximal oxygen uptake ($\dot{V}O_2max$), a parameter that is comparatively well defined and has been the focus of considerable study over 50 years or more (48). Researchers are now looking to determine the highest rate of muscular exercise attributable to aerobic metabolism that is practically sustainable. This rate is often called the anaerobic threshold, although there are persuasive arguments that it neither represents anaerobic metabolism nor displays threshold characteristics. One candidate for this intensity is that associated with both a progressive increase

in blood lactate (indicating a disturbance of acid–base homeostasis) and a disproportionate increase in pulmonary ventilation (presumptively attributable to the buffering of lactate by circulating bicarbonate).

There is little agreement over strategies to define this highest sustainable rate of aerobic metabolism (9, 14, 22, 26, 30). The capacity for exercise using aerobic metabolism is essentially limitless in that the energy reserves (as fat and carbohydrate) in even lean athletes are on the order of 55,000 kcal. At exercise intensities of 3 to 4 times resting (ordinary walking), this energy reserve could sustain exercise for about a week, but of course other factors, including dehydration, the need for sleep, and orthopedic limitations, make the theoretical impossible. Even at fairly high levels of exertion, such as marathon running, skiing, cycling, or skating, the maximal sustainable exercise duration is on the order of hours, supporting the notion that the capacity for aerobic metabolism is not limited in any practical sense.

Humans perform much of their exercise under circumstances that cannot be attributed solely, or even largely, to aerobic metabolism. Under conditions associated with the onset of exercise, there is a lag in the behavior of the oxygen transport system. The behavior of this lag, oxygen uptake kinetics, has been studied and appears to follow predictable rules (49). The result of this lag is that during the first several minutes of any rest-to-exercise transition, a considerable amount of the external muscular work accomplished cannot be attributed to aerobic metabolism; the work is accomplished anaerobically. The work during this period was labeled the oxygen deficit as long ago as 1913 by Krogh and Lindhard (32). Further, under conditions associated with exercise intensities greater than $\dot{V}O_2$max, the energy source for muscular contraction must also include anaerobic sources. Thus, anaerobic work may be attributable to a delay in the oxygen uptake kinetics at the beginning of work, to aerobic requirements greater than the peak rate of aerobic metabolism, or to both in combination. Work during periods of extensive anaerobic metabolism is associated with profound changes in intramuscular phosphagen and lactate concentrations (29).

Unlike the classical plateau of oxygen uptake, despite increases in the rate of external muscular work which led to the definition of $\dot{V}O_2$max (42), there has not been a single laboratory measurement historically associated with anaerobic work. The concept of the oxygen debt, the continued elevation of $\dot{V}O_2$ after exercise, was outlined in an early attempt to quantitatively model the magnitude of muscular work performed anaerobically (24, 35). But there are several problems with this model (7, 8), and the concept, particularly relative to describing the proportional contribution of aerobic and anaerobic energy production, is now largely discounted.

PERFORMANCE-BASED ANAEROBIC POWER TESTS

The dominant approach to determining both anaerobic power and anaerobic capacity has been to measure the rate and quantity of work performed under circumstances where aerobic metabolism is assumed to contribute very little. The concept of peak power production was originally developed by Margaria, Aghemo, and Rovelli (34), who developed the stair-climbing test. Although variations are possible and can be accounted for mathematically, the basic protocol involves ascending a staircase of about 1.75 m in height as rapidly as possible (e.g., taking two steps at a time). The preliminary run up to the staircase is variable, but 2 m has been the standard length of approach. A timing mat or photocell activated by the subject's passage simplifies timing and might reduce errors, because it takes only about 1 s to climb 1.75 m. The result is computed according to this formula:

$$\text{power (W)} = \frac{\text{mass (kg)} \times \text{vertical displacement (m)} \times 9.8}{\text{Time (s)}}$$

Normative data have been published and are reviewed by Bouchard et al. (5). Briefly, power can range from as little as 700 W (12 W/kg) in untrained females or female endurance athletes to as much as 1,500 W (18W/kg) in some male athletes.

The vertical jump test, often used as a measure of "explosiveness" in physical fitness testing, may also be used as an index of anaerobic power. The subject stands and reaches as high as possible, then jumps as high as possible. The vertical jump is the difference between standing height and jumping height. Generally three jumps are used, either from a crouched start or with a preliminary countermovement. More detail concerning this test is available in Fox and Matthews (20). Power is derived from this formula:

$$\text{power (W)} = 21.67 \times \text{mass (kg)} \times \text{vertical displacement (m)}^{0.5}$$

There are two cycle ergometer tests that are commonly used as measures of anaerobic power. In the widely employed Wingate anaerobic test (3), the power output during the early part (5-10 s) may be used as an index of anaerobic power. The test is usually performed on a mechanically braked cycle ergometer (Monarch). After warming up, the subject is instructed to pedal as rapidly as possible against zero resistance. The load is then applied (usually about 1 N/kg body weight) as quickly as possible. The process of loading usually takes 2 to 4 s. After the load is applied, the subject continues to pedal for 30 s, although less time could be used if peak anaerobic power is the measurement of interest. Flywheel revolutions are counted (often over a 5-s interval), ideally by a photocell that can resolve each flywheel revolution into 3 or 4 segments. Power is computed by this formula:

$$\text{power (W)} = \text{flywheel revolutions} \times 0.98 \times [60/\text{test duration (s)}] \times \text{resistance (N)}$$

Additional information regarding this test is presented in Bouchard et al. (5). Generally, peak power outputs will range from about 6 W/kg in young sedentary females to about 16 W/kg in some male athletes.

The Quebec 10-s test is another cycle ergometer approach to measuring peak power output. This test is also performed on a mechanically braked cycle ergometer (Monarch). It requires a photocell capable of resolving each one-third flywheel revolution and a potentiometer capable of sensing the momentary loading on the flywheel. The subject begins pedaling at about 80 rpm and the flywheel is loaded by the investigator (about 1 N/kg body weight). Remaining in a seated position, the subject then completes as many revolutions as possible in a 10-s period. The load on the flywheel is adjusted during the test to allow the subject to maintain a high pedaling rate. Power output is computed as the highest observed during any 1 s of the test. More information about this test is available (5, 6, 44, 45). Although about 1 N/kg body weight is the most commonly recommended flywheel resistance for a test of this nature, some authors have suggested a heavier load, particularly in athletes. Valuable discussion of the effect of loading variations is available (16, 17, 21, 43).

Withers et al. (50) have recently reported data on responses during heavy exercise on an air-braked cycle ergometer (Repco Ltd., Australia). Although they did not report very short-term peak power outputs, it would not be difficult to fit such an ergometer with a sensor for calculating power output per revolution of the flywheel (fan). This ergometer is arranged somewhat

differently, yet it is conceptually similar to the Air-Dyne ergometer (Schwinn) popular in the United States. The simplicity of the air-braked approach has much to offer over the relatively clumsy process of rapidly applying resistance to mechanically braked ergometers. The momentary power output is a simple function of the rpms. Resistance will vary, however, in relation to the local barometric pressure and the characteristics of the specific flywheel (fan). A correction for conditions other than 760 mmHg barometric pressure and 20 °C temperature can be computed on the basis of the following equation:

$$\text{corrected watts} = \text{observed watts} \times P/760 \times 293/(273 + T)$$

Interpretive standards are available for this instrument (51). This approach certainly deserves further study because of its simplicity.

More recently, instrumentation-intensive approaches to measuring muscular power output during very brief cycle ergometer (36, 37, 38) and treadmill (12, 13) exercise have been developed. Interpretive standards are available for the cycle ergometer protocol (33). These tests, which are not limited by acceleration of a heavy flywheel or delays in applying resistance, have been particulary valuable in that they have been able to demonstrate that (under optimal conditions) peak muscular power output is attained within the first 5 s of exercise and then follows a fairly predictable decay with continued exercise (Figure 6.1). This decay is based

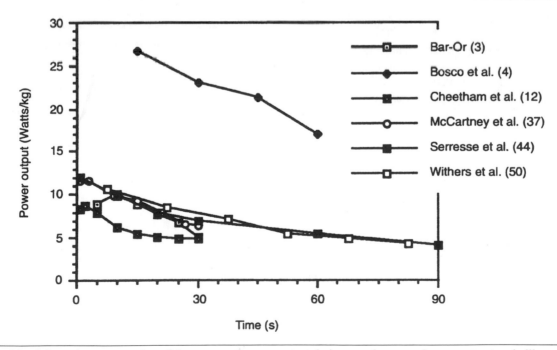

Figure 6.1 Schematic representation of the pattern of power output during very heavy cycle ergometer, treadmill exercise, or jumping exercise.

on the usual instructions for performance-based tests to go "all out" from the beginning of the test.

PERFORMANCE-BASED ANAEROBIC CAPACITY TESTS

Laboratory approaches to measuring anaerobic capacity and power using muscular performance tests have recently been well reviewed by Bouchard et al. (5). Significant discussion of issues related to the measurement of human muscular power output can be found in Jones et al. (28). Four tests merit specific description because of their wide use.

In the Wingate anaerobic test (3), the subject pedals a mechanically braked cycle ergometer at maximal possible rate against a heavy resistance of about 1 N/kg body weight for 30 s. Mean power output can be calculated from the following formula:

$$\text{power (W)} = \text{flywheel revolutions} \times 1.96 \times \text{resistance (N)}$$

Total work accomplished can be calculated from this formula:

$$\text{work (joules)} = \text{average watts} \times \text{duration (s)}$$

Normative data are available in Bouchard et al. (5).

The Quebec 90-s test is fundamentally similar to the Wingate anaerobic test, but continues longer. Based on data, presented later, concerning the relationship between work duration and anaerobic capacity estimated from accumulated O_2 deficit, the duration of the Quebec test may be much more suitable for estimating anaerobic capacity than the Wingate test. As indicated previously, the Quebec 90-s test is performed on a Monarch or other mechanically braked cycle ergometer. After warming up, the subject begins pedaling at 80 rpm while the work load is adjusted (usually to about 0.5 N/kg body weight). The subject then pedals as rapidly as possible for 90 s while the revolutions of the flywheel are counted by a photocell capable of resolving each one-third revolution, and the resistance on the flywheel is monitored from a potentiometer. During the test it is important to have the subject start very aggressively, with an initial pedaling rate of above 130 rpm for the first 20 s, and to adjust the resistance on the flywheel to maintain a high pedaling rate. Integration of the data can give moment-by-moment power outputs, give some information regarding the pattern of fatigue, and quantitate the total work done in 90 s, which may approach the anaerobic capacity. Normative data regarding this test are available (5, 6, 45).

A variation of the Quebec 90-s test has been presented by Withers et al. (50) using the Repco air-braked cycle ergometer. They have demonstrated that accumulated O_2 deficit and muscle lactate concentration peak after 60 s of exercise, given the premise that the subject goes "all out" from the beginning of the test. Their data argue that a 60-s version of either the Wingate anaerobic test or the Quebec test may be ideal, an option chosen by Szogy and Cherebetiu (47). Unfortunately, a significant amount of the work done during a test of even 30-s duration may be accounted for aerobically, so quantitation of anaerobic work for the purpose of calculating anaerobic capacity cannot be satisfactorily accomplished from the performance data alone.

Because it takes advantage of the potential for utilizing elastic energy storage in addition to chemical-mechanical energy conversion, the 60-s vertical jump test of Bosco, Luhtanen, and Komi (4) deserves some comment. A timer built into a mat is used to record cumulative flight time during the 60-s duration of the test. The subject is instructed to jump continuously, as high as possible on each jump, with knees preflexed to 90°, and with hands on hips to mimimize horizontal and lateral movement. The average power output during the trial can be computed as follows:

$$\text{power (W)} = \frac{9.8 \times \text{total flight time (s)} \times 60}{4 \times \text{number of jumps} \times [60 - \text{total flight time (s)}]}$$

As with other tests, the pattern of fatigue can be measured by observing the jumping pattern during convenient time intervals (every 15 s). In direct comparative studies, the calculated power output with the jumping test has been higher than during cycle ergometer tests of the same duration, although the pattern of decay in power output is similar to that observed during cycling (Figure 6.1).

ACCUMULATED O_2 DEFICIT

The validity of performance-oriented approaches to the measurement of anaerobic metabolism, particularly anaerobic capacity, can be challenged on at least three fronts.

First, performance-oriented tests usually involve very high rates of muscular power generation and substantial reductions in power output (fatigue) throughout the course of the test. Outside the laboratory, humans almost never work at their absolute maximal rate of momentary energy expenditure for more than about 5 s. There is usually some element of pace, designed to minimize the time required to complete a task. Certainly there are few examples in nature of the power output pattern associated with many of the contemporary tests of anaerobic power and capacity. Even athletic events as short as 20 s (running 200 m) involve some element of "relaxing and sustaining speed" so that the net duration of the task is minimized.

Second, under conditions of very heavy muscular work, the kinetics of the oxygen transport system are far from slow, and aerobic metabolism may account for a substantial portion of the energetic requirement in tests of as little as 30 s duration, which are frequently used as measures of anaerobic capacity. For example, aerobic metabolism has been shown to account for as much as 40% of the energetic requirements of the widely used Wingate test (25). This observation suggests that the assumption of a negligible oxidative contribution during tests of anaerobic power and capacity is fundamentally incorrect.

Third, the demonstration of considerable muscle lactate accumulation, even during very brief exercise (27), suggests that partitioning the alactic and lactic components of anaerobic work on the basis of time is intrinsically invalid. Further, the demonstration of significant rates of lactate production even at rest, the largely oxidative fate of produced lactate, and the importance of lactate turnover to the magnitude of lactate accumulation (1, 10, 47) suggest that the accumulation of muscle and blood lactate during heavy exercise is not a particularly good index of the contribution of anaerobic metabolism during any given exercise bout.

From the foregoing it may be justifiable to suggest that, although many of the widely used performance-based tests of anaerobic power and capacity might be useful indices of the peak rate of achievable muscular power output and of the quantity of muscular work achievable during comparatively brief periods of time, they might not satisfy their stated goal of measuring muscular power output and energetic capacity attributable to anaerobic metabolism alone.

Medbø et al. (39, 40, 41), following early suggestions by Hermansen (23) and Karlsson (29), have recently suggested that the magnitude of oxygen deficit accumulated during exhausting exercise may serve as a marker of anaerobic capacity. A modification of this concept, which includes the magnitude of blood lactate accumulation, has been proposed by Camus and Thys (11). The test may be conducted either on an electrically braked cycle ergometer or during treadmill running. Treadmill studies are often conducted up a rather steep grade (5%-10%) to provide for greater safety getting on the already moving treadmill.

We have found that a 2 mph (3.2 kph) greater velocity than that which the subject perceives as "hard" (or 5 on the category-ration scale of Borg) often gives a convenient test duration (unpublished results). If the accumulated O_2 deficit is to provide a satisfactory marker of the anaerobic capacity, at least three criteria

must be met. First, the accumulated O_2 deficit should level off with exercise duration. If there is a practical limit on the depletion of muscle phosphagens and the accumulation of metabolites from anaerobic metabolism, then the amount of work performed anaerobically should increase with exercise duration until some limit (the anaerobic capacity) is achieved.

To use a practical example, if one were to perform a single vertical jump (or even two or three jumps), the O_2 requirement might be very high (ultramaximal) relative to the $\dot{V}O_2$max, and the proportion of energy from anaerobic sources might be very high—but the total energy expenditure from nonoxidative sources would be very low, as the anaerobic capacity would not have been taxed. If one were to jump up and down for a minute, as suggested by Bosco, Luhtanen, and Komi (4), the O_2 requirements might be significantly in excess of $\dot{V}O_2$max (supramaximal), and the absolute amount of energy liberated from anaerobic sources would be high, although oxidative metabolism would also be important as a source of energy. However, if one were to jump up and down for several hours at a submaximal intensity, the oxidative contribution to the exercise bout would be very high and the net anaerobic energy release would in all probability not be greater than during 1 or 2 min of maximal jumping. The second criterion that must be met is that anaerobic capacity should be fundamentally independent from the $\dot{V}O_2$max. Given the different mechanisms involved in supporting aerobic and anaerobic metabolism, one would not expect much relationship between the two. The third criterion is that the measure of accumulated O_2 deficit should substantially agree with other methods of measuring the anaerobic capacity. Although the performance-based tests can be criticized relative to their ability to quantitatively partition aerobic and anaerobic contributions, they probably do measure to some degree the anaerobic capacity. The data of Withers et al. (50) and Szogy and Cherebetiu (47) provide this support.

Medbø et al. (39, 40, 41) have described an approach to measuring the accumulated O_2 deficit during heavy exercise. The magnitude of the accumulated O_2 deficit followed the relationship previously described, with maximal values observed at work loads causing exhaustion in 2 to 5 min. They have further demonstrated that the accumulated O_2 deficit is larger in sprint-trained athletes than in endurance-trained athletes or in the untrained, is larger in males than in females, and is responsive to training. Bangsbo et al. (2) have demonstrated a quantitative relationship between accumulated O_2 deficit and short-term changes in muscle metabolites during one leg exercise. Others have demonstrated the feasibility of this technique and have begun to describe normally expected values for the magnitude of the accumulated O_2 deficit, 30 to 80 ml O_2/kg (18, 19,

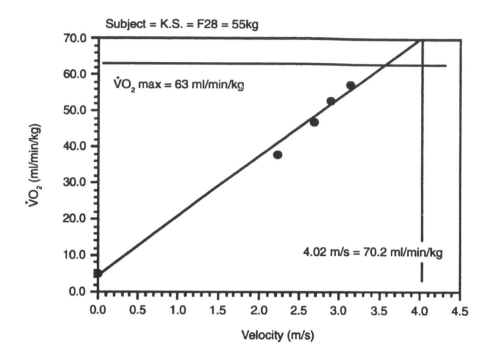

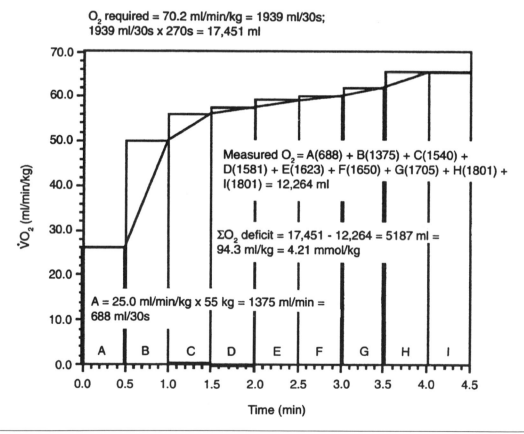

Figure 6.2   Sample calculation of accumulated O_2 deficit.

31, 50). An example test showing the computation of the accumulated O_2 deficit is presented in Figure 6.2. The O_2 requirement is first estimated based on several steady-state submaximal runs according to Medbø et al. (39). The subject then exercises to exhaustion at a fixed work load, with continuous measurement of $\dot{V}O_2$. Accumulated O_2 deficit is computed by subtracting the measured O_2 uptake from the O_2 required of a specific time interval (30 s, in the present example) and summating these measures.

One of the limitations of the accumulated O_2 deficit method as described by Medbø et al. (40) is the requirement that the subject continue an arbitrary work load to exhaustion. This is comparatively dependent upon the subject's level of motivation. We have had subjects perform a series of cycle ergometer tests where the total work requirement varied from 100 to 700 J/kg (19), and with instructions to finish the total work bout as quickly as possible (as in running a race). The pattern of accumulated O_2 deficit versus work accomplished followed the predicted relationship and was very similar to that earlier demonstrated by Medbø et al. (Figure 6.3). The temporal relationship also suggests that exercise durations of 2 to 5 min are associated with maximal values for the accumulated O_2 deficit (Figure 6.4). In a subsequent study (18), the accumulated O_2 deficit was compared

during a cycle ergometer ride to exhaustion at a power output requiring 110% of $\dot{V}O_2$max and during a 2-km time trial on a bicycle attached to a wind-load simulator (15). Accumulated O_2 deficit was similar during both trials (Figure 6.5). Reproducibility studies with both techniques suggested significant day-to-day variability in the accumulated O_2 deficit (Figure 6.6). These data suggest that these two approaches to measuring accumulated O_2 deficit can be used with more or less equivalent results.

There are several significant technical problems associated with the measurement of anaerobic capacity using the accumulated O_2 deficit approach described by Medbø et al. (40). Peak levels of power output cannot be measured as with the classical performance-oriented methods, thus no estimate of peak "anaerobic power" output can be made. However, combining the approach taken by the Quebec 90-s test (5) or using the air-braked ergometer as suggested by Withers et al. (50) might allow simultaneous measurement of peak power output over 1 to 2 s (anaerobic power) and accumulated O_2 deficit (anaerobic capacity).

The measurement of the accumulated O_2 deficit requires that the measured $\dot{V}O_2$ be subtracted from the required $\dot{V}O_2$ at several time periods during the work bout and that the measures of O_2 deficit be summated

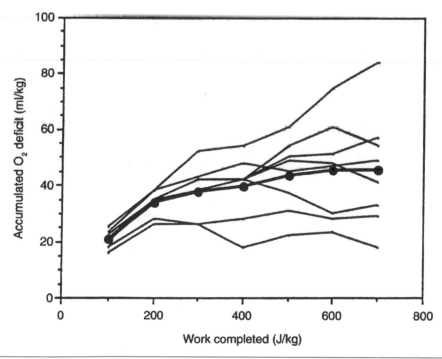

Figure 6.3 Increase of the accumulated O_2 deficit when differing amounts of total external muscular work are accomplished as quickly as possible, as in running a race. Exercise was performed on a mechanically braked cycle ergometer (Monarch) with a resistance setting of 3N. Total work accumulated depended on pedal revolutions completed. Beyond a given threshold of total work done (500 J/kg in the present example of well-trained subelite athletes), there is no increase in the magnitude of the accumulated O_2 deficit. The small dots and thin lines represent the responses of individual subjects. The large dots and bold line represent the mean value for accumulated O_2 deficit in relation to total work completed.

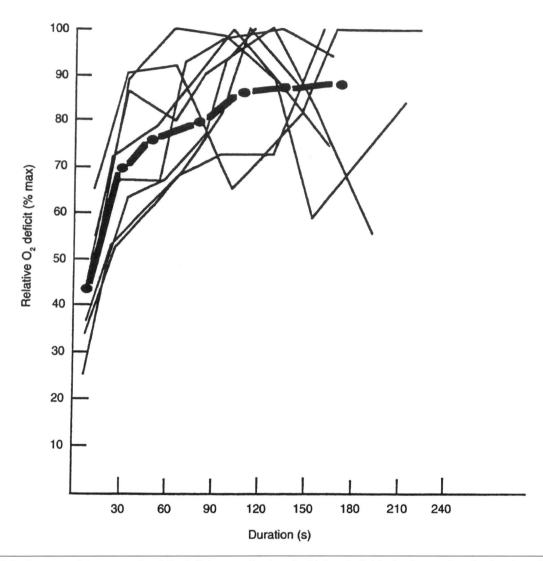

Figure 6.4 Increase of the accumulated O_2 deficit normalized to the highest individual values and to the duration of activity. Beyond an exercise duration of 120 s there is no further growth in the accumulated O_2 deficit. Data here are the same as in Figure 6.3; the subject was required to complete a fixed quantity of work in the shortest possible time. The small dots and thin lines represent the responses of individual subjects. The large dots and bold line represent the mean value for the relative O_2 deficit in relation to exercise duration.

(Figure 6.2). In our experience, measurement periods of 20 to 30 s usually give satisfactory results, although in principle either breath-by-breath measurements or a single collection could be made. It is important to remember that accumulated O_2 deficit is a quantity, not a rate. The raw data for $\dot{V}O_2$ required and $\dot{V}O_2$ measured are rates. If the collection period is exactly equal to 1 min, rate and quantity will be numerically the same. If, on the other hand, one uses 20-s collections, the deficit during that period is one third of the difference between the rate of $\dot{V}O_2$ required and $\dot{V}O_2$ measured. It is still easier for most to understand when the accumulated O_2 deficit is presented as an equivalent quantity of O_2 that was not consumed, normalized for the size of the individual, in milliliters per kilogram (ml/kg). However, the accumulated O_2 deficit is a quantity, so the more proper expression is in millimoles per kilogram (mmol/kg). This is obtained by normalizing liters of a gas to moles using Avogadro's principle. Computationally this is (O_2 deficit ml/kg)/22.4.

Medbø et al. (40) have discussed in some detail the importance and difficulty in estimating the $\dot{V}O_2$ required. Because the $\dot{V}O_2$ requirement is greater than $\dot{V}O_2$max, $\dot{V}O_2$ measured during submaximal steady-state exercise must be extrapolated considerably. Accordingly, even small measurement errors in submaximal $\dot{V}O_2$ can lead to considerable errors in computing $\dot{V}O_2$ required and, accordingly, in the summated O_2 deficit. In their original study, Medbø et al. performed approximately 20 submaximal measurements, each

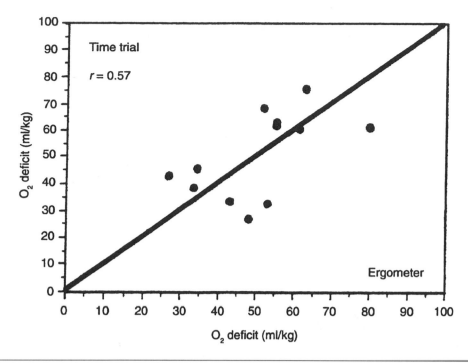

Figure 6.5   Comparison of accumulated O_2 deficit determined during a cycle ergometer ride to fatigue at a power output requiring 110% of $\dot{V}O_2$max and during a 2-km time trial on a bicycle attached to a wind-load simulator.

involving a 2-min collection of expired air at the end of a 10-min work bout, a laborious process to say the least. Medbø et al. have discussed an abbreviated approach to the computation of the O_2 requirement, which has been used by others (31), including ourselves (18, 19). The validity of the extrapolation method to compute aerobic requirements while using wind-load simulators that have nonlinear response characteristics, as is required for our "time-trial" method or for the air-braked ergometer method of Withers et al. (50), has not been independently verified. Similarly, suggestions that running may have nonlinear aerobic requirements at higher velocities present a problem for the use of running tests. The concept of steady-state $\dot{V}O_2$ is itself not a trivial problem. Wasserman et al. (49), in discussing the concept of the ventilatory anaerobic threshold, have suggested that above this exercise intensity there is a progressive increase in $\dot{V}O_2$ throughout the duration of a constant-power-output work bout. Accordingly, even if one uses rather long "steady-state" bouts as suggested by Medbø et al. (40), one either has to restrict the measurements to comparatively low intensities and assume the risk of a greater degree of extrapolation or has to accept the risk that "steady-state" measurements made above the "ventilatory anaerobic threshold" systematically underestimate the aerobic requirements and accordingly lead to underestimation in the subsequently calculated O_2 deficit.

The validity of using steady-state $\dot{V}O_2$ requirements to estimate the aerobic cost of the beginning moments

of exercise is far from clearly established. Medbø et al. (40) and Katz, Snell, and Stray-Gundersen (31) had subjects drop onto an already running treadmill. Are the aerobic requirements of accelerating to the velocity required to keep up with the treadmill accurately reflected by the $\dot{V}O_2$ requirement extrapolated from submaximal measurements? During studies on either the cycle ergometer or a cycle attached to a wind-load simulator, the torque requirements associated with accelerating to the required power output or velocity are subjectively very high. It is our impression that the assumed aerobic requirement during the first several seconds of exercise may be significantly less than that accounted for by the extrapolation method. With ergometer studies we have adopted the strategy of starting at a low power output and rapidly (within 5 s) increasing the power output to the required level. We have assumed that the average $\dot{V}O_2$ requirement during this period is 50% of the $\dot{V}O_2$ requirement for steady-state exercise at this power output. Whether this assumption is valid remains to be determined. With the time-trial studies, we have measured the average velocity over the first 200 m of the ride (about 20 s) and have used the steady-state $\dot{V}O_2$ requirement for this velocity in the computation of accumulated O_2 deficit. Our feeling is that this might underestimate the true requirement. Medbø and Tabata (41) have further discussed the necessity for correcting for desaturation of oxygen stores in the computation of accumulated O_2 deficit, although in practice many do not do this because of the necessity for making

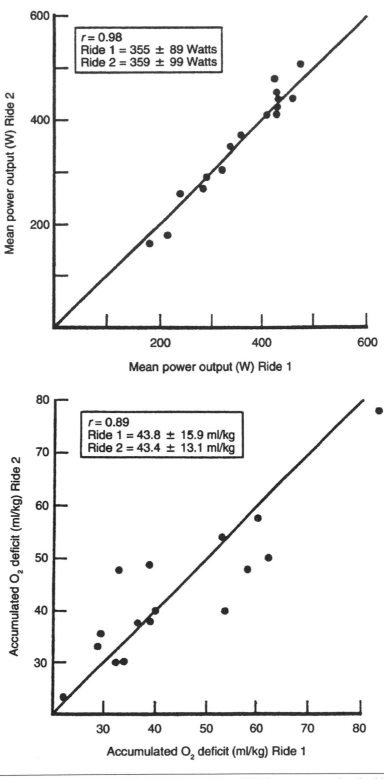

Figure 6.6   Reproducibility of accumulated O_2 deficit. Rides requiring 500 J/kg were completed with at least 48 hours between rides. Average power output was computed from the total work accomplished and the time required. Accumulated O_2 deficit was computed based on Figure 6.2 and the average power output during each segment of the ride.

assumptions about the magnitude of desaturation of oxygen stores. The O_2 stored in muscle and blood is thought to contribute approximately 10% to the maximal accumulated O_2 deficit.

CONCLUSION

The measurement of anaerobic power and capacity remains a difficult area. Several approaches, some as old as Margaria's stair-climbing test (35), may provide an estimate of the highest achievable muscular power output during very brief (< 5 s) time intervals (3, 5, 12, 13, 36, 37). If one is willing to accept assumptions regarding the lack of contribution from aerobic metabolism, it may be argued that these tests can provide reasonable estimates of anaerobic power. In view of the data of Jacobs et al. (27), partitioning this power output into alactic- and lactic-acid-dependent metabolic pathways may be inappropriate. With the development of nuclear magnetic resonance spectroscopy, perhaps this problem can be profitably readdressed in the near future.

Anaerobic capacity is more difficult to measure. Clearly most of the performance-oriented tests that have traditionally been used for this purpose have serious deficiencies relative to the basic assumptions that must be made for the test to be used. Attempts to estimate anaerobic capacity via the use of the accumulated O_2 deficit are conceptually attractive. There remain many technical problems with the collection of this data and with the assumptions necessary to claim that the accumulated O_2 deficit represents a meaningful estimate of anaerobic capacity. Combining the ergometric approach adopted in the Quebec 90-s test (5) or the air-braked ergometer as suggested by Withers et al. (50) with the accumulated O_2 deficit approach suggested by Medbø et al. (40) might offer the best compromise and allow reasonable simultaneous estimates of both anaerobic power and anaerobic capacity.

REFERENCES

1. Åstrand, P.O., Hultman, E., Juhlin-Danfelt, A., & Reynolds, G. (1986). Disposal of lactate during and after strenuous exercise in humans. *Journal of Applied Physiology*, **61**, 338-343.
2. Bangsbo, J., Gollnick, P.D., Graham, T.E., Juel, C., Kiens, B., Mizuno, M., & Saltin, B. (1990). Anaerobic energy production and O_2 deficit-debt relationship during exhaustive exercise in humans. *Journal of Physiology*, **442**, 539-559.
3. Bar-Or, O. (1987). The Wingate anaerobic test: An update on methodology, reliability and validity. *Sports Medicine*, **4**, 381-394.
4. Bosco, C., Luhtanen, P., & Komi, P. (1983). A simple method for measurement of mechanical power in jumping. *European Journal of Applied Physiology*, **50**, 273-282.
5. Bouchard, C., Taylor, A.W., Simoneau, J.A., & Dulac, S. (1991). Testing anaerobic power and capacity. In J.D. MacDougal, H.A. Wenger, & H.J. Green (Eds.), *Physiological testing of the high performance athlete* (2nd ed.) (pp. 175-221). Champaign, IL: Human Kinetics.
6. Boulay, M.R., Lortie, G., Simoneau, J.A., Hamel, P., Leblanc, C., & Bouchard, C. (1985). Specificity of aerobic and anaerobic work capacities and powers. *International Journal of Sports Medicine*, **6**, 325-328.
7. Brooks, G.A. (1971). Temperature, skeletal muscle mitochondrial functions and oxygen debt. *American Journal of Physiology*, **220**, 1053-1059.
8. Brooks, G.A. (1973). Glycogen synthesis and metabolism of lactic acid after exercise. *American Journal of Physiology*, **224**, 1162-1166.
9. Brooks, G.A. (1985). Anaerobic threshold: Review of the concept and directions for future research. *Medicine and Science in Sports and Exercise*, **17**, 22-31.
10. Brooks, G.A. (1991). Current concepts in lactate exchange. *Medicine and Science in Sports and Exercise*, **23**, 895-906.
11. Camus, G., & Thys, H. (1991). An evaluation of the maximal anaerobic capacity in man. *International Journal of Sports Medicine*, **12**, 349-355.
12. Cheetham, M.E., Boobis, L.H., Brooks, S., & Williams, C. (1986). Human muscle metabolism during sprint running. *Journal of Applied Physiology*, **61**, 54-60.
13. Cheetham, M.E., Williams, C., & Lakomy, H.K.A. (1985). A laboratory sprint running test: Metabolic responses of endurance and sprint trained athletes. *British Journal of Sports Medicine*, **19**, 81-84.
14. Davis, J.A. (1985). Anaerobic threshold: Review of the concept and directions for future research. *Medicine and Science in Sports and Exercise*, **17**, 6-18.
15. Dengel, D.R., Graham, R.E., Hones, M.T., Norton, K.I., & Cureton, K.J. (1990). Prediction of oxygen uptake on a bicycle windloaded simulator. *International Journal of Sports Medicine*, **4**, 279-283.
16. Dotan, R., & Bar-Or, O. (1983). Load optimization from the Wingate anaerobic test. *European Journal of Applied Physiology*, **51**, 409-417.
17. Evans, J.A., & Quinney, H.A. (1981). Determination of resistance settings for anaerobic power testing. *Canadian Journal of Applied Sports Science*, **6**, 53-56.
18. Foley, M.J., McDonald, K.S., Green, M.A., Schrager, M., Snyder, A.C., & Foster, C. (1991).

Comparison of methods for estimation of anaerobic capacity. *Medicine and Science in Sports and Exercise*, **23**, S34.

19. Foster, C., Kuettel, K., & Thompson, N.N. (1989). Estimation of anaerobic capacity. *Medicine and Science in Sports and Exercise*, **21**, S27.

20. Fox, E.L., & Mathews, D. (1974). *Interval training: Conditioning for sports and general fitness*. Philadelphia: W.B. Saunders.

21. Gastin, P., Lawson, D., Hargreaves, M., Carey, M., & Fairweather, I. (1991). Variable resistance loadings in anaerobic power testing. *International Journal of Sports Medicine*, **12**, 513-518.

22. Heck, H., Mader, A., Hess, G., Mucke, S., Muller, R., & Hollmann, W. (1985). Justification of the 4 mmol/l lactate threshold. *International Journal of Sports Medicine*, **6**, 117-130.

23. Hermansen, L. (1969). Anaerobic energy release. *Medicine and Science in Sports*, **1**, 32-38.

24. Hill, A.V. (1924). Muscular exercise, lactic acid and the supply and utilization of oxygen. *Proceedings of the Royal Society*, **96**, 438-455.

25. Hill, D.W., & Smith, J.C. (1989). Oxygen uptake during the Wingate anaerobic test. *Canadian Journal of Sport Sciences*, **14**, 122-125.

26. Jacobs, I. (1986). Blood lactate: Implications for training and sports performance. *Sports Medicine*, **3**, 10-25.

27. Jacobs, I., Tesch, P.A., Bar-Or, O., Karlsson, J., & Dotan, R. (1983). Lactate in human skeletal muscle after 10 and 30s of supramaximal exercise. *Journal of Applied Physiology*, **55**, 365-367.

28. Jones, N.L., McCartney, N., and McComas, A.J. (Eds.). (1986). *Human muscle power*. Champaign, IL: Human Kinetics.

29. Karlsson, J. (1971). Lactate and phosphagen concentrations in working muscle of man. *Acta Physiologica Scandinavica*, (Suppl. 358).

30. Karlsson, J., & Jacobs, I. (1982). Onset of blood lactate accumulation during muscular exercise as a threshold concept. *International Journal of Sports Medicine*, **3**, 190-201.

31. Katz, A.L., Snell, P., & Stray-Gundersen, J. (1989). A combined protocol for running economy, $\dot{V}O_2$max and anaerobic capacity. *Medicine and Science in Sports and Exercise*, **21**, S10.

32. Krogh, A., & Lindhard, J. (1913). The regulation of respiration and circulation during the initial stages of muscular work. *Journal of Physiology, (London)*, **47**, 112-136.

33. Makrides, L., Heigenhauser, G.J.F., McCartney, N., & Jones, N.L. (1985). Maximal short term exercise capacity in healthy subjects aged 15-70 years. *Clinical Science*, **69**, 197-205.

34. Margaria, R., Aghemo, P., & Rovelli, E. (1966). Measurement of muscular power (anaerobic) in man. *Journal of Applied Physiology*, **21**, 1662-1664.

35. Margaria, R., Edwards, H.T., & Dill, D. (1933). The possible mechanisms of contracting and paying the oxygen debt and the role of lactic acid in muscular contraction. *American Journal of Physiology*, **106**, 689-715.

36. McCartney, N., Heigenhauser, G.J.F., & Jones, N.L. (1983). Power output and fatigue of human muscle in maximal cycling exercise. *Journal of Applied Physiology*, **55**, 218-224.

37. McCartney, N., Heigenhauser, G.J.F., Sargeant, A.J., & Jones, N.L. (1983). A constant velocity cycle ergometer for the study of dynamic muscle function. *Journal of Applied Physiology*, **55**, 212-217.

38. McCartney, N., Spriet, L.L., Heigenhauser, G.J.F., Kowalchuk, J.M., Sutton, J.R., & Jones, N.L. (1986). Muscle power and metabolism in intermittent exercise. *Journal of Applied Physiology*, **60**, 1164-1169.

39. Medbø, J.I., & Burgers, S. (1990). Effect of training on the anaerobic capacity. *Medicine and Science in Sports and Exercise*, **22**, 501-507.

40. Medbø, J.I., Mohn, A.-C., Tabata, I., Bahr, R., Vaage, O., & Sejersted, O.M. (1988). Anaerobic capacity determined by maximal accumulated O_2 deficit. *Journal of Applied Physiology*, **64**, 50-60.

41. Medbø, J.I., & Tabata, I. (1989). Relative importance of aerobic and anaerobic energy release during shortlasting, exhausting bicycle exercise. *Journal of Applied Physiology*, **67**, 1881-1886.

42. Mitchell, J.H., Sproule, B.J., & Chapman, C.B. (1958). The physiological meaning of the maximal oxygen intake test. *Journal of Clinical Investigation*, **37**, 538-547.

43. Patton, J.F., Murphy, M.M., & Fredrick, F.A. (1985). Maximal power outputs during the Wingate anaerobic test. *International Journal of Sports Medicine*, **6**, 82-85.

44. Serresse, O., Lortie, G., Bouchard, C., & Boulay, M.R. (1988). Estimation of the contribution of various energy systems during maximal work of short duration. *International Journal of Sports Medicine*, **9**, 456-460.

45. Simoneau, J.A., Lortie, G., Boulay, M.R., & Bouchard, C. (1983). Tests of anaerobic alactacid and lactacid capacities: Description and reliability. *Canadian Journal of Applied Sports Science*, **8**, 266-270.

46. Stainsby, W.N., & Brooks, G.A. (1990). Control of lactic acid metabolism in contracting muscles and during exercise. In K.B. Pandolf (Ed.), *Exercise and sports sciences reviews* (Vol. 18) (pp. 29-64). Baltimore: Williams & Wilkins.

47. Szogy, A., & Cherebetiu, G. (1974). A one minute bicycle ergometer test for determination of anaerobic capacity. *European Journal of Applied Physiology*, **33**, 171-176.

48. Thoden, J.S. (1991). Testing aerobic power. In J.D. MacDougal, H.A. Wenger, & H.J. Green (Eds.), *Physiological testing of the high performance athlete* (2nd ed.) (pp. 107-173). Champaign, IL: Human Kinetics.

49. Wasserman, K., Hansen, J.E., Sue, D.Y., & Whipp, B.J. (1987). *Principles of exercise testing and interpretation*. Philadelphia: Lea & Febiger.

50. Withers, R.T., Sherman, W.M., Clark, D.G., Esselbach, P.C., Nolan, S.R., Mackay, M.H., & Brinkman, M. (1991). Muscle metabolism during 30, 60 and 90 s of maximal cycling on an air braked ergometer. *European Journal of Applied Physiology*, **63**, 354-362.

51. Withers, T.T., & Telford, R.D. (1987). The determination of maximum anaerobic power and capacity. In G. Gass (Ed.), *Physiological guidelines for the assessment of the elite athlete* (pp. 105-124). Canberra, Australia: Australian Sports Commission.

CHAPTER *7*

The Measurement of Human Mechanical Power

Everett A. Harman, PhD

U.S. Army Research Institute of Environmental Medicine

The purpose of this chapter is to describe the methodology for producing continuous records of the mechanical power generated during various human physical activities. The measurement of power at extremely short time intervals distinguishes such testing from common tests of anaerobic power, the scores of which represent power averaged over 1 s or longer. Because many movements critical to sport performance take place very quickly, high-speed power measurement is essential for the understanding of sport techniques.

It is widely recognized that the human body's capability for generating force is highly related to performance in most sports and other physically demanding activities (1, 2). Because the acceleration of an object is proportional to the force acting on it divided by its mass (3), an athlete who can generate high ground-reaction forces relative to body mass can change speed or direction quickly. Likewise, the ability to accelerate an external implement (e.g., golf club, baseball bat, javelin) is directly related to the ability to apply force to the implement. It is clear that the ability to exert force is critical to "explosive" sports (those in which acceleration is of primary importance).

It is logical to conclude that because acceleration is proportional to applied force and strength is the ability to generate force, "stronger" people should be faster. The fact that this is not necessarily true, particularly in sport activities involving high body-segment velocities (e.g., tennis, baseball pitching, football kicking), reflects the limitations of methods commonly used to measure strength. Strength is usually defined as the maximum force produced during an isometric exertion or as the maximum weight lifted in a particular movement (1, 4, 5). Yet the results of isometric and low-speed strength tests don't show the ability to exert force at high speeds. The latter ability is important because in many sports the body, body segments, or implements must be accelerated while they already are moving quickly.

That strength is commonly evaluated via isometric or slow weight-lifting tests most likely reflects the limited equipment available to physical educators, teachers, coaches, and others who commonly conduct strength testing. Even most sport science laboratories lack the equipment to measure force exerted at higher speeds. Defining strength in easily tested terms has allowed scientists and nonscientists alike to carry out strength testing. Unfortunately, the resulting strength scores have had limited usefulness for predicting sport performance.

Knuttgen and Kraemer (6) have suggested a broader definition of strength as "the maximal force a muscle or muscle group can generate at a specified velocity." According to this definition, testing would have to be conducted over a wide range of velocities, during both concentric and eccentric muscle action, to get a complete picture of a subject's strength. Relatively expensive or sophisticated equipment would be needed to either test strength at preset velocities or monitor limb velocities during lifting movements. Despite the difficulty and expense involved, such testing would provide a set of strength scores more meaningfully related to sport ability. A major implication of the new definition of strength is that most commonly used strength tests provide only a partial view of an individual's strength profile.

The limited applicability of strength test scores obtained at slow or zero speed has led to a heightened interest in "human power output" as a measurement of the ability to exert force at higher speeds. Outside of the scientific realm, power, as a physical attribute of living beings, is considered the same as "force, energy, strength, and might" (7). However, in the fields of science and engineering, power is specifically and precisely defined as "the time rate of doing work" (3). In the latter context, work is the product of the force exerted on an object and the distance the object moves in the direction in which the force is exerted. Work can also be calculated as the area under a curve of force versus distance, a method particularly useful when force varies rapidly.

The discrepancy between the general and scientific definitions of power has fostered misunderstanding and even conflict among sport researchers and practitioners. For example, the sport of power lifting is an athletic competition in which heavy weights are lifted without regard to the rate of lifting. It has been found that during power lifting (squat, dead lift, and bench press), considerably less mechanical power is generated than during Olympic lifting (snatch and clean-and-jerk) or several other sports (8). To avoid ambiguity, researchers should use the term *power* strictly in its scientific sense, while being tolerant of lay usage of the terms *power* and *powerful*.

It is unfortunate that the concepts of strength and power have become dichotomized, in the sense that "strength" is usually associated with slow speeds and "power" with high speeds of movement. *Strength* means maximal force, and both force and power can be measured at low speed, high speed, or any speed in between. Both reflect an individual's ability to do work at the speed tested. Power is a direct mathematical function of force and velocity. Therefore, if, at any instant, any two of the variables force, velocity, and power are known, the third can be calculated. If we say that, during

a test of maximal knee extension at 200°/s an individual can generate high force or high power, precisely the same ability is being described—that is, the ability to exert force at that particular movement speed. If Knuttgen and Kraemer's concept of strength were accepted, power could be calculated from the strength score as the product of the force measured and the velocity at which it occurred. Strength and power testing would thus be concurrent.

This chapter describes how mechanical power and force can be precisely and instantaneously measured during a wide variety of human activities through the use of electronic transducers, motion picture cameras, and computers. Power output tests that do not involve instantaneous measurement, such as the Margaria and Wingate tests (9, 10), involve calculation of power averaged over a few seconds, but lack the resolution to measure true peak power (11). These tests are described in chapter 6.

This chapter includes a description of the quantitative foundation of power output measurement, a discussion of the necessary instrumentation and data-processing procedures, and a number of examples of how power output during various physical activities has been measured.

THE QUANTITATIVE FOUNDATION OF POWER TESTING

The definitions of work and power in equation form are

$$\text{work} = \text{force} \times \text{distance} \tag{1}$$

and

$$\text{power} = \frac{\text{work}}{\text{time}} = \frac{\text{force} \times \text{distance}}{\text{time}} \tag{2}$$

Because Equation 2 can be rewritten as

$$\text{power} = \text{force} \times \frac{\text{distance}}{\text{time}} \tag{3}$$

power can also be defined as force times velocity,

$$\text{power} = \text{force} \times \text{velocity} \tag{4}$$

or, more precisely, as the product of the force exerted on an object and the velocity of the object in the direction in which the force is exerted. The same result is obtained when power is calculated as the product of the velocity of an object and the force exerted on it in the direction of its movement.

For the equations to be correct, it is necessary to use consistent units. In the Système International d'Unités (SI) (12), which is the worldwide standard for science and engineering, force is in newtons, distance is in meters, time is in seconds, work is in joules (newton · meters), and power is in watts (joules/second). When necessary, the appropriate input units can be obtained from those of other measurement systems using the factors listed in Table 7.1.

The preceding work and power equations apply to an object moving through space whose path is traced by the object's center of mass, a point at which all the object's mass could be concentrated without changing the path of the object in response to external forces. However, the generation of work and power doesn't require that the object's center of mass move through space at all, because work can result in rotation without translation. When force is applied to an object, translational work results if the object moves through space, and rotational work results if the object rotates. Both kinds of work can occur at the same time. If the object doesn't move at all, the applied force results in no work. The equation for rotational work is

$$\text{work} = \text{torque} \times \text{angular displacement} \quad (5)$$

where torque is the product of a force acting on the object and the perpendicular distance from the line of action of the force to the point about which the object rotates, and angular displacement is the angle through which the object rotates. The equation for rotational power is

$$\text{power} = \frac{\text{work}}{\text{time}} = \frac{\text{torque} \times \text{angular displacement}}{\text{time}} \quad (6)$$

Because the equation can be rewritten as

$$\text{power} = \text{torque} \times \frac{\text{angular displacement}}{\text{time}} \quad (7)$$

power can also be defined as the product of torque and angular velocity:

Table 7.1 Factors for Conversion of Common Measures to SI Units of Force and Distance

To get	Multiply	By
newtons	pounds	4.448
newtons	kilograms	9.807[a]
meters	feet	0.3048
meters	inches	0.02540

[a]The kilogram, a unit of mass, is frequently referred to as a unit of force. A kilogram reading on a spring or electronic scale is equivalent to 9.807 N of force. However, a kilogram of mass will register exactly 1 kg on such a scale only if the weighing occurs where the acceleration of gravity is 9.807 m/s[2].

$$\text{power} = \text{torque} \times \text{angular velocity} \quad (8)$$

In SI, torque is in newton · meters and angular displacement is in radians. Just as for translational movement, the work done in rotating an object is in joules, and power is in watts (12). Angles in degrees can be converted to radians by dividing by 57.30 deg/rad.

To calculate power output during translational movement, force and velocity must be either monitored directly or calculated. Force can be measured with various types of transducers described in the instrumentation section later in this chapter. Because velocity transducers are not as commonly available as are position transducers or accelerometers, velocity is usually calculated from position or acceleration.

INDIRECT CALCULATION OF PARAMETER VALUES

Calculating Velocity From Position or Acceleration

Position, velocity, and acceleration at any juncture can each be calculated from any of the others if position and velocity at the start of data collection are known. Velocity, a basic component of power, can be readily calculated from time records of position or acceleration, based on the facts that change in position divided by the time during which the position changes equals velocity, and change in velocity divided by the time during which the velocity changes equals acceleration.

$$\text{velocity} = \frac{\Delta \text{position}}{\text{time}} \quad (9)$$

$$\text{acceleration} = \frac{\Delta \text{velocity}}{\text{time}} \quad (10)$$

In the power output data collection system described later in this chapter, the time interval between successive data samples is known. Velocity throughout the movement can be easily calculated for each intersample interval using *position* transducer data and Equation 9. The calculation of velocity from *acceleration* data first involves rearrangement of Equation 10 to obtain the change in velocity over each intersample time interval.

$$\Delta \text{velocity} = \text{acceleration} \times \text{time} \quad (11)$$

The velocity at the end of each intersample time interval is the velocity at the start of the interval plus the change in velocity over the interval. It can be seen that, to calculate the velocity throughout the entire movement, the movement must start from a known velocity. The simplest way to start with a known velocity is to begin data sampling before the subject has begun moving, when the velocity equals zero.

Calculating Force From Acceleration

When the mass of an object is known, and the movement of the object can be accurately monitored, it is not necessary to directly transduce force exerted on the object. The applied force can be determined from Newton's second law, which states that

$$\text{force} = \text{mass} \times \text{acceleration} \qquad (12)$$

Calculating Acceleration From Force

If the mass of an object is known, and the magnitude and direction of force on the object can be measured, the acceleration of the object can be determined through rearrangement of Equation 12 to solve for acceleration:

$$\text{acceleration} = \frac{\text{force}}{\text{mass}} \qquad (13)$$

Determining Torque From Force

If the magnitude and direction of the force exerted on an object can be measured, the resulting torque about any pivot point of interest can be determined. For example, Figure 7.1 shows the force (F) exerted on a

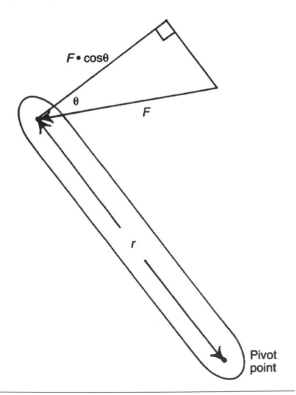

Figure 7.1 Variables used to calculate the torque resulting from an applied force (F). Torque about the pivot point is equal to $r(F \cdot \cos\theta)$.

pivoted lever. If r is a line from the point of application of F to the pivot point, torque about the pivot can be calculated as r times the component of F perpendicular to r, or $r \cdot (F \cdot \cos\theta)$. When it is more convenient to do so, torque can also be calculated as the product of the force acting on the object and the perpendicular distance from the line of action of the force to the point about which the object rotates.

Calculating Torque From Angular Acceleration

The angular equivalent to Equation 12 is

$$\text{torque} = (\text{moment of inertia}) \times (\text{angular acceleration}) \qquad (14)$$

Therefore, if the moment of inertia is known, and angular acceleration (in radians/s^2) is measured, torque can be calculated. There are standard methods for calculating the moment of inertia of a limb (18) or an object accelerated by a test subject (3).

TESTING STRATEGY

An electronic transducer is a device that produces an electrical signal, most often a voltage, proportional to the magnitude of a parameter of interest. To calculate power output for translational movements (e.g., jumping, running, and lifting), transducers are needed to monitor force and velocity. For rotational movements (e.g., cycling), transducers are needed to monitor torque and angular velocity. As described in the previous section, not all of these parameters need be measured directly.

The transducer output signal is passed through a signal conditioning device if amplification is necessary or to filter out unwanted electrical noise. If the transducer puts out a strong, clean signal, this stage is unnecessary.

The signal, coming directly from the transducer or from the signal conditioner, is converted by a computer interface device into information compatible with the computer. The interface device can be either a freestanding box connected to the computer by cable, or a board that plugs directly into an expansion slot of the computer. The better computer interface devices have some amplification capacity, which can eliminate the need for separate amplifiers in a signal conditioning stage.

Following the instructions of a computer program that incorporates the equations listed earlier, the microcomputer takes the converted information from the interface device and performs power output calculations. Results are displayed in tabular or graphic form on the computer screen or printer and stored on a computer disk.

TEST RESULTS

The system is set up to monitor, or "sample," all transduced parameters at known frequencies (e.g., 500 Hz [500 times per second]). The time interval between samples is the mathematical inverse of the sampling frequency (e.g., at a sampling frequency of 500 Hz, the intersample interval is 1/500 s). Using calibration coefficients, the computer converts the output of the computer interface device into real units of force, distance, and so on. Values of nonsampled variables are calculated from the values of the variables transduced at each point in time. The computer produces a history, rather than a single score, for power output, and, if desired, for the following variables as well:

Linear	Angular
Force	Torque
Linear position	Angular position
Linear velocity	Angular velocity
Linear acceleration	Angular acceleration
Force rate of change	Torque rate of change

Peaks and their times of occurrence can be determined for power and the other variables. Average magnitude for any of the variables can be calculated over an entire movement or for various movement phases (e.g., push-off phase of the vertical jump). In addition, linear and angular work can be calculated, and joint range of motion determined. Linear impulse (the area under the force-vs.-time curve) and angular impulse (the area under the torque-vs.-time curve) may be of interest as well.

INSTRUMENTATION

The following is a more detailed description of components that can be used to assemble the type of power output measurement system described previously. The compilation is not intended to be exhaustive. There are many electronic and mechanical components not mentioned that can be adapted for power output measurement. It is hoped that, after becoming familiar with the basic methodology, readers will be able to develop power measurement systems suited to their specific needs.

Transducers

The calculation of human mechanical power using Equations 4 and 8 requires knowledge of force and velocity for translational movement, and torque and angular velocity for rotational movement. Transducers must be able to directly monitor these variables or provide information from which they can be calculated.

General Considerations

Most transducers produce voltages proportional to the magnitude of the parameter being transduced. Following are some of the factors that must be considered when selecting a transducer.

Resolution

Resolution is the smallest change in the measured parameter that can be detected by the transducer. For human power output testing it is desirable to have a minimum resolution of 0.01% of full scale. For example, if a force transducer can measure up to 2,000 N, it should be able to distinguish changes in force as small as 2 N.

Measurement Range

The transducer must be able to register the minimum and maximum parameter value that might be encountered. It is safer to overestimate the range than to underestimate it. Transducers can be damaged or produce meaningless results when subjected to conditions beyond the range for which they are designed. On the other hand, the use of a transducer whose range is much greater than that expected can result in poor resolution.

Accuracy

Accuracy is the maximum amount the transducer signal can be expected to deviate from the correct output. Standards for accuracy are similar to those for resolution.

Thermal Effects

Thermal effects are changes in the output signal caused by variations in temperature rather than by changes in the measured parameter. If, within the range of temperatures expected under laboratory conditions (including the heat produced by the electronic measurement circuitry), the thermal effects are greater than the desired level of accuracy, special temperature compensation circuitry may be necessary. Frequently, plans for such circuitry come with the transducer. Temperature compensation circuitry might not be necessary under typical laboratory conditions where ambient temperature remains relatively constant, electronic devices are turned on at least an hour before the experiment to allow temperatures to stabilize, and any necessary calibration adjustments are made just prior to the experiment.

Excitation Voltage

Most transducers require a voltage source to excite them. It is convenient if the transducer accepts a voltage level typical of common power supplies, such as 5, 12, or 15 V. The lower the required voltage, the easier it is to use batteries instead of AC power. If batteries are used instead of a commercial power supply, some regulation circuitry is required to make sure the excitation voltage remains constant.

Output Voltage

It is most convenient if the full-scale transducer output signal comes close to but does not exceed 5 V, because the most common input voltage range for devices used to interface the transducer to the computer is ±5 V. If the transducer output can exceed the allowable input range of the interface device, then the signal must be reduced by a fixed percentage before being fed into the computer interface device. If the signal is much lower than the allowable input limit, it must be amplified or resolution will suffer. The better computer interface devices provide choices of various input voltage ranges that can be specified in software or by manipulating switches or jumper wires on the board itself, reducing the need for an extra stage for amplifying or reducing the signal.

Frequency Response

Frequency response is the highest rate at which the transducer is capable of "keeping up" with changes in the measured parameter. For power measurement, frequency response should be at least 100 Hz. "Response time," which is the mathematical inverse of frequency response, is sometimes used to describe the same characteristic (e.g., a frequency response of 100 Hz is comparable to a response time of 0.01 s).

Specific Transducers

The following are some transducers particularly useful for the measurement of human mechanical power. They either directly transduce the parameters needed for Equations 4 and 8 or transduce variables from which torque and velocity or torque and angular velocity can be calculated.

Load Cell

A load cell (Figure 7.2) is a small device that can measure tension and/or compression force exerted upon it. Two good sources of these are BLH Electronics (Canton, MA) and Tedea Huntleigh (Canoga Park, CA). Prices generally range from $250 to $500.

Force Platform

The force platform (Figure 7.3) is a standard tool in biomechanics research, most often used for gait analysis. A typical force platform provides voltage signals proportional to forces exerted on the platform's surface in the up-down, front-back, and side-to-side directions. Signals allowing the center of pressure to be located are usually provided as well. The devices are well suited to monitoring human power output during jumping. The most widely used force platforms are from Kistler (Amherst, NY) and AMTI (Newton, MA). Unfortunately, the expense of these devices (approximately $20,000 with accompanying electronics) puts them out of reach for many laboratories. AMTI sells software for calculation of power output during jumping or lifting activities. It is not difficult to write similar programs using the methods described throughout this chapter.

Strain Gauge

Some force platforms and most load cells are based on the strain gauge, which is a small, very inexpensive, foil-thin device that changes its electrical resistance as it is

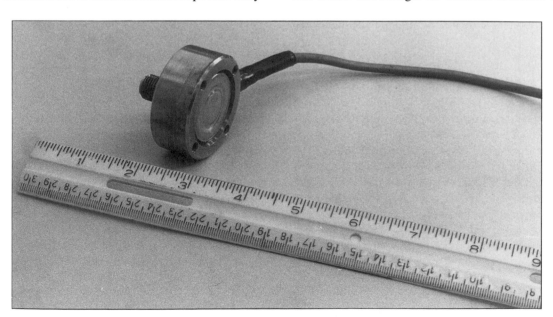

Figure 7.2   A load cell, which, when provided with electrical excitation, emits a voltage proportional to the tension or compression force to which it is subjected.

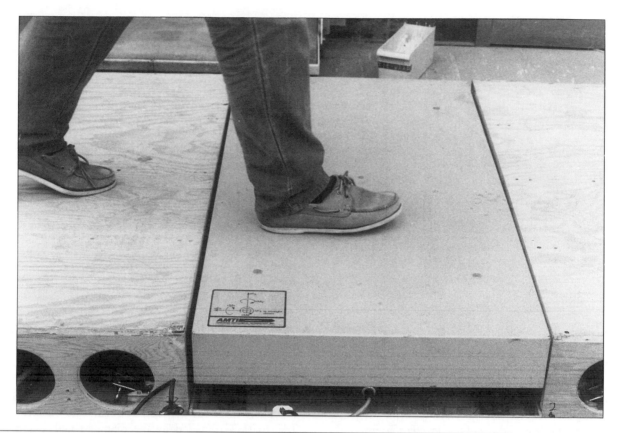

Figure 7.3 A force platform that emits 6 voltage signals proportional to the forces imposed upon it in the vertical, left-right, and fore-aft directions and torques about the three corresponding axes.

stretched or compressed. Scientists can have custom-tailored transducers made using the strain gauge, or order such devices ready-made (13, 14). A force transducer can be made by bonding the strain gauge to a piece of metal that bends slightly when force is exerted on it. The bending stretches or compresses the strain gauge, changing its electrical resistance. Specially designed electronic circuitry produces a voltage in proportion to the force exerted. Strain gauge implementation can be somewhat difficult, but proficiency can be developed with some effort and patience. BLH Electronics (Canton, MA), a prime supplier of strain gauges, provides very good instruction manuals. Advantages of making force transducers from strain gauges include low cost and great flexibility of design. Disadvantages include time and effort involved in development and difficulty in producing the same degree of precision found in commercial products.

The High-Speed Camera
High-speed cameras that can film at user-selectable rates of 500 frames per second and beyond are standard equipment in biomechanics laboratories. Systems that use video instead of movie film incorporate automatic image analysis and are available from companies such as Motion Analysis (Santa Rosa, CA), Peak Performance (Englewood, CO), and Ariel Dynamics (San Diego, CA).

The main advantage of video over 16mm film is the considerable time saving in automatic image processing versus the labor-intensive frame-by-frame processing required with film analysis. Researchers performing film analysis usually write their own programs, but the video-based systems come with well-developed software packages that make the systems usable for people without extensive training. Other advantages of video include avoidance of the delay and expense involved in film developing, and the lower cost of tape than of film. Disadvantages include the greater initial expense of the video system and the limitation of most video cameras to 60 frames per second. Faster video cameras are available at considerably greater expense.

The minimum cost of a film-based motion analysis system is about $20,000, and video systems start at about $30,000. These costs are high for a power output testing system that is not the major focus of a laboratory. However, such systems are often available in biomechanics laboratories for collaborative studies.

Angular Position Transducer (Electrogoniometer)
The angular position transducer (Figure 7.4) provides an effective and economical means of monitoring rotary movement (15). When affixed to either a device that rotates (exercise machine) or to a hinge-type body joint (knee,

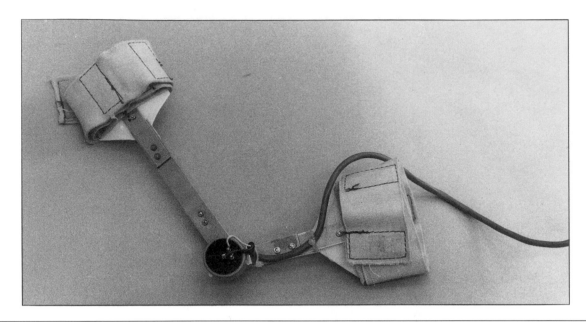

Figure 7.4 An angular position transducer (electrogoniometer) made from a rotary potentiometer. Voltage output is proportional to the angle between the device's arms. The elastic bands are used along with tape to secure the electrogoniometer about a body joint.

elbow), it can provide the angular-position information necessary to calculate angular velocity for power output determination. It is particularly adaptable for custom-designed power output testing and, as with film or video analysis equipment, it can be used without a force transducer to determine power output during the movement of an object of known mass and/or moment of inertia.

Although ready-made electrogoniometers are not generally available, they can be simply constructed from rotary potentiometers, which can be purchased in any electronics supply store. Rotary potentiometers are the familiar devices used to raise or lower volume on radios or make adjustments on other electrical implements by turning a knob. As its shaft is turned, the electrical resistance of the device changes. Radios use *audio taper* potentiometers, which are characterized by nonlinear relationships between electrical resistance and shaft knob position. The nonlinearity is needed because perceived loudness is not a linear function of sound energy. However, a *linear taper* potentiometer is preferable for goniometry because it is desirable for resistance to change by the same amount per degree of shaft rotation, no matter where in the range of motion the movement occurs.

Standard computer interface devices accept voltage input signals but are not designed to handle input from variable resistors. Thus a voltage signal proportional to the varying resistance must be obtained through application of Ohm's law (16).

$$\Delta voltage = current \times resistance \qquad (15)$$

The units for voltage, current, and resistance are, respectively, volts, amperes, and ohms. Using the ana-

logy of a fluid, voltage can be thought of as pressure, current as flow rate, and resistance as restriction to flow provided by the diameter and length of a pipe.

Figure 7.5 represents a rotary potentiometer. The curved zigzag line represents the resistor itself. The arrow represents a contact arm that rotates when the shaft is turned. The electrical current flowing from point A to point C doesn't change, because the resistance and voltage between the two points are constant. However, as the shaft is turned so that the arm contacts the resistor closer to or farther from C, the resistance and thus the voltage between B and C changes. The setup is called a *voltage divider* because the voltage drop between A and C is divided into one drop between A and B and another drop between B and C. The ratio of each of these voltage drops to the voltage drop across the entire resistor is the same as the ratio of the resistance across which the voltage drop is measured to the entire resistance. Because the resistance between B and C is directly proportional to the position of the potentiometer shaft, the position of the shaft can be determined from the voltage between B and C. For example, if the voltages at points A and C are constant at 10 and 0 V, respectively, a voltage reading at B of 3.8 V can be used to determine the potentiometer shaft angular position (θ) relative to the right horizontal, as follows:

$$\theta = 360° \times \frac{(3.8 \text{ V} - 0.0 \text{ V})}{(10.0 \text{ V} - 0.0 \text{ V})} = 136.8° \qquad (16)$$

In actuality, any standard potentiometer has a dead zone, which is an electrically nonconductive segment of the potentiometer's angular range. The dead zone occurs in the shaft angular range where potentiometer resistance changes from highest to lowest, and usually subsumes at least 3°. To find the extent of the dead zone, connect the potentiometer to a resistance meter to determine the angular range over which resistance actually changes (e.g., 354°). The actual range can then be substituted for 360° in Equation 16. If possible, the dead zone should be avoided. For example, for testing the knee extension movement, which cannot occur over more than 180°, the potentiometer can be arranged so that the dead zone is never crossed during the movement.

Angular position transducers are available that, for each angular position, emit the type of digital code described later in the section on analog-to-digital converters. They are highly precise and have no dead zones, but are expensive and more difficult to interface to the computer than rotary potentiometers. There is also a rotary transducer with an internal disk of alternating light and dark bands. As the shaft is turned, the transducer puts out a pulse each time a band is passed.

When connected to a frequency-to-voltage converter (described later), this type of transducer is good for monitoring angular velocity. However, it is not easily used for encoding absolute angular position.

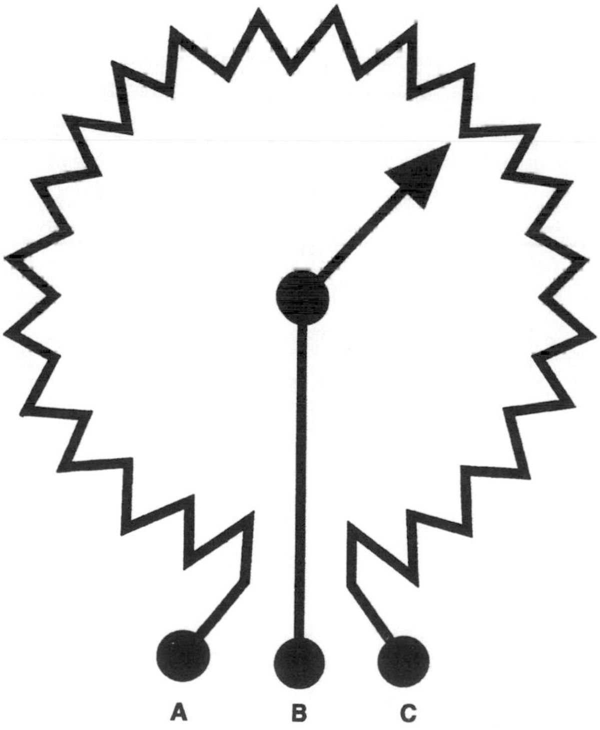

Linear Position Transducer

A very useful series of position transducers is made by Celesco (Canoga Park, CA; Figure 7.6). The basic device costs about $500 and consists of a small box containing a spooled, thin, flexible steel cable, the end of which protrudes from a hole in the box. The device puts out a voltage proportional to the distance the cable is pulled out. A spring on the spool keeps enough tension on the cable so that it recedes back into the box when it is not being pulled on by an external force. The device can easily be used to monitor the location of anything moved in a straight line. Where cost is a factor, a similar device can be constructed based on an inexpensive linear taper potentiometer, described earrlier, and a cable wrapped around a spring-loaded spool. However, it can be difficult to obtain

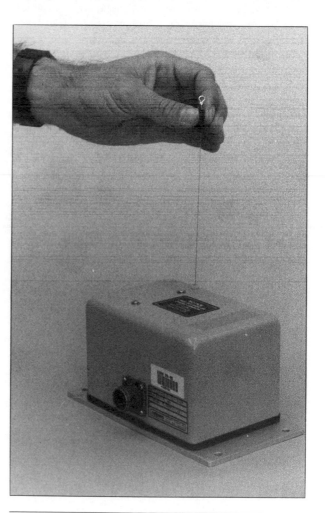

Figure 7.5 A linear taper rotary potentiometer used as an angular position transducer. Because the electrical resistance between B and C is directly proportional to the position of the potentiometer shaft, the voltage between B and C can be used to determine shaft position.

Figure 7.6 A linear position transducer that outputs a voltage signal proportional to the distance the cable is pulled out.

the same level of precision and durability in a homemade transducer as in a commercially produced unit.

Accelerometer

When provided with excitation voltage, an accelerometer (Figure 7.7) produces a voltage proportional to the acceleration it experiences. The accelerometer is usually less than 1 cu. in. in size and contains a mass supported by a small beam. When the container is accelerated, the inertia of the mass bends the beam in proportion to the acceleration. A strain gauge circuit translates the bending into a voltage. High-quality, but expensive ($500-$2,000), accelerometers are available from Entran (Fairfield, NJ). IC Sensors (Milpitas, CA) produces very small, light, and inexpensive ($80) accelerometers that work well when used according to the manufacturer's instructions.

Velocity Transducer

Transducers are available that produce voltage proportional to velocity. For power output determination the advantages of transducing velocity directly rather than calculating it from position data include (1) reduction in computer programming requirements, (2) faster production of results, and (3) greater accuracy. One source of velocity transducers is Celesco (Canoga Park, CA). Also, Lakomy (35) reported that an electrical generator can be used as a velocity transducer. He observed excellent linearity of response, with an r^2 of 0.998 for the generator's output voltage versus the angular velocity of its shaft.

Signal Conditioning Devices

If a transducer produces a strong, clean signal, no signal conditioning is necessary. However, a low amplitude transducer signal must be boosted to the input range of the analog-to-digital converter board, and a signal with significant electronic noise must be filtered. Whenever possible, it is best to avoid the need for conditioning by selecting transducers with desirable specifications and shielding them and their connecting wires from sources of electronic noise.

Each transducer that requires signal conditioning must be attached to its own amplifier and/or filter. This might necessitate three or more amplifier/filters. Multi-channel chart recorders with built-in amplifier/filter units are often available in laboratories. They can be used to condition transducer signals without using the chart recorder itself. Companies producing such units include Western Graphtec (Irvine, CA) and Hewlett-Packard (Palo Alto, CA).

A good way to avoid buying expensive filter/amplifiers is to perform filtering in software rather than hardware and to use small, low-cost, single-chip instrumentation amplifiers. Computer software libraries that contain digital-filter or cubic-spline routines that can be used to smooth somewhat noisy data are available from various sources, such as IMSL (Houston, TX) or Quinn Curtis (Needham, MA). Instructions are provided that show how the routines can be called from the user's program. Filtering in software rather than hardware has the advantages of (1) allowing the experimenter to keep the unfiltered raw data, (2) providing great flexibility in degree and type of filtering, and (3) costing less than hardware. Instrumentation amplifiers on a chip, from a source such as Analog Devices (Norwood, MA), are very economical (under $40) and effective. To make these units functional, some electronics experience is

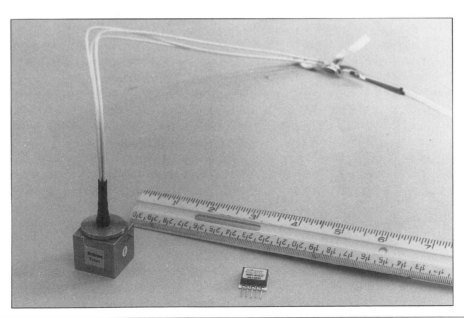

Figure 7.7   Two types of accelerometers. The one on the left is a precision triaxial version; the right one is a small, low-cost, uniaxial type.

helpful for assembly of the chip, power supply, and connectors.

Computer Interface Devices

Information is transmitted to and received from the computer via interface devices, the most common of which are keyboards and monitors. Because the entry of long streams of data into computers via keyboards is prohibitively slow and labor-intensive, other interface devices have been developed to meet the needs of a modern scientific laboratory. The interface devices described in the following paragraphs greatly enhance the speed and facility of entering data from experimental devices and, given the appropriate experimental setup, allow for immediate processing and feedback.

Analog-to-Digital Converter

The analog-to-digital converter (A/D) translates a voltage into a numerical value that can be read by the computer. The device is an essential component of a computerized laboratory, because a great majority of transducers put out voltage signals proportional to measured parameters. Although these are available in the form of a freestanding box that connects to the computer by cable, a more economical and compact form is that

of a board that plugs directly into the expansion slot of a desktop computer (Figure 7.8). The plug-in boards are fully functional and as a rule are more compact and less expensive than the stand-alone units.

In a *digital* computer, the most prevalent kind, information is transmitted and processed in *bits*, including all information entering or exiting the computer. Each bit can assume only two possible values, represented by either a higher or a lower voltage on an electrical wire. The two voltage levels are logically represented as "0" for low and "1" for high. In a typical microcomputer, a character is coded by 8 bits and an integer number by 16 bits.

The voltages on a set of x wires can be represented by a binary (each digit is either a one or a zero) number, x bits long. The number of possible combinations of x ones and zeros is 2^x. For instance, 16 bits can form $2^{16} = 65,536$ different combinations of ones and zeros. Most desktop computers today transmit bits in groups of 16 or 32. The computer can handle very large numbers, and numbers requiring many decimal places of precision, by using more than one group of bits to encode a number. The analog-to-digital converter serves the function of converting a voltage, which can vary in infinitely small increments, into a binary number that can be read by the computer. Table 7.2 shows how some numerical values are represented in the computer.

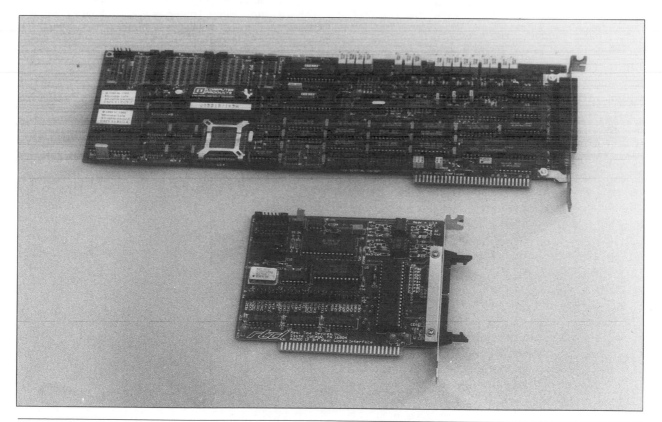

Figure 7.8 Two types of analog-to-digital converter boards capable of being plugged into an expansion slot of an IBM PC compatible computer. The larger board is more expensive than the smaller one, and has a number of additional features.

Table 7.2 Binary (Base 2) Equivalents of Decimal (Base 10) Numbers

Decimal	Binary
1	0000000000000001
2	0000000000000010
3	0000000000000011
4	0000000000000100
5	0000000000000101
6	0000000000000110
7	0000000000000111
8	0000000000001000
9	0000000000001001
10	0000000000001011
.	.
.	.
.	.
65,535	1111111111111111

Note. For the binary values, each 1 represents a bit at a higher voltage and each 0 represents a bit at a lower voltage. A 1 in the nth bit from the right has the value $2^{(n-1)}$.

The following are some characteristics that should be considered when purchasing an analog-to-digital converter board:

• Number of inputs—The number of transducers that can be connected to one board generally ranges from 1 to 16. For general use, it is best to have 16 channels. If economy is an important consideration for a dedicated system involving only one transducer, a single-channel board may be appropriate.

• Data collection speed—This is the overall speed at which the board can sample and translate voltages. For example, each of 8 transducers connected to a board rated at 10,000 Hz can be sampled as fast as $10,000 \div 8 = 1,250$ times per second. For most laboratory testing, each transducer need not be sampled more than 500 times per second, so that a board with an overall speed of 5,000 Hz can adequately monitor 10 transducers.

One advantage of a very fast board is that all transducers can be sampled almost simultaneously. For instance, with a 50,000-Hz board, the time between sampling of adjacent channels can be as little as 1/50,000 s. A convenient way to use such a fast board is to sweep all the channels at maximum speed, but wait 1/100 s between sweeps. Because the time between sampling of adjacent channels is only 1/500th as long as the time between successive sweeps of the channels, the different channels can be considered to be sampled simultaneously. Faster but more expensive boards are available if needed.

When a relatively slow board is used, the time delay between sampling of the different channels becomes significant, and mathematical interpolation should be incorporated into the analysis program to determine what the values of all the transduced variables would have been had they been sampled simultaneously.

• Input voltage range—The more flexibility a board has in allowable voltage input, the better. A basic board might have only a single input voltage range, say 0 to 5 V; a more flexible board could have multiple ranges including −5 to +5 and −10 to +10 V.

• Resolution—This may be the most important consideration in a board. Resolution is defined in bits. For example, 8 bits of resolution means that the full range of input voltage is translated into $2^8 = 256$ discrete numbers. For example, when a transducer that emits 0 to 5 V in response to 0 to 5,000 N of force is connected to an 8-bit A/D board with a 0 to 5 V input range, the smallest change in force that can be registered is 5,000 N ÷ 256 = 19.5 N. If the board's input range is −10 to +10 volts, then only one fourth of the range would be used, so that resolution would be limited to 5,000 N ÷ (256 ÷ 4) = 78.1 N. For most laboratory purposes, it is best to buy an A/D board with 12 bits of resolution, which translates the input voltage into 2^{12} or 4,096 discrete numbers. Also, to make the best use of the board's resolution, the transducer's voltage output range should match the board's voltage input range. More precisely, the highest and lowest voltages expected in the experiment should be fairly close to the highest and lowest voltages the board could translate.

• Overvoltage protection—Even if care is taken, it is not unusual to accidentally expose a board to a higher input voltage than it can translate. It is thus desirable to have a board that can withstand input at least 50% above the highest translatable voltage without being damaged.

• Gain—This allows the input signal to be amplified to match the input range of the board. This feature does not exist on a basic board. A full-featured board might be able to multiply the input signal by 1, 10, 100, or 1,000. In combination with multiple input voltage ranges, this gives the experimenter much flexibility and greatly reduces the chance that separate amplifiers will be needed.

• Digital input/output—Several boards have the additional capability of sensing and emitting the digital numbers described previously. This is useful for allowing the computer to sense when an event marker switch is tripped or to turn on an external device at a particular time.

• Input impedance—A voltage measuring device with a high input impedance allows only a tiny amount of current to flow into its inputs. This is important because the greater the flow of current into the measuring device, the greater the error in the measured voltage. In general, an input impedance of at least 1 megohm is desirable.

• Triggering—A board starts sampling and translating voltages as soon as it is triggered. Some boards can be triggered only by a computer program. Others can also be triggered by an external switch. External triggering is a useful feature because it allows more flexibility in setting up an experiment or testing device and facilitates automation. An experimenter may wish to configure a light-beam switch or contact pad so that the test subject's movement triggers data collection.

Some companies producing analog-to-digital converter boards for PC compatible computers are Data Translation (Marlboro, MA), whose boards are very widely used; Microstar (Bellvue, WA), which produces a board with many "intelligent" functions; and Real Time Devices (State College, PA), which sells some very economical boards (as low as $149), which work well but have few frills and might require some extra programming. Most of the full-function boards cost from $1,000 to $1,500, including software that is sometimes required.

Film Digitizer Tablet

To get information from the film record of an activity into the computer, the film is projected frame by frame onto a digitizing table (Figure 7.9). When the researcher places a cursor or stylus over each point of interest in the film image and pushes a button, the x and y digitizer coordinates of the point are fed to a computer. The computer file containing the x and y coordinates of all points digitized in every frame can be processed by a program to produce histories of various parameters, including power output.

Sources of digitizing tables include Numonics (Montgomeryville, PA), Altek (Silver Spring, MD), and Science Accessories (Stratford, CT). Prices range from $400 to $10,000, depending mainly upon the tablet's surface area and accuracy. One particularly useful feature is translucence of the tablet surface, which allows images to be projected from behind the tablet rather than from above, avoiding shadows cast by the operator's hand or body.

Frequency-to-Voltage Converter

A frequency-to-voltage converter puts out a voltage proportional to the rate at which the input signal switches cycles between a higher and a lower level. This is useful for translating the output of pulse-emitting transducers, such as the light-and-dark-band rotary transducer described earlier, into a voltage to be fed into an analog-to-digital converter. The faster the rotary

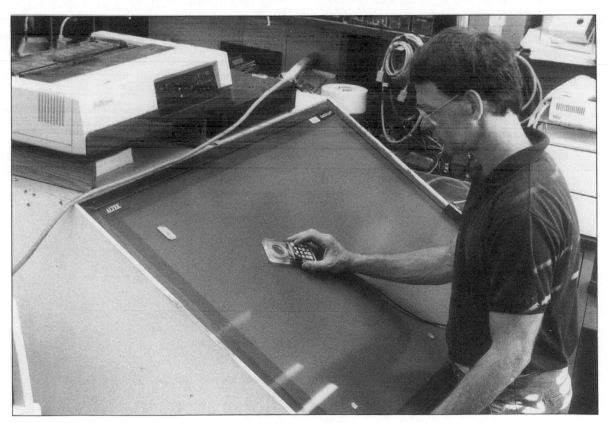

Figure 7.9 A film digitizing table.

transducer's shaft is turned, the higher the frequency of output pulses. The frequency-to-voltage converter can be used to monitor velocity in any experimental setup where the testing equipment is designed to put out one pulse for each specific increment of movement. It is not difficult to instrument cycles, rowing ergometers, and other devices in this way. The frequency-to-voltage converter is available as a flexible, ready-to-use device (Western Graphtec) in the $500 range, or as a very economical (under $10) microchip, from companies such as Cherry Semiconductor (East Greenwich, RI), that requires a small amount of additional circuitry to make it operational.

Mathematical Circuitry

Velocity, a convenient quantity for power output determination, is often calculated indirectly from position or acceleration. Although not difficult, such calculations do require computer time. In cases where very rapid turnaround is needed, the translation of position or acceleration data to velocity can be accomplished in hardware. Velocity can be obtained from position data through mathematical differentiation, or from acceleration data through integration. There are very simple circuits described in electronics texts, that accomplish both differentiation and integration using an inexpensive and widely available electronic component called an operational amplifier (16).

The Computer

There has been a steady increase in the number of computer hardware and software options available to the scientist, many of which are aggressively marketed. However, only a limited number of these options are appropriate for laboratory testing of human power output.

Hardware

Any computer capable of being interfaced to transducers can be used for power output testing. However, a mainframe computer is usually a poor choice because it generally has multiple users, which can slow the system below the speed required for data collection, and it can't be moved, requiring long electrical cables between it and the experimental site. Microcomputers are clearly preferable and are available from a wide variety of suppliers. IBM PC compatible computers are particularly appropriate for general laboratory use because of their power, low cost, established user base, and vast amount of available software. If possible, the computer should have at least a 486 central processing unit to ensure high processing speed and the ability to use innovative software. At least 8 MB of memory and a

200 MB hard disk are also recommended. Such computers are available from a number of manufacturers for about $1,500. A less powerful computer already in a laboratory may be used when very high speed is not required.

Software

Limited commercial software is available for human power output calculation, and is generally sold along with expensive video motion analysis or force platform systems. However, it is not difficult to write the necessary programs using the steps described later in this chapter.

Data Collection

The A/D board manual must be read carefully to determine the programming steps needed to communicate with the board. The program usually transmits information to the board by sending character strings to the board's address. Generally, the program must first send setup instructions to the board that tell it (1) which channels are to be sampled, (2) the order of sampling, (3) the degree of amplification of each channel, (4) the sampling speed, (5) the total time of sampling, and (6) the type of triggering. Less-expensive boards have fewer setup options and require more programming steps for controlling the data collection process; more-expensive boards provide a greater number of options and reduced programming requirements. Some of the companies producing boards sell extensive software to simplify data collection.

Data Analysis

When experimental data collection is triggered, the A/D board samples voltages from the specified channels and converts them to binary-coded integers to be read by the computer. A file is produced in which the number of values equals the number of channels times the sampling rate per channel (Hz) times the total sampling time (s). Files can become quite large. For example, if two channels are sampled at 500 Hz each for 3 s, the data file contains 3,000 numbers. The most convenient way to arrange the data file is to have each column represent a different transducer and each row a time point.

It is easiest to analyze the data in terms of power output when (1) the transducers directly monitor force and velocity, (2) the transducer signals emit negligible electronic noise, and (3) the A/D board is set up to take readings from the two transducers virtually simultaneously. In such a case the computer program need only implement a loop structure to read each succeeding line, convert the A/D board output units into meaningful values of force and velocity, and calculate power at each time point as the product of force and velocity.

If position is transduced instead of velocity, the program must determine the velocity between each pair of successive positions as the change in position divided by the change in time. Each resulting velocity can be considered to occur at a time midway between the times corresponding to the two positions from which it was calculated. For example, if force and velocity were monitored at 100 Hz, the data file would contain values for both variables at 0.000 s, 0.010 s, 0.020 s, 0.030 s, etc. The velocity calculated between 0.020 s and 0.030 s would be considered to occur at 0.025 s, which is a time at which force was not measured. Adjacent velocities would have to be averaged to get velocities corresponding to times at which force was actually measured. For example, the velocities for times 0.015 s and 0.025 s would be averaged to get the velocity at 0.020 s. As an alternative to averaging, curve-fitting and nonlinear interpolation are sometimes used to find the velocities at the desired times, but this is unnecessary for rapid rates of data collection.

Electronic noise is to be avoided if possible by careful selection of transducers. However, some degree of noise can be eliminated in software through mathematical smoothing. Descriptions of the programming steps needed to write a digital filter smoothing routine are available (17). Alternatively, inexpensive computer subroutine libraries with filtering capabilities can be obtained from companies already mentioned. The subroutines are segments of program code that can be called from the user's program to perform mathematical operations.

If the transducers are not sampled virtually simultaneously, linear or nonlinear interpolation can be used to estimate what the transducer readings would be if all transducers were sampled at the same time. For example, if channels are sampled at the times depicted in Table 7.3, then interpolation would result in values for all channels occurring at 0.020, 0.050, 0.080 s, and so on. Channel C is actually measured at those times and does not require interpolation. Using linear interpolation, the reading for channel A at 0.020 s would be two thirds of the way between its readings at 0.000 and 0.030 s. The reading for channel B at 0.020 s would be one third of the way between its readings at 0.010 and 0.040 s. The same steps would produce simulated simultaneous readings over the entire sampling period except for very short periods at the start and end of data collection lost in the interpolation process. The small data loss is no problem, because data collection always starts before and ends after the monitored activity. Alternatively, for nonlinear interpolation, a curvilinear equation can be fit to the data from each channel and used to solve for readings at the desired times.

Table 7.3 An A/D Board Sampling Pattern Requiring Interpolation for Simulation of Simultaneous Sampling

Time(s)	Channel
0.000	A
0.010	B
0.020	C
0.030	A
0.040	B
0.050	C
0.060	A
0.070	B
0.080	C
.	.
.	.

Computer Languages

The programming languages most widely used on microcomputers are Basic, Pascal, and C. There is somewhat of a trade-off between simplicity of programming and speed of program execution. Basic is usually the slowest language of the three but the easiest to learn and use. C is the fastest, but requires more understanding of the computer. Pascal is intermediate in speed and ease of programming, and is designed to be logical in structure and easy to read. Of the three, C provides the greatest power and flexibility, and is recommended except to those for whom simplicity is the most important factor.

It is possible to perform data collection and analysis without knowledge of computer programming. Software for data collection can generally be purchased along with an analog-to-digital converter board. The resulting computer data file can be processed to produce meaningful information using commercially available spreadsheet programs such as Lotus (Cambridge, MA) 1-2-3, Borland (Scotts Valley, CA) Quattro Pro, or Microsoft (Redmond, WA) Excel. The latter is highly recommended because it has far more analytical functions than any of its competitors.

In the experimental data file, each column usually corresponds to a different transduced variable, and each row corresponds to a point in time. The spreadsheet analysis consists of specifying mathematical formulas that define new columns of data in terms of existing columns. Such processing can be used to produce records of force and power from the transduced data.

System Calibration

Some transducers are precisely calibrated in the factory. Often, each individual transducer comes with its own set of factors for conversion of output to meaningful units. For example, an accelerometer might output 5.8 mV per g of acceleration per volt excitation. Another one with the same model number might output 6.1 mV · g⁻¹ · V. The different figures result from limitations in the precision of the manufacturing process. Factory calibration of transducers is useful because companies usually have the resources to provide elaborate and accurate calibration devices, the user is spared the time and effort of calibration, and factories have the capability to perform dynamic calibration, while most laboratories are only equipped for static calibration. Dynamic calibration is best because, for power measurements, transducers must monitor rapidly changing phenomena.

The following example shows how to develop an equation for translation of transducer output into meaningful units if factory-calibration figures are provided. Let us say that the force transducer used in a particular experiment is factory-calibrated at 15 microvolts per newton. The particular 12-bit A/D board has user-connectable jumper wires that allow it to accept voltage ranges of 0 to 5, 0 to 10, −5 to +5, or −10 to +10. It can also multiply the signal amplitude by either 1, 10, 100, or 1,000. If the maximum force anticipated in the experiment is 5,000 N, then the maximum transducer output voltage would be $5,000 \times 0.000015$ V = 0.075 V. Choosing a board amplification of 100 would bring the maximum signal to 7.5 V. It would then be best to set the board's input voltage range to 0 to +10 V, which would most closely match but not be exceeded by the anticipated input. Twelve bits encode $2^{12} = 4,096$ binary numbers. However, only part of the input voltage range is used. The following equation can be used to produce a factor to convert from the A/D board output values read by the computer, which are in machine units (μ), to actual units of force:

$$\frac{5,000 \text{ N}}{7.5 \text{ V}} \times \frac{10.0 \text{ V}}{4,096 \text{ }\mu} = 1.63 \text{ N} \cdot \mu^{-1} \qquad (17)$$

The resulting number is both the resolution of the system and a conversion factor. To calculate the force in newtons exerted on the transducer, the program has to multiply the μ values read by the computer by 1.63. For example, a computer value of 1,756 μ corresponds to a force on the transducer of (1.63 N/μ)(1,756 μ) = 2,862 N.

Where transducers must be calibrated by the user, trials are carried out in which known input is provided to the transducer over its entire range. The set of real and machine unit pairs are processed by a statistical regression program to produce a conversion equation with slope and intercept. It is best to have a zero intercept, so that the machine units need merely be multiplied by a constant to produce meaningful results, as is generally the case for factory-calibrated transducers. If the correlation between real and machine units is high (above .98), then a linear equation is appropriate. Nonlinear output requires curve-fitting, which is beyond the scope of this chapter. If at all possible, a transducer should be designed to have a linear response.

Sometimes a transducer is known to be highly linear, but has a slope and intercept that might vary slightly. In such a case, calibration should be performed before each testing session, with only two calibration measurements needed to determine the equation needed to convert machine units into meaningful values. The calibration procedure involves subjecting the transducer to two known stimuli, one at the low end and one at the high end of the anticipated measurement range, and recording the machine unit readings. The equation to convert from machine units to real values is then

$$Q_t = Q_L + \frac{\mu_t - \mu_L}{\mu_H - \mu_L} \times (Q_H - Q_L) \qquad (18)$$

where:

Q_t = real quantity measured at time t
Q_L = real quantity to which transducer is subjected during low calibration measurement
Q_H = real quantity to which transducer is subjected during high calibration measurement
μ_t = machine unit reading at time t
μ_L = machine unit reading during low calibration measurement
μ_H = machine unit reading during high calibration measurement

The equation must be used to convert each μ value into meaningful units. It can be seen that each conversion involves an addition, three subtractions, and a multiplication. Because the computer may have to convert thousands of values, processing can be slow. To speed up the calculations, it is best to rearrange the equation into the slope and intercept form below so that only one multiplication and one addition need be done per conversion. The program must be written so that the slope and intercept are not recalculated each time a μ value is converted, but calculated only once, before the loop structure in which the μ's are converted.

$$Q_t = \left(\frac{Q_H - Q_L}{\mu_H - \mu_L}\right)\mu_t + \left(Q_L - \frac{\mu_L(Q_H - Q_L)}{\mu_H - \mu_L}\right) \qquad (19)$$

SPECIFIC APPLICATIONS

The components and procedures I have described can be used to measure power output in a wide variety of human activities. Following are some samples of how the techniques can be applied.

Film or Video Analysis of Human Movement

The power transmitted to a sport implement, such as a baseball or javelin, is easily determined from film or video analysis. Force on the implement need not be measured directly, because it can be determined from acceleration of the implement's known mass.

The first step is to locate the implement's center of mass as the point at which the implement balances no matter how it is turned. For a typical ball, this point is at dead center. Then determine the object's mass, preferably using a kilogram balance scale, which accurately measures mass no matter what the location.

Using a spring or electronic scale, which actually measures force rather than mass, results in up to 0.5% error in measurement of mass on the earth's surface, due to local variations in the earth's gravitational force, an error level generally considered acceptable for this type of measurement. However, precision mass measurement can be carried out anywhere on earth using a spring or electronic scale by first calculating the object's weight in newtons from the pound or kilogram scale readings using the factors in Table 7.1. The object's mass in kilograms is then determined as the weight in newtons divided by the acceleration of gravity in m/s² at the location of testing (Table 7.4). For experimentation in space scales cannot be used at all, and special devices must be employed to measure mass.

A record of the velocity and acceleration of the throwing implement's center of mass while the implement is

Table 7.4   Acceleration Due to Gravity at Sea Level by Latitude

Latitude	Acceleration due to gravity (m/s²)	Sample locations
0	9.780	Ecuador, Kenya
15	9.784	Philippines, Guatemala
30	9.793	Texas, Israel
45	9.806	Oregon, France
60	9.819	Alaska, Sweden
75	9.829	Greenland, Antarctica
90	9.832	North Pole, South Pole

Note. Gravitational variations are largely accounted for by the earth's equatorial bulge. A more complete table can be found in the *Handbook of Chemistry and Physics* (43).

in contact with the hand is obtained through the film or video analysis procedure described earlier. For the time corresponding to each film or video image, net force applied to the implement is calculated from the implement's mass and acceleration, using Equation 12. The *horizontal* force exerted by the hand equals the net horizontal force calculated from the implement's mass and horizontal acceleration. The *vertical* force exerted by the hand is equal to that calculated from the vertical acceleration plus the implement's weight. Power transmitted to the implement at each instant is then calculated as the product of the component of force applied in the direction of the implement's travel and the implement's velocity.

A test was developed in our laboratory to determine the external force and power generated during very rapid elbow flexion and extension. While lying supine, subjects were videotaped at 60 Hz as each horizontally threw balls of 0.91, 1.81, 3.63, and 5.44 kg at maximal speed. Physical restraint ensured that either elbow flexion or elbow extension was the only movement used.

Using the video images of the ball and reflective markers on the shoulder, elbow, and wrist, APAS video analysis software (Ariel Life Systems, La Jolla, CA) calculated, at 1/60 s intervals, the ball's x and y position, velocity, and acceleration, and the elbow joint angle. A commercial spreadsheet program was used to calculate power output from the APAS data file. First the ball's direction and absolute velocity during each video frame were determined from its x and y velocities. Then the acceleration in the direction of ball travel was determined from the x and y accelerations. Force in the direction of ball travel was calculated as the product of acceleration and ball mass. Power on the ball was the product of the ball's velocity and the force in the direction of ball travel. Figure 7.10 shows ball velocity, joint angular velocity, and force and power exerted on the ball during an elbow flexion throw of the 0.91-kg ball.

The total power output of the human throwing the implement can be considerably greater than the power transmitted to the implement itself, because of the work required to move the athlete's body. One can calculate the power generated during body movement by digitizing the film or video image locations of all the major body joint centers and processing the resulting file of x and y joint coordinates using standard biomechanical methodology (18). A computer program calculates for each film or video image the location of each body segment's center of mass, using standard body proportions. The location of the total body's center of mass is the average of the locations of the individual segment centers of mass weighted according to the mass of each segment. From the resulting record of total body center of mass position, curves of velocity and acceleration are derived. The net force propelling the body during

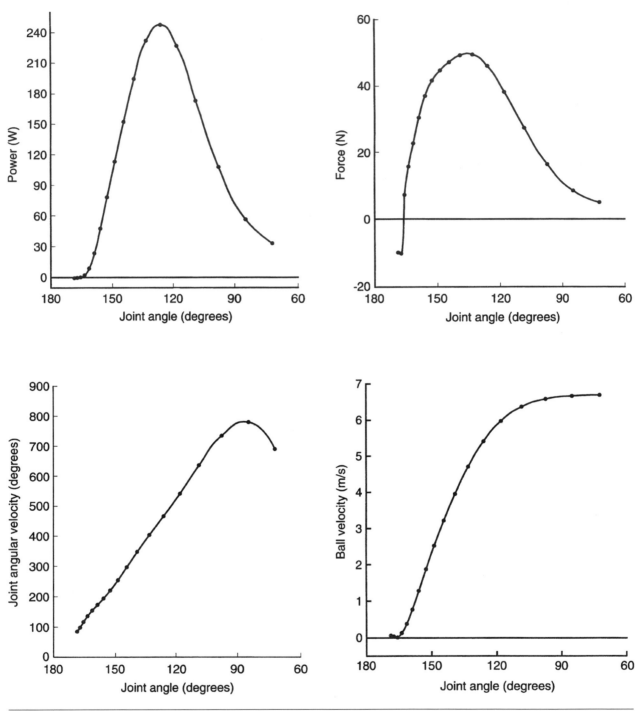

Figure 7.10   Power, force, and velocity generated by a supine subject throwing a .09-kg ball horizontally using elbow flexion only. Extraneous body movements were prevented by physical restraint.

each interframe time interval equals the body's mass times the acceleration of its center of mass. When the force of gravity is taken into consideration, force and power exerted on the body's center of mass can be calculated, as in the analysis of the implement described previously. More complex analyses are sometimes used to take into account the energy transferred within and between the body segments (19, 20).

Major advantages of film or video analysis for the determination of power output are that they can be used to monitor a wide range of physical activities and need not interfere with performance. Disadvantages include high system cost and time needed to digitize the film or videotape.

Single-Joint Free-Weight Lifting

A system was developed in our laboratory to test power output during various body movements. The subject, wearing an electrogoniometer on the knee or elbow, held a dumbbell or wore a weighted iron shoe (21). The body was stabilized so that movement could occur only about the joint in question. On cue, the subject raised the weight as quickly as possible.

Angular velocity was calculated from the transduced joint angle. Power output was calculated as the product of joint angular velocity and torque. Torque at all time points was calculated as the sum of torque attributable to gravity and the torque attributable to acceleration of the weight and limb. Figure 7.11 depicts the power output test results. Figure 7.12 and the following equations explain these calculations for the dumbbell lifts.

$$T_g = (W_f r_f + W_d r_d)\cos\theta \qquad (20)$$

where

T_g = torque attributable to gravity (N · m)
W_f = weight of the forearm-and-hand (N)
r_f = distance from the elbow joint-center to the center of mass of the forearm-and-hand (m)
W_d = weight of the dumbbell (N)
r_d = distance from the elbow joint-center to the center of mass of the dumbbell (m)
θ = angle of the forearm relative to the horizontal (radians)

$$T_a = (I_f + I_d + m_d r_d^2)\alpha \qquad (21)$$

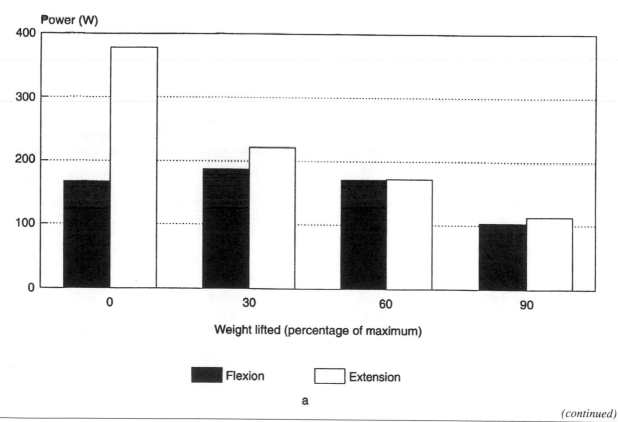

Power (W)

Weight lifted (percentage of maximum)

■ Flexion   □ Extension

a

(continued)

Figure 7.11 Single-limb peak power generated by 21 male subjects flexing and extending (a) the elbow and (b) the knee at maximal speed against the resistance of a dumbbell and an iron shoe, respectively. Each of the four movements was tested using a different body position so that the weight always provided resistance in the appropriate direction. Different patterns for flexion and extension are evident.

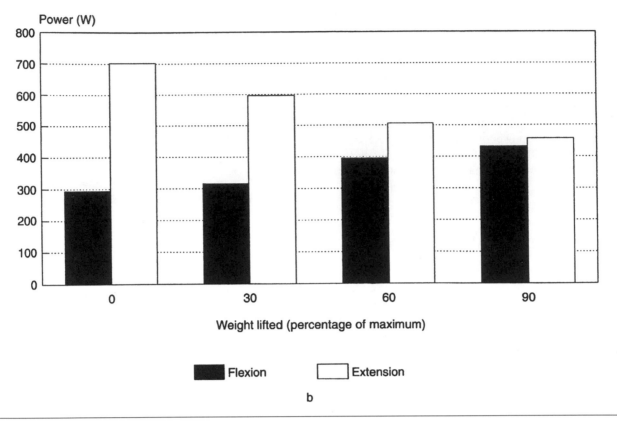

Figure 7.11   *(continued)*

where

T_a = torque attributable to acceleration (N · m)
I_f = moment of inertia of the forearm-and-hand (kg · m²)
I_d = moment of inertia of the dumbbell (kg · m²)
m_d = mass of the dumbbell (kg)
α = angular acceleration of the limb and dumbbell

Because it is more accurate, the reaction board method (22) was used to estimate limb weight, rather than calculating limb weight as a proportion of total body weight using standard tables. The reaction board method involves laying the subject on a horizontal board supported at one end by the scale, and taking scale readings when the limb is held both horizontally and vertically. Based on the change in the scale reading, and measurement of body position relative to the board, the limb's weight can be calculated. The limb moments of inertia needed for the equations were calculated according to a method described by Winter (18). Moments of inertia of the weights were estimated from their shapes and masses using standard equations (3).

Weight-Stack Machine Lifting

A linear position transducer was used as part of a system (Figure 7.13) used to monitor power output produced by a subject while lifting on a leg extension weight-stack machine (23). A model PT-101 Celesco linear position transducer was placed on the floor. Its cable was drawn up and connected to a custom-made arm protruding from the top of the weight stack of a Universal (Cedar Rapids, IA) leg extension machine. The transducer produced a voltage linearly related to the height of the stack above the floor. Custom-machined adapters allowed a BLH load cell to be affixed between the weight stack and its supporting cable to detect any forces exerted on the stack. Another custom-made device was used to take up the slack in the cable caused by the addition of the load cell. Power output throughout a lift was calculated as the velocity of the stack times the concurrent cable force.

The addition of an electrogoniometer at the lifter's knee allowed calculation of net instantaneous muscle torque. Assuming negligible friction in the moving parts of the well-lubricated exercise machine, power at the knee had to approximate power at the stack. Thus

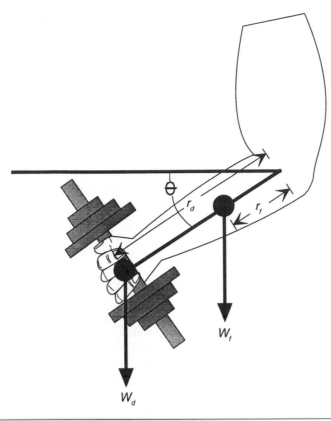

Figure 7.12 Variables used to calculate muscle torque during a dumbbell lift. The total torque is the sum of torque attributable to gravity and the torque attributable to acceleration of the weight and limb.

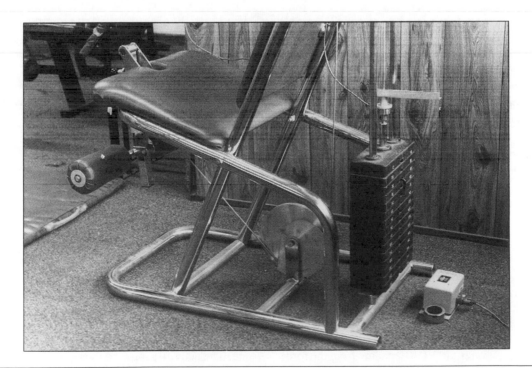

Figure 7.13 A leg-extension weight-stack machine instrumented for power output measurement. The load cell is attached between the weight stack and its supporting cable. A thin wire, not visible in the photograph, extends from the linear position transducer box on the floor to the end of the horizontal bar positioned just above the load cell, allowing the vertical position of the stack to be monitored.

$$\text{power}_{knee} = \text{power}_{weights} \qquad (22)$$

$$\text{torque}_{knee} \times \text{angular velocity}_{knee} = \qquad (23)$$
$$\text{force}_{weights} \times \text{velocity}_{weights}$$

$$\text{torque}_{knee} = \frac{\text{force}_{weights} \times \text{velocity}_{weights}}{\text{angular velocity}_{knee}} \qquad (24)$$

If the mass of the stack is known, the force transducer is not really necessary, because force can be derived, using Equation 12, from the stack's mass and acceleration (determined from position transducer data). However, the masses of plates in weight-stack machines have been found both to be variable and to differ from labeled values. The force transducer makes it unnecessary to disassemble exercise machines upon which the system is mounted to weigh each plate in the stack.

Vertical Jumping

The force platform has been used to measure human power output during the vertical jump (24-28). The procedure involves calculation of power as the product of force and velocity, the latter two of which are obtained from the force platform data. Contractile force exerted by the jumper's muscles results in vertical ground reaction force (VGRF) at the feet, which is mirrored by voltage at the force platform's vertical force channel. The VGRF can be considered to act at the total body center of mass (TBCM) to accelerate the body upwards. Instantaneous jumping power is the product of VGRF and TBCM vertical velocity (TBCMVV).

Although VGRF can be obtained continuously from force platform output, TBCMVV has to be calculated, using the principle that impulse equals change in momentum, or force multiplied by time equals change in the product of mass and velocity. In jumping, body mass doesn't change while force is applied, so that

$$\text{force} \cdot \text{time} = m \cdot \Delta V \qquad (25)$$

and

$$\Delta V = \text{force} \cdot \text{time/mass} \qquad (26)$$

Thus, change in TBCMVV during each sampling interval equals the net vertical force acting on the body multiplied by the intersample time period (*t*) divided by body mass (BM). The force used for the vertical velocity calculation is the VGRF reading from the force platform minus body weight (BW), because it is *net* vertical force that results in changes in vertical velocity of the jumper's body, and VGRF acts in the direction opposite to the force of gravity:

$$\Delta \text{TBCMVV}_{m/s} = (\text{VGRF}_N - \text{BW}_N) \cdot t_s / \text{BM}_{kg} \qquad (27)$$

Absolute TBCMVV is updated at the end of each time interval by adding ΔTBCMVV to the velocity at the start of the interval, starting at zero velocity at the beginning of the jump. Instantaneous power is calculated throughout the jumping movement as the product of VGRF and the calculated TBCMVV. Equation 27 is equivalent to calculating TBCM vertical acceleration as VGRF-minus-body-weight divided by body mass according to Equation 13, and calculating ΔTBCMVV as the product of acceleration and time (24, 25, 26).

Figure 7.14 shows VGRF, TBCM vertical position and velocity, and muscle power output during a jump. During the landing phase, as in any eccentric muscle activity, muscle power output is negative because the muscles *absorb* power generated by gravity. Table 7.5 shows the power generated by 18 physically active male subjects performing maximal vertical jumps from a force platform with and without arms and countermovement. The nocountermovement jumps began with the knees bent, and no initial downward body movement was allowed. During the no-arm jumps, the arms were kept down at the sides.

The jumping power experimentation in our laboratory showed that the Lewis formula, widely used for estimation of power output during the vertical jump (29, 30, 31), does not accurately reflect either peak or average power produced by a jumper. For 17 young male subjects, vertical jump height and body weight were found to provide good prediction of peak power and fair prediction of average power using the following regression-derived formulas:

$$\text{peak power (W)} = 61.9 \text{ [jump height (cm)]} +$$
$$36.0 \text{ [body mass (kg)]} - 1{,}822 \qquad (28)$$

$$\text{avg. power (W)} = 21.2 \text{ [jump height (cm)]} +$$
$$23.0 \text{ [body mass (kg)]} - 1{,}393 \qquad (29)$$

Equations based on the test results of a relatively small group of subjects cannot be considered definitive. Testing of a large and diverse population would determine if one set of equations could be effectively applied to various types of subjects.

The force platform can be used to calculate power output during many activities other than vertical jumping. The activities must be those in which (1) the mass of the athlete (and any implement) is known, and (2) the athlete or implement is not in contact with any surface other than the force platform during the power measurement. Garhammer (8) did extensive research

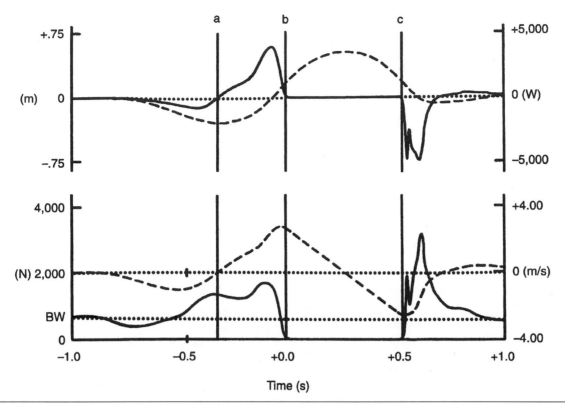

Figure 7.14 Position, velocity, force, and power during a vertical jump with countermovement. The lower graph shows vertical ground reaction force (solid line) and vertical velocity of the body's center of mass (dashed line). The upper graph shows vertical position of the center of mass (dashed line), and power output (solid line). The vertical lines: a = jump low point, b = take-off, c = landing.

Table 7.5 Peak Power Output and Peak Ground Reaction Force

	No countermovement		Countermovement	
	No arms	Arms	No arms	Arms
Power (W)	3,262±626	3,804±684	3,216±607	3,896±681
Force (N)	1,562±219	1,687±205	1,697±308	1,725±218

on power output during weight lifting using a force platform.

Isokinetic Dynamometry

Isokinetic dynamometers produce records of torque generated during constant-velocity movements. A record of power output can be determined by multiplying the torque value by the constant angular velocity selected by the operator. Unfortunately, the machines are geared for clinical, rather than research, use. They usually come with integral computers and cost at least $30,000. The output information is limited, and it is difficult to modify

the internal programs to provide additional processing or to make the raw data available for transfer to another computer for further calculations.

Older Cybex II (Ronkonkoma, NY) isokinetic dynamometers are amenable to custom computerization. Although they are no longer sold new, thousands of the machines remain in laboratories and physical therapy facilities. These systems weren't sold with integral computers, and output signals were fed to chart recorders. The heads of the devices frequently came with connectors for monitoring voltages corresponding to angular position and torque. We passed these output signals through the amplifier/conditioner stage of the standard Cybex chart recorder before sending them to an A/D converter and computer for analysis. Signals were sampled at 500 Hz. A program determined angular velocity from the angular position data and calculated power as the product of torque and angular velocity. Peak torque and power were determined, as were the torque and power produced at selected joint angles. Figure 7.15 depicts peak power produced during isokinetic knee extension at various speeds of movement. Perrine and Edgerton found a similar positive association of power output and isokinetic test speed, but with more leveling-off of power at the higher test speeds (32). Based on additional experimentation, they reported an *r* of .87 between vertical jump height and peak isokinetic leg power normalized for body mass among collegiate volleyball players, and similar correlation between leg power and sprint speed among women track athletes (33).

Nonmotorized Treadmill Running

Lakomy (11, 34) employed a small electrical generator in conjunction with a load cell to measure horizontal propulsive power during sprint running on a nonmotorized treadmill (Figure 7.16). The test subject, rather than a motor, propelled the running surface. The system was based on the fact that, in order to keep the runner from accelerating horizontally, the strap connecting the runner to the load cell had to exert a force on the runner equal in magnitude to and opposite in direction from the horizontal force of the treadmill belt on the runner's feet. Horizontal power output was calculated as the product of the instantaneous force registered on the load cell and the treadmill belt velocity. The method required the assumption that errors due to the following were negligibly small: (1) force and velocity were not measured at the same point; (2) the tether strap deviated from the horizontal during running; and (3) the strap had some elasticity, which could have had a damping effect.

Lakomy (35) used an electrical generator in a similar way to measure power output during ergometer cycling. His study showed that the Wingate test, by averaging power over 5 s and not taking flywheel acceleration into account, underestimated peak cycling power by a mean of 51% and overestimated the time needed to reach peak power by 3.8 s.

Cycling

Cycle ergometers have been instrumented in various ways to continuously monitor the mechanics of pedaling (36-42). Most cycle force transducers have incorporated strain gauge technology and have been custom-made for each laboratory. When strain gauges are mounted on the crank arm (39, 40), they are capable only of measuring forces perpendicular to the crank arm. When strain gauges are mounted on the pedals, they have been able to monitor forces perpendicular and parallel to the pedal surface (36-42).

In our system seven cycle parameters are continuously monitored:

- The crank angle relative to the cycle frame
- Forces exerted by the feet in the following directions

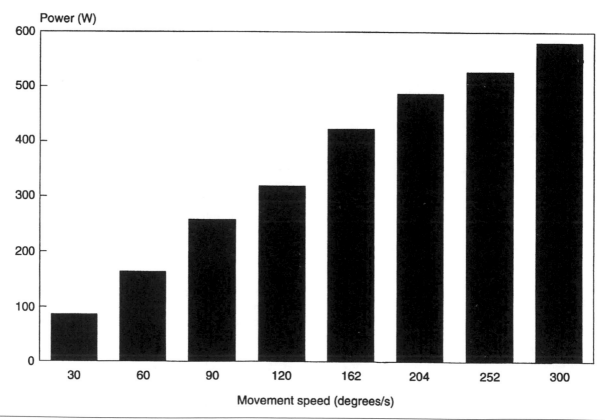

Figure 7.15 Peak power (W) generated by 13 male subjects during isokinetic single-leg knee extension at various movement speeds.

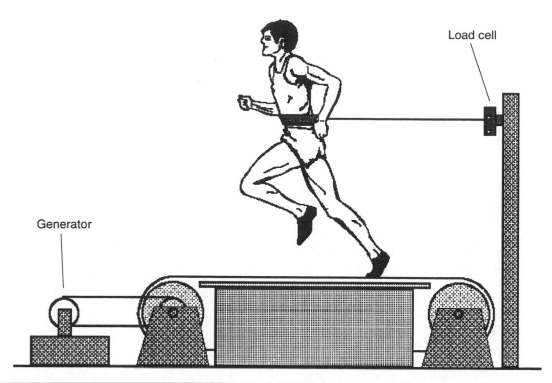

Figure 7.16 Experimental apparatus for measuring running power on a nonmotorized treadmill. Force and velocity are transduced, respectively, by a load cell and by an electrical generator.
From "Measurement of Human Power Output in High Intensity Exercise" by H. Lakomy. In *Current Research in Sports Biomechanics* (pp. 46-57) by B. Van Gheluwe and J. Atha (Eds.), 1987, Basel, Switzerland: Karger. Adapted by permission of S. Karger.

Perpendicular to the left pedal surface
Parallel to the left pedal surface
Perpendicular to the right pedal surface
Parallel to the right pedal surface
• The angle of the left pedal relative to the left crank arm
• The angle of the right pedal relative to the right crank arm

Details of the methodology have been presented elsewhere (36). The component of pedal force perpendicular to each crank arm, the only component that can result in power generation, is calculated from the transduced forces and pedal angle. Pedaling torque is determined as the product of the force exerted perpendicular to the crank arm and the length of the crank arm. Angular position data from the crank arm is processed to produce a record of angular velocity. Power application throughout the entire pedal cycle is determined as the product of torque and angular velocity.

At 40 rpm, maximal power averaged over one full crank revolution was 3.07 ± 0.40 W per square centimeter of midthigh muscle cross-sectional area for a group of 17 physically active males; at 100 rpm, maximal power was 4.68 ± 0.81 W per square centimeter (42). McCartney et al. (40) reported peak instantaneous 100-rpm cycling power of 1,626 ± 102 W for 8 male university students.

SUMMARY

A wide variety of electronic equipment is available today that can be applied to the measurement of human mechanical power. The financial resources and expertise needed to set up such systems are available to most laboratories. The procedures described herein can be applied to the measurement of power output during diverse human activities. It is hoped that readers will go beyond the examples described in the chapter to develop systems suited to their specific needs.

REFERENCES

1. Jensen, C., & Fisher, A. (1979). *Scientific basis of athletic conditioning* (2nd ed.). Philadelphia: Lea & Febiger.
2. Komi, P., & Hakkinen, K. (1988). Strength and power. In A. Dirix, H. Knuttgen, & K. Tittel (Eds.), *Encyclopaedia of sports medicine: Vol. 1. The Olympic book of sports medicine* (pp. 181-193). Boston: Blackwell Scientific.
3. Meriam, J. (1978). *Engineering mechanics: Vol. 2. Dynamics*. New York: Wiley.

4. Atha, J. (1981). Strengthening muscle. In D. Miller (Ed.), *Exercise and sport sciences reviews: Vol. 9.* (pp. 1-73). Philadelphia: Franklin Institute.

5. Enoka, R. (1988). *Neuromechanical basis of kinesiology.* Champaign, IL: Human Kinetics.

6. Knuttgen, H., & Kraemer, W. (1987). Terminology and measurement in exercise performance. *Journal of Applied Sport Science Research,* 1(1), 1-10.

7. Mish, F. (Ed.). (1984). *Webster's ninth new collegiate dictionary.* Springfield, MA: Merriam-Webster.

8. Garhammer, J. (1989). Weight lifting and training. In C. Vaughn (Ed.), *Biomechanics of sport* (pp. 169-211). Boca Raton, FL: CRC Press.

9. Margaria, R., Aghemo, P., & Rovelli, E. (1966). Measurement of muscular power (anaerobic) in man. *Journal of Applied Physiology,* 21(5), 1662-1664.

10. Bar-Or, O., Dotan, R., Inbar O., Rothstein, A., & Tesch, P. (1980). Anaerobic capacity and muscle fiber type distribution in non-athletes and in athletes. *International Journal of Sports Medicine,* 1, 82-85.

11. Lakomy, H. (1987). Measurement of human power output in high intensity exercise. In B. Van Gheluwe & J. Atha (Eds.), *Current research in sports biomechanics* (pp. 46-57). Basel, Switzerland: Karger.

12. *Le système international d'unités (SI)* (3rd ed.). (1977). Sevres, France: Bureau International des Poids et Mesures.

13. Sargeant, A., & Davies, C. (1977). Forces applied to cranks of a bicycle ergometer during one- and two-leg cycling. *Journal of Applied Physiology,* 42(4), 514-518.

14. Harman, E. (1989). An axial force transducer for a weightlifting bar. *Proceedings of the American Society of Biomechanics 13th Annual Meeting,* 216-217.

15. Chaffin, D., & Andersson, G. (1984). *Occupational biomechanics.* New York: Wiley.

16. Diefenderfer, J. (1979). *Principles of electronic instrumentation* (2nd ed.). Philadelphia: Saunders.

17. Press, W. (1988). *Numerical recipes in C.* New York: Cambridge University Press.

18. Winter, D. (1979). *Biomechanics of human movement.* New York: Wiley.

19. Winter, D. (1978). Calculation and interpretation of the mechanical energy of movement. *Exercise and Sports Sciences Review,* 6, 183-201.

20. Winter, D. (1979). A new definition of mechanical work done in human movement. *Journal of Applied Physiology,* 46, 79-83.

21. Rosenstein, M., Harman, E., Frykman, P., & Johnson, M. (1989). An inexpensive method for measurement of torque and power output during accelerative movement. *Journal of Applied Sport Science Research,* 3(3), 77.

22. Hay, J. (1978). *The biomechanics of sports techniques.* Englewood Cliffs, NJ: Prentice Hall.

23. Frykman, P., Harman, E., Rosenstein, M., & Rosenstein, R. (1989). A computerized instrumentation system for weight machines. *Journal of Applied Sport Science Research,* 3(3), 77.

24. Davies, C., & Rennie, R. (1968). Human power output. *Nature,* 217, 770-771.

25. Davies, C. (1971). Human power output in exercise of short duration in relation to body size and composition. *Ergonomics,* 14(2), 245-256.

26. Davies, C., & Young, K. (1983). Effect of temperature on the contractile properties and muscle power of triceps surae in humans. *Journal of Applied Physiology,* 55(1), 191-195.

27. Harman, E., Rosenstein, M., Frykman, P., & Rosenstein, R. (1990). The effects of arms and countermovement on vertical jumping. *Medicine and Science in Sports and Exercise,* 22(6), 825-833.

28. Harman, E.A., Rosenstein, M.T., Frykman, P.N., Rosenstein, R.N., & Kraemer, W.J. (1991). Estimation of human power output from maximal vertical jump and body mass. *Journal of Applied Sport Science Research,* 5(3), 116-120.

29. Fox, E., & Mathews, D. (1981). *The physiological basis of physical education and athletics* (3rd ed.). Philadelphia: Saunders.

30. Fox, E., & Mathews, D. (1974). *Interval training: Conditioning for sports and general fitness.* Philadelphia: W.B. Saunders.

31. Kirkendall, D., Gruber, J., & Johnson, R. (1987). *Measurement and evaluation for physical educators* (2nd ed.). Champaign, IL: Human Kinetics.

32. Perrine. J., & Edgerton, V. (1978). Muscle force-velocity and power-velocity relationships under isokinetic loading. *Medicine and Science in Sports,* 10, 159-166.

33. Perrine, J. (1986). The biophysics of maximal muscle power outputs: Methods and problems of measurement. In L. Jones, N. McCartney, & A. McComas (Eds.), *Human muscle power* (pp. 15-22). Champaign, IL: Human Kinetics.

34. Lakomy, H. (1984). An ergometer for measuring the power generated during sprinting. *Journal of Physiology,* 354, 33P.

35. Lakomy, H. (1986). Measurement of work and power output using friction-loaded cycle ergometers. *Ergonomics,* 29(4), 509-517.

36. Harman, E., Knuttgen, H., & Frykman, P. (1987). Automated data collection and processing for a cycle ergometer. *Journal of Applied Physiology,* 62(2), 831-836.

37. Patterson, R., & Moreno, M. (1990). Bicycle pedalling forces as a function of pedalling rate and power output. *Medicine and Science in Sports and Exercise*, **22**(4), 512-516.

38. Hull, M., & Davis, R. (1981). Measurement of pedal loading in bicycling: Instrumentation. *Journal of Biomechanics*, **14**(12), 843-856.

39. Daly, D., & Cavanagh, P. (1976). Asymmetry in bicycle ergometer pedalling. *Medicine and Science in Sports*, **8**(3), 204-208.

40. McCartney, N., Spriet, L., Heigenhauser, G., Kowalchuk, J., Sutton, J., & Jones, N. (1986). Muscle power and metabolism in maximal intermittent exercise. *Journal of Applied Physiology*, **60**(4), 1164-1169.

41. Frykman, P., Harman, E., & Kraemer, W. (1987). The effects of all-running, all-lifting, and mixed training on power output at two different speeds. *Journal of Applied Sport Science Research*, **9**(4), 59.

42. Harman, E., Frykman, P., & Kraemer, W. (1986). Maximal cycling force and power at 40 and 100 RPM. *National Strength and Conditioning Association Journal*, **8**(4), 71.

43. Weast, R. (Ed.) (1973). *Handbook of chemistry and physics* (54th ed.). Cleveland: CRC Press.

CHAPTER 8

Strength Testing: Development and Evaluation of Methodology

William J. Kraemer, PhD

The Pennsylvania State University

Andrew C. Fry, PhD

University of Memphis

That the expression of muscular strength is a fundamental property of human performance is readily apparent from the large amount of empirical and scientific literature devoted to its development and evaluation. The evaluation of physiological responses and adaptations (e.g., cardiovascular, endocrine, neural, metabolic) associated with force production in humans has allowed us to gain a greater understanding of the various systems under conditions of high-threshold motor unit recruitment. In evaluating the effects of training, muscular fatigue, injury rehabilitation, muscular balance, or the functional abilities of different individuals, strength testing provides important information regarding human performance. This chapter will consider the different testing modalities, individually and as they share aspects. The purpose of this chapter is to give an overview of the various factors involved in understanding, developing, implementing, and evaluating strength-testing protocols.

WHAT IS STRENGTH?

Let us start with a definition: *Force* is what changes the state of rest or motion of a body, measured by the rate of change of momentum. In other words, force = mass × acceleration of the object as a result of the force. Of particular interest for our purposes is the peak force or peak torque of a particular muscular activity. There are, however, a number of contributing factors in the development of strength. For the purposes of this chapter, *strength* will be operationally defined as the maximal force a muscle or muscle group can generate at a specified or determined velocity (88).

Atha (10) presented and Enoka (41) endorsed a definition of strength as ". . .the ability to develop force against an unyielding resistance in a single contraction of unlimited duration." This definition of strength as an isometric or static measure avoids consideration of the complex interaction of force development and the velocity of muscle action, shortening, or lengthening. By limiting the definition in this manner, only static activity is evaluated and all dynamic force development is ignored. Though this definition appears to make the task of strength evaluation simpler, it involves the confounding factor of avoidance of dynamic force production so prevalent in human performance.

Force will vary depending upon the velocity of the movement. The expression and ultimate quantification of strength is dependent upon the conditions of the test. Because of the number of variables or conditions involved, the strength of a muscle or muscle group must be defined as the maximal force generated at a specified velocity (88). The velocity may be zero (i.e., isometric action) or may involve a range of velocities of shortening and lengthening for concentric and eccentric actions, respectively. For comparative purposes, the force and torque measurements must be performed when the muscle or muscle groups are at similar lengths. The force measurements can be obtained directly from the muscle or its tendons, from a particular point on one of the body parts, or as torque developed on a testing device. However, the muscles may perform in either isometric, dynamic concentric, or dynamic eccentric muscle actions.

Different power outputs are associated with the force–velocity characteristics of the movement. Maximal muscular power of a joint or muscle group should not be confused with maximal aerobic power, which relates to the cardiorespiratory ability of the body to deliver and utilize oxygen.

The term *isotonic* is frequently and improperly used to indicate dynamic muscle activity when the external resistance is constant. The term actually denotes a dynamic event in which the muscle generates the same amount of force throughout the entire movement. Such a condition occurs infrequently, if at all, in human performance, due to a combination of differences in force generation by muscle at various lengths and the changes in mechanical advantage at different joint angles. Therefore, the term *dynamic constant external resistance* (44) will be used herein to describe the testing of muscle activity using specific external resistances, such as free weights. This type of exercise includes both concentric (shortening) and eccentric (lengthening) muscle activity.

WHY IS THE MEASUREMENT OF STRENGTH IMPORTANT?

Probably the most important reason for monitoring strength performance is to help in the evaluation and progression of resistance-training programs. Presently, resistance-training programs are being used by almost every segment of the population, from children to adults well into old age. The programs, as well as the goals for training, are quite diverse. The amount of strength

development is dependent upon the exercise prescription, time available, and objectives of the program. Regular assessment of strength capabilities allows the exercise prescription to be properly evaluated and changes to be made in the exercise program when appropriate.

Strength development does not continue at a constant rate of increase or magnitude of change over long-term training programs. Decisions have to be made regarding the exercise prescription for each exercise movement as to the cost-benefit ratio of putting continued attention, time, and effort into strength improvement. In certain circumstances small changes in strength require large amounts of training time as the "window of adaptation" is close to the theoretical genetic ceiling. This means that, instead of 3 sets for an exercise movement, 6 sets might be required for an increase to occur. Furthermore, the increase observed may be less than 5% compared to the higher percentage gains observed earlier in a person's training history. Such small gains may be the difference between winning and losing in certain types of elite athletic competition but may be of less importance for other situations. The increased time needed to obtain small gains in strength might not be the best use of available training time, unless the small gains are directly related to needed performance abilities. For example, a 5% gain by a competitive lifter in a competitive lift could mean the difference between winning and coming in 25th in a competition. Conversely, an individual with good biceps strength might not need to put in the extra time to make a 5% gain in arm curl strength and might better use the extra training time to train another exercise movement. That is, she or he might need a "strength cap" for that particular exercise: maintaining the present level of training and not increasing the dose of exercise to elicit further strength changes. Thus, so-called clinical judgments often have to be made regarding the exercise prescription. This requires a solid knowledge of the individual's strength profile for a variety of muscles. Furthermore, one must understand the basic physiological adaptations associated with strength-training programs.

PHYSIOLOGICAL ADAPTATIONS ASSOCIATED WITH STRENGTH TRAINING

The review of physiological adaptations related to resistance training have been previously reviewed in great detail (42, 90, 92, 95). We will give a brief overview of some of the major training adaptations. Table 8.1 is a list of some basic physiological adaptations due to strength training.

Table 8.1   Muscle Fiber Adaptations With Resistance Training

Variable	Muscle's adaptational response
Muscle fiber myofibrillar protein content	Increase
Capillary density	No change/decrease
Mitochondrial volume density	Decrease
Myoglobin	Decrease
Succinate deyhdrogenase	No change/decrease
Malate dehydrogenase	No change/decrease
Citrate synthase	No change/decrease
3-hydroxyacyl-CoA dehydrogenase	No change/decrease
Creatine phosphokinase	Increase
Myokinase	Increase
Phosphofructokinase	No change/decrease
Lactate dehydrogenase	No change/increase
Stored ATP	Increase
Stored PC	Increase
Stored glycogen	Increase
Stored triglycerides	Increase?
Myosin heavy chain composition	Slow to fast

Note. Specific changes are dependent upon the exact type of exercise program utilized, and variability of response may be due to the differential effectiveness of various types of heavy resistance training programs.

Rehabilitation and Safety of Strength Training

For over 60 years, resistance training has been used to effectively intervene in postinjury rehabilitation programs to enhance patient recovery (109, 135). Evidence now indicates that important benefits of strength-training programs include improving individuals' injury risk profiles (92, 145). Although injuries can occur due to a strength-training program itself, injury is rare, and injuries are often attributable to improper exercise technique and unsupervised training (22, 132). In fact, the injury profiles for resistance training and strength testing are among the lowest for strenuous forms of exercise and sport. In a 4-year study, resistance training has been shown to be safe (0.13 injuries per 1,000 hours of athlete exposure, or 0.35 per 100 players per season), regardless of the training methods used (149).

Psychological Benefits

Strength-training programs have resulted in improvements in self-concept and self-esteem for both athletic

and patient populations (22, 23). In the athletic community, strength testing is often used as a motivator (3). Furthermore, it allows for quantification of specific training goals. In general, the benefits of a properly designed resistance-training program are many and have practical applications for many populations (45).

Evaluation of Strength-Training Programs

The roles of a strength-training program are many. An optimal training program requires periodic assessments of the variables to be trained. This in turn requires accurate and objective methods of evaluating strength, which also allows one to predict athletic performance (30), evaluate physical performance in an industrial setting (104), assess strength fitness (51, 72), identify the physical capabilities associated with varying levels of performance (27), and characterize physical demands and characteristics of various occupations or athletic positions in a particular sport (78). Furthermore, changes in muscular strength during an injury rehabilitation program can be closely followed (109, 135). We will now examine some of the testing modalities used in strength testing.

TESTING MODALITIES

Free Weights

Perhaps the most common tools for assessing strength are free weights—barbells, dumbbells, Olympic-style weights, and related types of equipment. Interpreted broadly, free weights can also include body weight when used as resistance in calisthenic-type activity (e.g., push-ups, chin-ups). In strength tests using free weights, the velocity of movement is typically not controlled but could be determined via laboratory methods (e.g., video analysis) (9, 10, 41, 73). When more than one repetition (e.g., 5 RM) is performed in a strength test, each subsequent repetition is slower, until the subject is unable to complete another repetition (88). Demanding a specific power-output performance during multiple-repetition strength tests by implementing a specific time interval for the performance of the movement creates another type of strength test for a given number of repetitions.

With free-weight strength tests, the movements involved can be somewhat similar to those found on the athletic field or in other areas of human motor performance, due to the fact that a constant external resistance is involved that requires balance. Free weights present a number of different testing conditions compared to weight machines (45, 113). Free weights require greater motor coordination than do machines (113, 124), primarily because free weights must be controlled through all spatial dimensions, whereas machines generally involve control through only one plane of movement (45). This can be an advantage or a disadvantage, depending on whether the development of motor capabilities associated with various exercises is being taken into consideration. Therefore, the test specificity of free weights may be more appropriate for certain tasks being evaluated (45, 123). Another more practical reason for using free weights is their low cost and ready availability. This may be important for many testing situations, especially when strength tests are used to assess training-related improvements. Test and training-mode specificity are vital for optimal expression of true strength gains.

Total body strength is also easier to assess with free weights, because multiple joint movements (e.g., squat, power clean) require recruitment of a larger amount of the total muscle mass. Conversely, isolated single-joint motions (e.g., leg curls, arm curls) can be performed more strictly with the use of a machine when isolated muscle function is of interest. Free weights also involve both concentric and eccentric muscle activity. Eccentric muscle activity is not possible on some weight-training machines (e.g., typical hydraulic machines) or with certain isokinetic (i.e., controlled constant velocity) dynamometers (113). Recent advancements by various manufacturers have made an eccentric option available on more recent models of isokinetic dynamometers. Free weights almost always allow the desired range of motion, whereas other strength-testing modalities can be somewhat limited if it is not possible to get a proper fit between the subject and the machine configuration (45).

Familiarization

It is important to get a baseline value for muscular strength at the start of a program or scientific investigation, and to familiarize individuals with each type of strength-testing protocol. Without base line data, values for strength gains can be inflated and not representative of the true physiological adaptations that have occurred from training. This problem is often seen in studies that perform no familiarization process and conduct only pre- and posttraining tests. Before testing begins, all subjects must be thoroughly instructed in the proper lifting method to be used (130, 137). Certain free-weight exercise movements (e.g., power clean) may require a relatively long familiarization period prior to 1-RM testing, to eliminate learning effects. Furthermore, some training is absolutely needed for certain exercises, such as the complete Olympic-style power clean and snatch lift, before testing is performed to determine 1-RM strength levels. Subjects must have had previous experience with the testing apparatus and know how to perform the exercise to be strength-tested. This is true even

with highly trained subjects, especially if their lifting form in training deviates from what will be used for testing. Two weeks of resistance training, including four training sessions for each exercise and practice of the tests to be performed, will achieve appropriate familiarization and reliability for maximal strength testing (52). A training effect from testing alone is rarely observed if the number of maximal efforts and volume of exercise are kept to a minimum (52).

This familiarization period is even more important if the subject has no prior experience with resistance exercise or if several exercises wil be tested. Subjects must learn how to produce a maximal effort in the test, and this requires proper familiarization. Proper familiarization also avoids increases in performance that are due solely to improved motor coordination, a phenomenon commonly observed when using free-weight exercises with inexperienced subjects. This is especially important if treatment effects (e.g., physiological training responses) are to be evaluated. Familiarization is crucial in some populations, such as children or older adults. Patient populations often require specialized teaching to learn how to best perform a strength test. For example, cardiac patients are capable of performing maximal strength tests if properly instructed (43). Blood pressure increases in healthy individuals with an acute bout of heavy resistance exercise are normal and demonstrate from a positive perspective the plasticity of the system (90). Still, it is important to be consistent about whether subjects should hold their breath during a strength-test procedure.

The conditions of the test are always unique to the methods used and developed for the population being evaluated, and the familiarization period must have specific goals related to achieving the type of strength test needed for the individual. This period of time is also important for the development of a professional rapport between the testing staff and the individual subject. The level of motivation and encouragement can be established during this period of time. Furthermore, prior to establishing any test profile, the test-retest reliabilities (e.g., the *r*-value correlation coefficients) for each exercise to be tested should be determined with the sample population to be used in the investigation or program.

Familiarization includes the following:

1. Practice of the exercises
2. A "dry run" through the test protocol
3. Repeated practice of the test protocol under actual test conditions and maximal efforts until a stable, reproducible base line for strength performance is achieved

Safety Considerations

Safety is an important consideration when performing strength evaluations, including those with free weights.

All equipment being used must be in proper working order (49, 79). This includes properly rotating Olympic barbells, properly functioning barbell collars, and solidly secured weights (on both barbells and dumbbells). Any related equipment used (benches, weight racks, etc.) should be properly functioning and capable of withstanding the use of maximal resistance. Each test session should be preceded by a thorough inspection of all equipment to be utilized (79). Included in the initial inspection should be a calibration of all weights to be used. Posted weights are not always correct and have been known to be off by 10% or more. This usually occurs with weights made from cast metals; weights that have been machined are generally more accurate. Any equipment malfunctions can lead to accidental injury.

The lifting environment is also made safer by the presence of properly trained spotters (49, 137, 141). Even if safety equipment such as power racks and other specially designed devices are available, an adequate number of spotters must always be present. Injury and accidents are improbable during strength testing, but spotters must be aware of the potential dangers of the test protocols. Emergency procedures should be formulated before testing is performed (93). It may seem that an excessive number of precautionary measures have been suggested, but it is imperative that all possible steps be taken to insure the safety of your subjects, athletes, or patients. Prudent methods and procedures will help avoid unwanted litigation due to negligence and enhance approval of strength-testing protocols by human use review boards. Maximal strength tests have been shown to be quite safe if proper technique is used and if the investigators know how to perform the exercise movements. It should be emphasized here that these safety considerations are by no means limited to the use of free weights, but concern all strength testing modalities (weight machines, isokinetic dynamometers, etc.).

Proper Positioning With Free Weights

Proper positioning of the subject is an often overlooked variable that can affect test-retest reliability. Factors such as grip position (e.g., wide vs. narrow), grip style (e.g., thumbless, thumbs around, hook grip, use of wrist straps), foot stance (e.g., wide vs. narrow, heels elevated vs. heels flat, toes straight ahead vs. toes flared out), and bar position (e.g., high trap vs. low trap for barbell positions in the squat) can all affect the mechanics and results of the lift. In these respects, the expression of strength can be influenced by the biomechanical aspects of the lift.

The starting position of the limbs is also very important. In the bench press, an eccentric movement of the musculature (lowering the weight to the chest) can

be performed before the concentric phase (upward movement of the weight from the chest) of the exercise. Conversely, the subject can start with the concentric phase, first lifting the weight from the chest. Whether one has muscle lengthening (i.e., the eccentric phase) prior to muscle shortening (i.e., the concentric phase) or vice versa is a very important characteristic of the test and needs serious consideration in the development of a strength-test protocol. The actual positions used should be standardized and controlled over all testing situations (61, 96, 98).

Consistency of test procedures is vital for establishing good test reliability. The use of free weights can make reliability difficult to attain if confounding variables are not controlled. Test-related variations for 1-RM evaluations have been reported as ranging from 1.5% to 20% (137). Emphasizing the importance of precise testing procedures is vital to accurate assessments.

Resistance Exercise Machines

Much of the information (e.g., familiarization concepts) already presented in this chapter for the development of strength-testing protocols using free weights can also be used in the development of strength tests using weight machines. Although many different types of resistance-training machines are currently available, this section will focus on machines that use a movable external resistance such as a weight stack or plate-loaded apparatus. Isometric, isokinetic, and "isokinetic-like" machines will be addressed in later sections. In general, these machines are somewhat like free weights in that the external resistance (weight stack, plates, etc.) is constant. Under certain circumstances specific quantification of the actual forces involved with the movement may require more advanced evaluation of the machine. If needed, the actual forces produced beyond a plate number or stack weight will involve more sophisticated analysis and breakdown of the machine (e.g., weighing the stack plates, determining friction coefficients, determining the movement patterns for gravity corrections) (39, 96, 98).

Safety and Test Specificity of Machines

Many machines alter the resistance encountered by the muscles with a system of cams, levers, or pulleys, resulting in a variable-resistance system. Even more interesting is that the weight lifted up in some machines is not the same amount of weight lowered in the exercise movement, due to mechanical variations in the direction of movement and the method of loading for the machine (39). Some manufacturers attempt to increase the resistance during a range of motion in an attempt to mimic the human strength curves of various joints or physical movements. Strength curves, however, are quite variable, and in some instances the strength curves of the machines are not identical with those of the human body (46). Machines of this nature can be useful training tools, but they may be inappropriate for testing unless their unique characteristics are taken into account.

Depending on the nature of the evaluation, strength testing with machines may or may not be appropriate. If training has been performed with a different modality or if the strength curve encountered on a particular machine is quite different from the normal human strength curve (46), such a machine may not be appropriate as an evaluation tool. For example, if one is training using a free-weight squat exercise, strength-testing the leg press exercise would not be appropriate, as it is not a training-specific test, and vice versa. On most variable-resistance machines, the actual resistance to the muscles is modified via levers, pulleys, or cams. This can create highly variable movement velocities over the range of motion, and these are magnified during maximal testing when the strength curve of the machine differs from the test subject's actual strength curve. Thus, it is imperative that a smooth movement be performed by the subject or athlete for a particular exercise. Exercise test movements that are ''jerky'' or have noticeable ''micro stops'' during their performance should not be performed on a variable-resistance machine. This is especially noticeable at the slow speeds (i.e., close to $0° \cdot s^{-1}$) that are typical in 1-RM testing. Because the increase may ''kick in'' at different phases of the range of motion in different people, a true 1-RM value may be difficult to assess. Such individual equipment incompatibility should be screened for in the familiarization phase prior to testing. Still, an important concept for strength testing is that if a subject trains with a particular machine, the testing should typically be performed on the same device. Which movements are tested is based on the clinical judgment of the professional who evaluates all of the risks and benefits of the test.

There are other considerations for the use of weight machines. Most machines operate in only one plane of motion (45), due to their controlling nature, resulting in different requirements for motor coordination (113, 124) and lifting technique (45, 93). By ruling out technique factors, strength testing with machines may more accurately assess pure strength changes if the proper movement pattern and exercise form are strictly maintained. This consideration is important when evaluating subjects who have had little resistance-training experience. Even with machines, it is possible to show improved strength performance simply with better motor patterns—without any changes ocurring in the size of a muscle's protein contractile unit (128). Thus, screening and familiarization are vital in every mode of strength testing to ensure accurate results.

Because only one plane of motion is involved in most machine exercises, there is no guarantee that the optimal direction of force has been applied to the device. For example, in performing a machine bench-press exercise a person needs to apply force only in a generally upward direction to elicit movement of the resistance. If an improper plane of movement were used with free weights the barbell likely would not be under control, resulting in a missed lift. How much of this synergistic control of movement is desired in a specific test is a major consideration in choosing the training and testing modalities.

Another factor is that machines are readily available at many facilities, even though their cost may be prohibitive. A popular aspect of machines for many is perceived increases in safety, although this has never been empirically demonstrated. Generally, spotters are not needed, although someone knowledgeable in the operation of the equipment should always be present (45). Just as with free weights, the equipment must be closely inspected for unnecessary breakdowns that can interfere with testing or cause injury to the subject (49, 79). It is also imperative that the machines are operating smoothly; improper lubrication or a misalignment of the device may add unknown resistance to the machine. If the devices are always in optimal operating condition, test reliability is enhanced.

Subject Positioning in Machines

Weight machines often can isolate muscle groups or joints while minimizing extraneous body movements. This is dependent on a proper fit for each subject, which may be a problem with certain populations. Children and small adults (e.g., female gymnasts) might not be able to adjust to the dimensions of a machine (111). Currently, many manufacturers make adjustable machines or even design their equipment specifically for use by children or adults of various sizes (from small to large). However, simply adjusting seat positions cannot always account for differences in limb lengths in relation to various machine lever lengths. Even with properly adjusted equipment, the subject must be positioned each time according to a predetermined protocol developed by the investigator to meet the needs of the specific strength test. Small position deviations on a machine can affect resultant force production (105). All such positional data must be quantified for each test.

Starting positions of the machine during strength testing can also affect test results. For example, during a 1-RM machine bench-press test, the exercise is usually initiated with the machine handles in the lowest position. This eliminates the eccentric part of the lift. If the test is initiated with the arms fully extended, eccentric muscle activity during the lowering of the machine handles precedes the concentric muscle activity of the actual lift. This procedure enhances performance by making greater use of the stretch-shortening cycle via recovery of stored elastic energy and activation of the stretch reflex. Although either procedure is acceptable, all tests should be consistent. Furthermore, when comparing different test protocols, these factors must be taken into consideration.

The weight increments possible with some machines may also be a limiting factor. When evaluating subjects who are relatively weak or activities where low levels of force production are possible (e.g., injury rehabilitation), an increase of 10 lb, as is commonly found with many weight stacks, may be too great. Adaptations to the equipment must be made to allow an accurate assessment of the actual strength capabilities for the activity. If a weight stack is utilized, it might be necessary to attach smaller weights to the stack, thus allowing for smaller incremental changes.

STRENGTH-TEST PROTOCOLS FOR REPETITION MAXIMUMS

Tests using free weights and machines for evaluation of muscular strength are commonly cited in the scientific literature (4), but, in the past, procedures were seldom reported in any great detail. The methods used can also be employed for many, if not all, weight machine strength tests. Complete descriptions of test methodology for both free weights and machines have become standard to methodological write-ups in the scientific literature (55, 96, 130, 137). Usually a 1-RM effort is the "gold standard" for evaluating strength, although RM testing can involve any number of repetitions (89). Also, some studies have attempted to predict maximal strength from submaximal efforts, but this has resulted in mixed effectiveness. It is a common myth that higher RM testing is safer than a 1-RM evaluation or that it tests the same element of force production capabilities. This, however, is not the case (71). A modification of the 1-RM methods of Stone and O'Bryant (137) and Kraemer and Fleck (93) results in the following basic steps for 1-RM testing:

1. A light warm-up of 5 to 10 repetitions at 40% to 60% of perceived maximum.
2. After a 1-min rest with light stretching, 3 to 5 repetitions at 60% to 80% of perceived maximum.
3. Step 2 will take the individual close to the perceived 1 RM. A conservative increase in the weight (i.e., mass) is made, and a 1-RM lift is attempted. If the lift is successful, a rest period of 3 to 5 min is allowed. One of the most costly errors is not allowing enough rest before the next maximal attempt. One hopes to find the 1 RM within 3 to 5 maximal efforts. This process of titrating the increases in weight up to a true 1 RM can be enhanced by the prior familiarization tests that have already made an initial determination of the 1 RM, and with this prior data the likelihood of undershooting or overshooting an individual's capabilities is reduced. This process continues until a failed attempt occurs. (Important: Rest-period length will determine recovery.)
4. The 1-RM value is reported as the weight of the last successfully completed lift.

It is very important that a great deal of communication take place between the subject being tested and the testing staff. "How do you feel?" "Are you ready to go?" "How close to your 1 RM do you think you are?" "Can you lift about 2 more pounds?" These types of questions and others are vital to the interaction with the test subjects as they attempt to exhibit their best functional performance. Showing concern for the subject as the test is under way is also vital to getting a maximal effort. The purpose of this type of test is to determine the 1 RM, and other factors should not confound this goal.

A vital consideration is the length of the rest period. The number of preliminary repetition attempts (warm-up) is also important. To some extent these factors need to be individualized. Thus, sufficient recovery for enhanced maximal performance needs to be given during the test. Some individuals may require 5 to 7 min rest between attempts. Typically, the goal of a 1-RM test protocol is to achieve the 1 RM within 3 to 5 attempts beyond the warm-up phase. If rest time appears restrictive and elongates testing protocols, testing can often be performed with more than one subject. This allows one subject to be lifting while another is resting. If a greater number of repetitions is to be attempted, such as a 5 or 10 RM, it is suggested that fewer warm-up sets be used. Procedures for determination of a 6 RM will be outlined in the numbered list that follows and can be adapted to other RMs greater than 1. For all tests of this type, it is essential that the number of lead-up repetitions be adequate for proper warm-up but be few enough so as not to fatigue the subject before a maximal effort is attempted (18). It is recommended that strength training of children utilize no greater loads than a 6 RM (111), but 1 RM can be determined in children if appropriate procedures are used (93). Often, 6-RM tests or greater can be used to assess strength in children and can be gained directly from training logs. Previous training can give valuable insight for the expected test performances, but familiarization data still provide the best insights as to what one might expect. The following protocol is suggested for testing a 6 RM and could be modified to test other RM numbers (e.g., 5 RM, 10 RM) (93).

1. Subject warms up with 5 to 10 repetitions with 50% of the estimated 6 RM.
2. After 1 min of rest and some stretching, the subject performs 6 repetitions at 70% of the estimated 6 RM.
3. Step 2 is repeated at 90% of the estimated 6 RM.
4. After a 2 min rest, depending on the effort required for the previous set, 6 repetitions are performed with 100% to 105% of the estimated 6 RM.
5. After a 2 min rest, if Step 4 is successful, increase the resistance by 2.5% to 5% for another 6-RM attempt. If 6 repetitions were not completed in Step 4, subtract 2.5% to 5% of the resistance used in Step 4 and attempt another 6 RM.
6. If all sets performed through Step 5 were successful, retesting should occur after 24 hours of rest, because performing more sets would be greatly affected by fatigue. If weight was removed for Step 5, and 6 repetitions were performed, this is the subject's 6 RM. If the subject was not successful with this reduced resistance, retesting should occur after 24 hours of rest.

Testing procedures for RMs on machines are essentially the same as for free weights. In many situations, the test may be faster, because a simple adjustment of a weight stack is all that needs to be done. A sample of machine-test protocols has been compiled by Altug et al. (4). Special care must be taken with machine testing to make sure proper technique is used at all times. When the velocity of the movement slows down with heavy resistances, there is a tendency to alter the lifting form in an attempt to complete the lift. For example, in the seated cable row, a "break in form" can occur toward the end of the range of motion as the torso is extended posteriorly in an attempt to complete the lift, thus increasing the risk of injury. It is important not to be lulled into complacency when strength testing with machines.

ISOMETRIC TESTING

Another method of assessing strength is isometric testing, where the length of the active muscle remains constant. Isometric testing removes variation in the velocity of movement, as all tests are performed at $0° \cdot s^{-1}$. Factors such as the angle to be evaluated, anatomical point force recordings, standardization between subjects, feedback, and motivation all make isometric testing as demanding as any other strength-testing procedure.

Devices for isometric strength assessment have been in existence for many years. Early work in this area commonly used devices such as the hip and back dynamometer to test multijoint isometric capabilities (31); these devices are still in use (5). Strength of muscles of isolated joints can be tested using cable tensiometers. Still popular is the handgrip dynamometer, which is simply a variation of a dynamometer designed specifically for grip force evaluation. Modern technology has developed force transducers (load cells) and strain gauges that allow interfacing with computerized data storage and analysis systems. Furthermore, isokinetic devices can be used for isometric testing by simply selecting a velocity of zero.

Many test protocols have been developed for isometric testing (4). Although peak force assessment is often the primary purpose for isometric testing, other data have been generated. The rate of isometric force development is important, as it provides information as to the functional abilities of the neuromuscular units being tested and it also reflects physiological characteristics of the muscle fibers (e.g., fast- vs. slow-twitch fibers). It can be quantified in several ways (130). Provided the testing equipment has a timing mechanism, the time to peak force can be measured in milliseconds. This is sometimes made difficult by the oscillations found in the resulting strength curve. If an isokinetic dynamometer is used for the test, the damping control can be set to filter out these oscillations. An alternative method is to select an arbitrary percentage of the peak force of an individual (e.g., 50% maximal force production) as the cutoff for timing.

For various reasons, some test protocols call for a gradual increase of force, in which case the time to peak force measures would be inappropriate. It should be noted that the rate of force production may affect the resulting peak force, with faster muscle actions eliciting slightly greater peak values (16). Furthermore, it is suggested that the isometric muscle action must be held for at least 5 s to allow a maximal effort. Shorter time periods might not permit a maximal effort. Whatever protocol is selected, be sure that all subjects are clearly instructed in and are allowed to practice the appropriate procedures to assure a high test-retest reliability.

Fatigue Tests

Fatigue tests are also commonly used with isometric devices to assess local muscular endurance. These tests generally involve maintaining a muscular force over a specified period of time (e.g., 60 s). If a fatigue curve is to be developed, it is important that the subjects go "all out" and do not pace themselves, as this makes interpretation of the fatigue curve difficult and cheating is possible. Evaluation of the mean force over a specific time period (e.g., 30 or 60 s) does provide for a measure of isometric endurance and the total amount of fatigue. Mean force over the selected time period can give valuable information that can be better compared among subjects. Other isometric performance tests can be quantified in several ways, with fatigue being defined as the time interval for which the subject can maintain a certain percentage of the maximum voluntary isometric muscle action. The percent decline can also be determined over a set time period. This is simply calculated as the percentage of initial force that is being maintained at the end of the selected time period.

Pretest Considerations

Before testing begins and at periodic intervals, the isometric testing device should be calibrated with known masses. Calibration should be performed through the entire range of measurement of the device, because a nonsignificant error at light resistances might be magnified at greater resistances (130). Before testing, have all subjects warm up with activities using the musculature to be tested. Take care not to fatigue the subject; therefore, use activity with little or no resistance. The actual test requires only 2 or 3 maximal voluntary efforts (130). Generally, the peak force for the highest trial is recorded because averaging the scores does not improve the reliability and penalizes the subject for a top voluntary effort (2).

Body Position, Test Specificity, and Visual Feedback

For every test protocol it is important to properly isolate the joint and position the subject. For isometric testing, positioning must be carefully quantified with regard to the specific joint angles used in each individual subject setup. This enhances the reliabilities of isometric strength tests. First, each subject must be comfortable, as discomfort may lead to a submaximal performance (130). This means that all surfaces being pushed against must be comfortably padded because very large forces may be produced at those sites. Care must be taken, however, to not use too much padding, which can result in less than maximal forces due to absorption of the forces by the padding material. The subject must also be securely stabilized in the desired position. Otherwise the data might be contaminated, because different body positions can result in different forces (105).

During maximal isometric efforts, restraining straps have been known to give way or shift, resulting in altered body positions. An often overlooked consideration is that of the angles of nontested joints. For example, although a test may be concerned only with knee extensor capabilities, the associated hip angle can affect the resulting knee extension forces (112) due to the effects of different levels of muscle stretch on force production (140).

All isometric testing is specific to a velocity of zero, so it is not always appropriate to compare these results with those of dynamic testing (53, 55). The concept of specificity of testing must be considered. Research that utilizes dynamic training, but assesses strength changes only with static methods, is not evaluating specific dynamic training improvements (5). The testing tool must be identical to the training tool in order to serve as a valid assessment of functional changes due to the mode-specific training. For example, studies that utilize static strength testing to evaluate dynamic training programs are only viewing improvements in force production from the static perspective and need to include dynamic mode-specific test data.

Isometric testing can provide valuable joint-specific data to evaluate various sport-specific movement angles. Furthermore, it can help evaluate joints in rehabilitation when dynamic movements are not possible. Isometric tests can also provide information on carryover effects from dynamic training. Thus, the magnitude and pattern of strength changes at the various joint angle forces can be compared to 1-RM strength-testing data. Additionally, unique isometric tests can be developed to help evaluate injury and sport-specific gains in muscular strength. In a recent study, sport-specific volleyball tests for the two-arm overhead block, two-arm underhand bump, and single straight-arm dig were developed and shown to be sensitive to dynamic training and detraining (52). It is important to properly integrate and not misuse isometric testing in a strength test battery. No doubt, isometric test data can provide valuable information on force production characteristics of muscles in various joints and should not be overlooked in a testing profile.

Subjects in an isometric test should be provided concurrent feedback concerning their performance. This is especially important for unfamiliar tasks (60). It has also been observed that local muscular endurance may decrease in the absence of feedback (60). Typically, visual feedback is the most important type of feedback, but verbal cues of the magnitude of force can also be given along with encouragement. Verbal cues are important in many maximal efforts where subjects may have the tendency to close their eyes during exertion. Here again, familiarization and specifics of the test protocol must be spelled out as such test characteristics as visual cues, verbal cues, and breathing pattern are accounted for. These factors can contribute to optimal reproducibility of isometric tests. Reproducibility has been reported to be quite good with many types of isometric performance characteristics, such as maximum force, plateau force, inflection force, and maximal rate of force increase. However, variables such as time to percent maximum force and force curve shapes have greater variability, resulting in poor reproducibility (58). Methods of testing must, thus, be precise and appropriate.

Physiological Responses to Isometric Testing

Physiological responses to static strength measures are a further consideration for isometric testing. It has been shown that heart rate and blood pressure increase during tests of this type (110). Interestingly, these increases were independent of time of muscle activity, but were dependent on the magnitude of force produced and the muscle mass involved. Valsalva maneuvers can also affect these variables. All subjects should be instructed not to hold their breath during tests of long duration, such as isometric fatigue tests. The health profiles of the subjects to be tested must be carefully inspected to avoid any testing that might be harmful to them, such as testing of cardiac patients who are not clinically stable (43).

ISOKINETIC TESTING

Testing performed with a dynamometer that maintains the lever arm at a constant angular velocity is called "isokinetic" (130). This type of strength evaluation accounts for velocity of movement that is uncontrolled with free weights and machines, and that is lacking in isometric evaluations. A brief review of isokinetic testing has been previously presented by Sale and Norman (130), and an in-depth review of isokinetic muscle activity and evaluation has been prepared by Osternig (115). Isokinetic assessments have become quite popular in recent years, and a wide variety of protocols are being used (4).

Isokinetic testing is performed on specially constructed dynamometers that control the velocities of the dynamometer's lever arm movement and therefore are thought to keep limb velocity constant. Technological advances over the past several decades have greatly enhanced the capabilities of these testing machines. The cost of an isokinetic dynamometer can be prohibitive, but many laboratories, training rooms, and clinical facilities now have them. Similar to machine testing and different from the use of free weights for assessing strength, isokinetic testing does not monitor changes in

motor coordination, because the subject is restricted to the direction of movement dictated by the isokinetic instrument. Furthermore, for years isokinetic dynamometers involved no eccentric muscle activity. Now various isokinetic dynamometers include isokinetic eccentric testing capabilities.

Due to the complex nature of isokinetic assessments, there are a number of important considerations. Of primary importance is the specificity of angular limb velocities. The accepted SI unit for angular limb velocity is radians per second (rad · s^{-1}). It is common, however, to report the velocities in degrees per second with 1 rad · s^{-1} = 57.29578° · s^{-1} (130). The velocity used for concentric testing should be carefully considered, because the resulting forces can increase with decreasing velocities (30, 53, 55, 144). In addition, isokinetic performance may be related to fiber characteristics of the involved muscles (92), although recent evidence indicates that this relationship is weak (118). These factors can all have marked effects on variables such as muscle balance characteristics where various muscle groups are being compared relative to each other. As the velocity of assessment changes, the characteristics of the two muscles or muscle groups can result in variable ratios. For example, hamstring-to-quadricep ratios increase with greater velocities (53, 112), whereas internal-to-external rotator ratios are not as affected because torque for internal rotator muscles is not affected by limb velocity (144). It is also important to note that different training programs can have differing effects on the shape of the torque curve (26). This effect can be due to the training velocity, the range of motion, or the motor patterns used in training. Each of these variables is controlled for with isokinetic testing, so the results could easily be biased. This specificity of testing to training can also explain why isokinetic performances can lag behind other strength performances in a training program (52).

The specificity of the joint being tested is also an important factor. It has been shown that different muscle groups exhibit different isokinetic performance characteristics (30). This makes it difficult to compare data from different joints or muscle groups. These variable characteristics are readily seen when muscle balance data are collected, with each joint having its own muscle balance ratio (119).

The reliability of the testing device must be high for acceptable data to be collected. Some isokinetic dynamometers have exhibited a high day-to-day reliability of $r = 0.99$ when assessed with inert weights (115). All isokinetic dynamometers should be calibrated according to the manufacturer's guidelines on a regular basis. They should also be monitored for test-retest reliability to assure accurate data (132). Data from two different brands or models of dynamometers cannot always be compared, because their results may be significantly different (47). Furthermore, the actual testing apparatus, such as the mechanism to anchor the limb to the machine, can also affect the results (42). With the newer eccentric-capable dynamometers, greater test error has been recorded for eccentric muscle activity when compared to concentric activity (147). The eccentric error increases slightly with increased limb velocity.

Body Positioning for Isokinetic Testing

Proper positioning of the subject is essential for accurate testing. As with other types of strength testing, various limb positions can result in altered torque production (105). Joints that have extremely large ranges of motion in many directions, such as the shoulder, must be carefully secured in the proper position. For example, assessments of internal and external rotator cuff torques are dependent on the position assumed at the shoulder (144). Generally only one joint is tested at one time, so it is necessary to stabilize all body parts that may affect the torque measurement. A test of the knee extensors and flexors requires stabilization at the ankle, the thigh, the hips or waist, and the upper torso; but it is not necessary to stabilize the nontested limb, because this does not affect the results (117). All straps used for securing must be snug but comfortable, without interfering with the proper range of motion of the exercise. All securing devices should be regularly inspected as a safety precaution. It is not unusual for devices such as velcro straps to wear out with usage. Some test protocols have required subjects to grasp handles by their sides (26, 38). Newer dynamometer models are now equipped with more elaborate stabilization capabilities, thus negating the need for gripping. However, if this procedure is chosen, it should be consistent for all subjects. Another problem with subject positioning occurs when utilizing chairs and devices, such as an upper body exercise table, that are not directly attached to the dynamometer. Very large or strong subjects can cause the whole device to move, resulting in altered joint angles. It is imperative that the subjects be completely stabilized in these instances.

An additional consideration for positioning the subject is that of angles of related joints. Muscle stretch can affect the force capabilities of a muscle (140). In tests of muscles such as the knee extensors, one of the involved muscles, the rectus femoris, also crosses the hip joint. Therefore, the angle of the hip can affect the amount of stretch of the rectus femoris, and possibly the resulting torques at the knee. Thus, the positions of all related joints should be constant. It is also important to note that muscle activity during isokinetic exercise is not facilitated by a concentric action of the antagonist muscle (100), suggesting that activity of the opposing

muscles should not affect isokinetic performance of the agonist muscle.

Isokinetic Test Protocols

Numerous protocols have been suggested for isokinetic testing. Although rest intervals between efforts are often approximately 1 min in length, rest intervals as short as 10 s between sets (26, 38, 40) or as long as 3 min between single repetitions (33) have been used. It is important for full recovery to occur between efforts, but 3-min rests between repetitions did not enhance recovery when compared to 3 consecutive repetitions (33). Some dynamometers allow test subjects to observe their performance results as they actually do the test. This type of feedback may be beneficial (60), but all subjects should be made aware of the feedback in advance of each test. This helps assure similar efforts for each test. There are a number of "isokinetic-like" devices (e.g., hydraulics) available on the market. Although these machines are able to control velocity of movement to a certain extent, they are not identical to an isokinetic dynamometer. The reliability of hydraulic devices has been found to be acceptable (101), but their results are unique and specific to the instrument and should not be confused with those of true isokinetic modalities (75). There are also devices on the market that are isokinetic in nature but utilize multiple-joint movements. As a result, exercise velocities are quantified by the speed of the machine lever arm rather than the subject's joint angular limb velocity. Therefore, in multiple-joint tests, various joint and limb velocities are differential through the movement. Results from this type of strength testing cannot be compared with classical standard isokinetic testing where limb velocity is controlled for one specific joint.

Once the isokinetic test has been appropriately performed, there are many performance measures that can be monitored, including peak torque, angle-specific peak torque, mean torque, total work (area under the curve), time to peak torque, angle of peak torque, and torque at various time intervals. Fatigue tests can be performed, with a greater number of repetitions resulting in a fatigue index (final torque/initial torque) or percent decline (130). The variables available will depend on the brand and model of dynamometer used as well as the software package accompanying it. Therefore, when shopping for isokinetic equipment, be aware of the needs of your testing.

Although many options are available for quantifying the test data, many situations require only a few variables. Peak torque is not significantly different from the mean torque of 3 successive repetitions (12). Similarly, for peak torque and total work, as indicated by the area under the curve, relationships of $r = 0.86$ to 0.97 have been observed (108). Although a number of measures can be made, care must be taken to avoid redundancy. In some research settings, customized software may be necessary, because the clinical software provided by the manufacturers may not provide the needed information.

Gravity can have a very large effect on some isokinetic tests (142). Correcting for gravity is performed in some studies (119) because the results can be dependent on gravitational effects. Most new machines have gravity correction capabilities. Errors of over several hundred percent have been documented in flexion at the knee in certain situations (142). Because this enhances results for only one of the muscle groups tested, muscle balance characteristics can also be greatly altered (7). However, some tests, such as fatigue tests, might not require this correction factor, because absolute torque development is not of primary concern (130).

The determination of muscle balance ratios is an area full of potential pitfalls. Both agonist-antagonist muscle strength ratios and bilateral muscle balance characteristics can be determined. These properties are dependent on the test conditions and will vary considerably between different joints and different individuals. For example, the value of 0.60 for hamstring/quadricep torques is widely accepted, yet is dependent on limb velocity and joint angle (53, 106). Some of the original data collected were not even at a constant angle (106). This topic will be discussed in greater detail later in this chapter.

Several important aspects of isokinetic assessments are often overlooked. Early phases of an isokinetic effort are characterized by large oscillations of the strength curve (40, 115). This is primarily due to the mechanics of the dynamometer as it makes constant adjustments to assure the preset velocity is attained. Velocities of up to 200% of the selected speed have been recorded during the initial acceleration (131). To avoid this problem area of the curve, some investigators have measured torque only at a later point in the strength curve, such as 20° to 50° of knee flexion (26, 38). The use of the damping control will smooth out this portion of the curve, but care must be taken not to filter out other important characteristics of the curve as it shifts the torque curve to the right. Furthermore, the damping must be set consistently from one test to the next.

Another factor is that although limb angular velocities are constant, the muscle contractile velocities are not (9, 115). This can be affected by the joint mechanics and the anatomical characteristics of the muscle itself. Therefore, isokinetic performances are dependent on more than joint angle considerations. Three phases have been associated with each isokinetic effort: an acceleration phase where the machine makes adjustments for the preset limb velocity, a constant velocity phase where

torque measurement occurs, and a deceleration phase (115). These are affected by limb velocity and range of motion, with faster velocities requiring longer acceleration (116) and deceleration phases. Some experts have utilized a protocol where maximal effort was delayed until approximately one half the range of motion had passed, which resulted in consistently greater torques (40). Although attributed to a fatigue effect (115), this phenomenon may be influenced by the muscle fiber contraction velocities or dynamometer characteristics as well. It should also be noted that a decreased range of motion for maximal effort or an increased limb velocity would also decrease the constant-velocity portion of the curve, thus making it more difficult to measure torque during this phase. An increased limb velocity has also been associated with a decreased angle of peak torque for extension at the knee (142). It was theorized that this was due to the time necessary for muscle contractile force to reach its maximum, which at greater limb speeds lagged slightly behind the time to reach the anatomically optimal joint angle (115). Care must also be taken to avoid measuring torque during the deceleration phase, late in the range of motion. In general, angle-specific torques can provide valuable information for isokinetic testing. The review of isokinetic exercise by Osternig addresses this issue (115).

The actual test itself should be preceded by several submaximal warm-up efforts. Although these do not necessarily enhance the resulting performance (115), they are suggested as a safety precaution to avoid injury to the subject (115, 130). During these warm-ups, be sure the subject exerts enough force to actually engage the dynamometer at the desired speed. For the actual test, subjects should be instructed to perform their repetitions as forcefully as possible as quickly as possible (130) unless using the delayed effort protocol previously suggested. It is not unusual to see the greatest torques on the second or third repetition (130).

OVERVIEW OF TESTING CONSIDERATIONS

RM Testing

Testing of maximal effort with resistance exercise usually involves assessment of a subject's 1 RM for a desired number of repetitions. This procedure has been utilized for a number of years (31) and is usually associated with 1-RM testing (17), but it can involve any number of repetitions. As previously described, 1-RM testing involves several 1-repetition efforts with increasing resistance until failure. Multiple-RM testing, such as 5 or 10 RM, is more difficult to assess, because the subject will often be able to perform greater or fewer repetitions. Furthermore, the greater number of repetitions involved can contribute to the onset of fatigue, making more than one effort at 5 or 10 RM exhausting and with a greater chance for error. Highly trained subjects, however, will generally be able to self-report their 5- or 10-RM capabilities, making this type of testing easier with this population (56). Two days of 1-RM testing have been used in some cases, with the best performance of the two recorded (70). This helps eliminate random poor performances and helps establish greater reliability.

Estimating RM

Many test situations simply estimate 1-RM capabilities from a multiple-RM performance. This procedure is attractive from an administrative standpoint, but its validity can be seriously questioned. Conversion factors have been developed that allow, for example, a 10-RM resistance to be equated with a 1-RM resistance (1, 103, 122), but these can lead to erroneous results, because different individuals and different exercises exhibit variable relationships when comparing 1-RM capabilities with multiple-repetition tests (71). For field settings involving large numbers of athletes or untrained subjects with little resistance-training experience, a weak case may be made for this type of estimation of a 1 RM, but definitely not for research purposes. Such scales can help target the actual 1-RM test.

Muscle Endurance

Local muscle endurance tests are performed specifically to evaluate repetitive muscular capabilities of the subjects. Although there is some relationship between 1-RM capabilities and muscle endurance (18), it is generally poor. This is the rationale against using multiple-RM testing for 1-RM estimation. Some settings, however, such as industrial and military (104, 134), are interested primarily with local muscular endurance. Lifting endurance tests have even been used to estimate $\dot{V}O_2$max with satisfactory results (134). An important consideration is what resistance to use. Relative loading is based on a percentage of the subject's RM capability (e.g., 60% 1 RM), whereas absolute loading has the same resistance for all subjects and all tests (e.g., 50 kg or 100% of body weight) (6, 19). For most individuals, the relationship between strength and absolute muscular endurance is positive, whereas the relationship between strength and relative endurance is negative (19).

A good example of absolute load testing is the 225-lb bench-press test currently performed by professional American football scouts as they evaluate prospective players. The efficacy of such a test remains to be demonstrated, and performance on this type of test is quite dependent on the training program used (6). The 1-RM bench press has the best predictive value for playing ability (51). Thus, careful consideration must be given to the purpose, validity, and appropriateness of this type of test for football players.

Females have been shown to fatigue less with relative loads (32, 127), while males fatigue less with absolute loads (32). Verbal feedback and encouragement should be provided to the subject during such tests to ensure optimal performance (60). The lifting cadence can be controlled to provide similar test conditions for all subjects and to eliminate unwanted body movements such as ''bouncing'' the bar during a bench press (130). But it is important to realize that such speed control during dynamic constant external resistance exercise will produce different results than tests where no lifting cadence is used.

Training Status of Subjects

For a strength-testing protocol, the training status of the subjects is of primary importance (63). Previous training can affect the functioning of the nervous system (129), motor coordination (113, 124), and the hormonal profile (99). These effects are all dependent on the type (84, 139), intensity, and duration of previous training (6). Different intensities and durations of exercise provide different physiological stresses (64).

Furthermore, fiber-type composition can contribute to physical performance (61). The effect of prior training differences can be seen in the different muscle-performance characteristics of various athletes (7, 35). Different strength profiles are also evident in similarly trained subjects of various calibers (27, 51). Even motivational factors may contribute, with highly trained subjects affected most (83). Depending on the variables being measured, short-term prior training may (129) or may not (54) affect the monitored variables.

The amount of strength improvement exhibited by a subject is greatly dependent on pretraining status. Therefore, one must temper athletes' expectations about training and test performances as strength gains from training slow down as the performance level increases. Increasing such awareness among athletes, coaches, and parents will reduce the pressure some athletes feel to use performance-enhancing substances (e.g., anabolic steroids) because of reductions in strength gains.

Age

The role of age on muscle strength is a topic receiving increasing attention. Most interest is centered on youth and resistance training (93, 95, 111), but older age groups are beginning to be focused on it as well in light of the many positive health benefits (36, 143). It has recently been demonstrated that males 60 to 72 years of age can still attain increases in muscular strength and hypertrophy (48). In the past, it was believed that preadolescents could not increase strength apart from maturational increases, due to their immature hormonal profiles (136). However, it has been shown that strength increases can be achieved via resistance training with this age group (93, 126). It is believed that factors such as increased fat-free mass (76, 95) and neural development (77, 95) can contribute to such strength gains in youth. When compared with adolescents, preadolescent males exhibit different muscle forces and contraction times; but they are able to fully activate their motor units as early as 6 years of age (15).

It has also been observed that muscle balance characteristics, including velocity specificity and joint specificity, are similar for youth and adults (146). Reliability of strength-testing young age groups has not been a problem (58) but must be carefully controlled. Injury to young subjects is an important concern during strength testing, but recorded injuries are few and most often occur during unsupervised training (22, 111). Older subjects have also been monitored, and some normative data are available (36). Although it appears possible to increase strength at increasing ages (23, 48), strength tends to decrease due primarily to inactivity and decreased fat-free body mass (143). When testing older subjects, care must be taken concerning their physical capabilities and any preexisting disease states. Joint ranges of motion may be diminished, as may their kinesthetic awareness. Bone mineral density decreases associated with osteoporosis might also have to be considered when designing strength-testing protocols (34).

Finally, motivation factors may be different with older subjects—they may require more encouragement to achieve maximal efforts. Regardless of the number of precautions that must be taken, it is evident that resistance training and its associated positive health benefits will necessitate the need for strength testing in individuals who are young or old.

Gender

Strength performance differences due to gender must be carefully considered when comparing sexes (10). Although males typically exhibit greater absolute strengths, it has been shown that upper body strength differences between males and females are greater than lower body strength differences (20, 69). This is most likely due to fat-free mass levels, which have been reported to account for 97% of the gender strength differences (20). It may also explain why upper body strength is sometimes more difficult to develop and maintain in women (52). Also, as previously mentioned, women have a different muscle fatigue pattern, with greater muscle endurance with relative loads, and poorer muscle endurance with absolute loads (32, 127). Other variables, such as muscle balance characteristics, are similar for both genders (36). There may be some neural or structural differences, because the integrated electromyographic activity and peak torque is associated with different knee joint angles for males and females (24). Some evidence also exists for anatomical gender differences contributing to altered lifting technique with untrained subjects (50).

Mode of Muscle Activity

An often overlooked aspect of strength testing is what type of muscle activity is tested—concentric, eccentric, or isometric. This becomes an issue of specificity of testing. Some types of training, such as isokinetic, might not have an eccentric component (113), thus affecting tests that do include eccentric activity (80). It should also be remembered that eccentric activity generates greater peak torque than does concentric activity (121). If different types of muscle activity are used for testing, as compared to training, the test may not be sensitive to the physiological alterations that have occurred (52, 55). Therefore, extensive familiarization and practice is needed if nontraining-specific tests are used. Training using one mode of muscle activity should typically be assessed with an identical type of muscle activity within a strength-testing profile.

Joint Angle

The angle of each joint will determine the amount of muscle stretch. Outside factors, such as the type of equipment used for testing (e.g., isokinetic dynamometer), can affect the joint angles to be monitored (26, 38, 40). Factors, such as biomechanical joint characteristics, can also affect muscle force development (53) and the levels of muscle stretch. The mechanics of the contractile elements, as well as neural factors, can be involved (140). All joint angles need to be monitored and kept constant for all testing. Changing joint angles can alter the contribution of various muscles or muscle groups, affecting the results (144). Although the exact relationship is not clear, gender differences in joint-angle characteristics may exist (24). Testing that does not involve eccentric muscle actions of antagonistic muscles (e.g., some isokinetic or hydraulic instruments) can also affect force production, because the stretch-shortening cycle is not emphasized (100).

Velocity of Movement

Some test modalities, such as isokinetic or isometric, control the velocity of movement, whereas dynamic constant external resistance exercise (inappropriately termed "isotonic") does not. In order to select the appropriate velocity at which to test, several important factors should be considered. Velocity characteristics of prior training can affect velocity-specific test results (26, 38), with the greatest improvements occurring at the training-specific velocities (139). Peak torque will vary at different limb velocities, within a subject (29), with increasing velocities eliciting decreased torque (53, 55) but increased power (121). Concentric muscle activity is affected by this more than is eccentric activity (62). Greater limb velocities for training have been associated with preferential development of fast-twitch fibers (138), which may explain why the velocity at which torque decreases is related to fiber composition (61). Velocity considerations are also important when determining muscle balance characteristics (53, 87). Still, not all muscle groups exhibit altered torque production with different limb velocities (35, 144). When using fixed-velocity testing, do not confuse machine lever arm velocities with actual velocities of muscle shortening or lengthening.

Test Specificity

An essential consideration in strength testing is test specificity. Various types of exercise impose different demands; exercise of less than 15 s duration stresses different physiological systems than does exercise of greater than 15 s duration (64). Different types of muscle actions will also have specific effects. For example, dynamic constant external resistance ("isotonic") exercise will increase "isotonic" strength more than isometric strength and may have little effect on peak power production (55, 123). Conversely, in other subjects dynamic constant external resistance exercise training will increase isometric strength more than "isotonic" strength (52). Such variability in strength relationships to training underscores the need for the inclusion of tests specific to the mode used in training. Therefore, proper assessment of a training program should include a similar type of muscle action, not a different type as some investigators have used (5). Different muscle actions may not be sensitive enough to training adaptations if familiarization and practice are less than the training mode (53, 55). They may be helpful for determining the carry-over effects and relationships of

certain muscle action types to one another. Adaptations are also specific to limb velocity in training (84). Training velocities will preferentially affect specific portions of the force–velocity curve as well as specific populations of muscle fibers (139). This is somewhat evident from the increases in low-velocity isokinetic strength resulting from dynamic constant external resistance training (113). Other training modalities, such as hydraulic machines, will also present different physiological stresses and cannot always be equated with dynamic constant external resistance or isokinetic exercise (75, 80). Therefore, it is essential that strength assessments be performed in a modality similar to that in which the training occurred.

Technique

Some types of strength evaluations require using a specific movement pattern. This is not a typical concern for machine testing, as the machine usually dictates the movement pattern, but proper positioning is required (93, 105). Regardless of whether free weights or machines are used, proper exercise technique is required for the safety of the subject. Lifting injuries are often associated with unsupervised exercise sessions (22, 111) and are often avoidable with knowledgeable supervision. Proper exercise technique also insures that an appropriate range of motion is used (45). Changes in the range of motion used can affect test results. For example, norms developed for females performing a half squat (86) are much greater than would be expected for subjects performing a parallel squat. Proper exercise technique is a prerequisite for valid testing as well as for subjects' safety. If proper technique is not utilized, the test should be terminated. Criteria for termination of the test should be established prior to the testing. For example, a bench-press test may be terminated if the subject raises the buttocks off the bench or if excessive twisting motion of the body is evident. Good technique is essential for any strength-testing exercise and has been previously described in detail (93).

Pretest Exercise and Ambient Temperature

The scientific efficacy of exercise prior to performance is not completely clear, but subjects typically perform some type of warm-up exercise before actual strength testing occurs. Most protocols utilize the specific mode of testing at submaximal efforts (i.e., warm-up repetitions) to accomplish this prior to the test. This familiarizes the subject with the test. It is also known that there is an optimal muscle temperature for force and power development (8). Whether all pretest exercise accomplishes this objective remains unknown. Temperature of the surrounding environment can also affect subject performance (107) and should be held constant for all subjects and test sessions. Additional measures should be taken when testing in an uncontrolled environment such as the outdoors, including extra warm-up clothing or cancellation of testing due to variable conditions.

Breathing and Blood Pressure

Although a seemingly simple matter, the role of breathing during resistance exercise is of major concern (11). Beginning exercisers are often instructed to breathe continuously during resistance training, but more advanced lifters have found that breath holding during certain phases of some lifts may enhance their performance on maximum efforts (11). Breath holding results in a Valsalva maneuver, with extremely high blood pressures resulting in some instances (106). The amount of blood pressure increase is dependent in part on the resistances used, with greater weights and forces eliciting greater pressure increases (67, 110). The increased blood pressure is related to increased abdominal and thoracic cavity pressures, thus contributing to body stability (67). The use of a weight belt will also contribute to this effect (81). The amount of muscle mass used in the exercise (110) as well as the lifting cadence (56) can contribute to the blood pressure response. For the monitoring of cardiovascular variables during resistance exercise, breathing patterns must be constant for all subjects and compatible with health considerations.

Rest Intervals

Adequate recovery time must be allowed for all subjects. The time required will depend on the amount of musculature involved and the forces developed during the exercise. Thus, high-velocity, low-force activity (e.g., high-velocity isokinetics), may require shorter recovery times than low-velocity, high-force activity (e.g., 1-RM barbell squat). Rest intervals as short as 10 s have been successfully used between isokinetic efforts (38, 40, 61). Rests of up to 3 min between single repetitions for isokinetic leg extension and flexion testing have resulted in no significant performance differences compared to 1-min rests between sets of 3 repetitions (33). Rest intervals during free-weight exercise may be more critical. Rests of 5 min between 90% and 100% of 10-RM back-squat exercise appeared adequate and necessary (56). Consistency of the rest interval may be important for some types of strength testing, especially if related physiological parameters are also being monitored (e.g., blood pressure, heart rate).

Arousal and Encouragement

It is important to give thorough instructions to all subjects prior to the actual strength test (130). Performance on strength tasks can be enhanced if the subjects are optimally aroused (19). Verbal encouragement is suggested for all strength testing to help ensure optimal results. Care must be taken that the form of this encouragement is consistent for all subjects. For some tests, such as isometric, isokinetic, or fatigue tests, simultaneous visual feedback should be provided concerning subject performance (60). Factors such as a subject's yelling during a strength task or prior training experience can all affect arousal and the resulting strength scores (83). Such factors need to be considered and kept consistent in all testing.

Familiarity of the Exercise

Performance on a strength test can be enhanced when subjects are familiar with the task. If prior testing or training has not occurred on the test apparatus, practice sessions should be scheduled to familiarize the subjects with the testing modality and protocol (39, 52). Some studies have utilized only subjects with previous experience on the testing apparatus (38, 40), but this is not always possible. The role of feedback may be more important in these situations (60). Prior training experience may also contribute to strength-test performance. For example, sprinters may have an advantage over distance runners in tests of high power and velocity, due to the nature of their training and mental set for the activity. In general, the more complex the exercise or the less experienced the subject, the greater the need for familiarization (39).

Reliability

Test reliability is the ability of a strength test to repeatedly give the same results for identical performances. This should not be confused with the *validity* of the strength test utilized—that is, whether the test can actually assess the desired variable. Reliability is determined from several test sessions with similar test performances using the same subjects and conditions, or using calibration weights. Test-retest reliability is quantified by the standard deviation or method error of repeated trials. The coefficient of variation (SD/X) is also used as an indicator of reliability. Further information is provided by the correlation coefficient (r) of repeated trials (130). Before testing begins, all equipment should be evaluated for reliability (96, 101, 132, 135). Furthermore, reliability cannot be assured among different types of equipment and their various attachments (42, 47). The reliability of test technicians should also be periodically monitored to insure that their methods and techniques are similar. Although reliability may have been established for certain measures of a strength test, the reliability may not extend to other variables of the same test (58). Factors such as type of muscle action and limb velocity can affect testing error (147).

Muscular Balance

A variable often monitored is muscular balance, where strength levels of antagonistic muscles are assessed relative to each other. A great amount of research has been performed in this area and is summarized in a review by Nosse (112). Attempts have also been made to identify the muscle balance requirements of a variety of subject populations (68). Muscle balance characteristics are not different when comparing prepubertal males to adults (146), but age may be a factor for other populations (138). Other subject characteristics to consider include gender (28) and body size (120) of the subject.

The strength ratios (agonist-antagonist) are affected by limb velocity (53, 62, 114), because different muscle groups have different force–velocity characteristics. Thus, limb velocities of muscle balance properties must be identified (87). The ratios are also joint-angle specific (53, 144), which is an important consideration when using angle-specific isokinetic torques or isometric testing. Furthermore, different joints have their own unique muscle balance ratios (35, 62, 119).

Some investigations have corrected for the effects of gravity (119), which can greatly affect the ratios (7). Therefore, when comparing data, check to see if this factor has been accounted for. Muscle balance ratios are also specific to the population, with prior training affecting the results (37, 78, 119, 120). The value of 0.60 for hamstring/quadricep torques is widely accepted (112) but is dependent on all the previously stated variables. Training programs may affect muscle balance characteristics, but durations of greater than 8 weeks appear to be necessary (54).

Bilateral differences are also sometimes observed due to usage patterns (35, 62) and can be monitored by testing both right and left limbs for contralateral asymmetries. Differences of 10% to 15% in the bilateral strength values are indicative of a muscle imbalance (25, 114), although acceptable values may actually be higher (59). When comparing muscle balance data, a variety of testing conditions must be identified.

Ergogenics

Methods and materials used to improve performance can be classified as *ergogenics*. Needless to say, this is a very broad category, including items such as lifting belts and wraps, wrist straps for enhancing grip, various types of lifting apparel, mental preparation techniques, dietary manipulations, and of course performance-enhancing drugs. The use of any of these can affect performance, and careful consideration must be given to whether to allow these items when testing. Some of these are easily controlled, such as the use of various lifting apparel. Others, such as performance-enhancing drugs, are more difficult to screen. Using acceptable drug-testing procedures can help control this factor but might not be foolproof. If acceptable, equipment such as lifting belts should be made available for all subjects. The use of performance-enhancing drugs should be screened for as carefully as possible and their use discouraged by realistic attitudes toward strength-training gains, use of effective training programs, elimination of inappropriate pressures, and changes in value systems.

Units of Measure

The International System of Units (SI) includes the accepted units of measure for strength testing. The SI unit for force is the newton (130). In the everyday world, pounds (1 lb = 4.44822 N) and kilograms (1 kg = 9.80665 N) are often reported as units of force. Testing for research purposes should always use SI units, but for field testing—for example with athletic teams or with large populations for fitness assessments—it may be beneficial to use pounds and kilograms. Several good discussions on appropriate units of measure can be found in the literature (9, 88, 130). See Table 8.2 for a list of some commonly used SI units.

Table 8.2 Common Units of Measurement Used in Strength Testing

Measure	SI unit	Common conversions
Force	newton (N)	1 lb = 4.44822 N
Mass	kilogram (kg)	1 lb = 0.45359237 kg
		1 kg = 2.2046 lbs.
Power	watt (W)	1 hp = 746 W
Work	joule (J)	1 ft-lb = 1.355818 J
Torque	newton meter (N · m)	1 ft-lb = 1.355818 N-m
Velocity	meters per second (m · s^{-1})	1 mph = 0.44704 m · s^{-1}
Acceleration	meters per second squared (m · s^{-2})	
Angle	radians (rad)	1 rad = 57.29578°
Angular velocity	radians per second (rads · s^{-1})	1 rad · s^{-1} = 57.29578° · s^{-1}
Distance	meter (m)	1 foot = 0.3048 m

Correction for Body Mass

Strength performances can be influenced by the individual's body mass. Therefore, correction factors for body mass have been developed. Some methods involve coefficient tables based on body weights (137), which are quite popular with the competitive lifting sports. An easier method is to simply correct for body weight by dividing the strength score by body weight or fat-free mass. This method allows for comparisons between genders (20), as well as across chronological ages, both intrasubject (76, 77) and intersubject (143).

Total Work

An important consideration in comparing training programs is total work as measured in joules (see Table 8.2). Although sometimes defined as the area under a torque curve (108), work is actually "force expressed through a distance but with no limitation on time" (88). Therefore, if one is trying to equate training programs, the forces of each repetition and the distances moved must be carefully monitored to control for total work (96, 98).

Normative Data

The development of normative strength data is very difficult due to many of the previously mentioned factors. Strength performances are very population-specific and are dependent on the testing equipment and methodology used. With a large enough sample size, you can develop norms specific to your own particular needs. A small sampling of available strength data includes testing of large population groups (13, 14, 31, 51, 66), more specific age and gender studies (36, 76, 77, 86, 119, 143), as well as a compilation of muscle balance characteristics (112).

SUMMARY

As is evident from the preceding material, accurate strength testing must take many considerations into account. Care must be taken to design and develop a test protocol that controls variables important to the particular testing situation. Simple field tests for general fitness appraisals might not appear to be very involved, but they require careful consideration of all the variables mentioned in this chapter for accuracy and clinical viability. When strength testing is used as a highly defined research tool, the procedures can be quite elaborate. Table 8.3 lists variables that must be addressed in many

Table 8.3   Basic Considerations Checklist for Strength Testing

_____   Is muscle strength or muscle endurance to be tested?
_____   RM testing procedures
_____   Training status of subjects
_____   Age of subjects
_____   Gender of subjects
_____   Type of muscle activity to be tested:
  ___ Concentric
  ___ Eccentric
  ___ Static
_____   Type of resistance to be used:
  ___ Dynamic constant external resistance
  ___ Variable resistance
  ___ Isokinetic
  ___ Isometric
_____   Starting position of the resistance
_____   Joint angles
_____   Velocity of movement
_____   Test specificity:
  ___ Follows movement patterns used in training
  ___ Metabolically specific
_____   Proper technique utilized
  ___ Subject properly positioned
  ___ Equipment fit
_____   High reliability of equipment and testers
_____   Adequate instructions given
_____   Familiarization with the test protocol provided
_____   Test practice sessions
_____   Proper warm-up provided
_____   Proper breathing patterns used
_____   Adequate rest intervals allowed
_____   Consistent encouragement and verbal feedback to all subjects
_____   Appropriate and consistent visual feedback
_____   Proper units of measurement used
_____   External aids (ergogenic) controlled
_____   Determine if body weight or total work correction needed

test situations. Careful consideration of each of these will help you develop a protocol appropriate for your individual needs.

Ackowledgments
The authors would like to express thanks to Drs. Howard G. Knuttgen and Robert V. Newton for their time, counsel, insight, and helpful comments in the writing and revision process of this manuscript. The authors would also like to thank Ms. Joann Ruble and Ms. Carol Glunt for their help in the preparation of this manuscript.

This chapter was supported by the Robert F. and Sandra M. Leitzinger Research Fund in Sports Medicine at Penn State.

REFERENCES

1. Abdo, J.S. (1985). Weight training percentage table. *National Strength and Conditioning Association Journal*, **7**(1), 50-51.

2. Alderman, R.B., & Banfield, T.J. (1969). Reliability estimation in the measurement of strength. *Research Quarterly*, **40**(3), 448-455.

3. Allerheiligen, B., Arce, J.H., Arthur, M., Chu, D., Lilja, L., Semenick, D., Ward, B., & Wozcik, M. (1983). Coaches roundtable: Testing for football. *National Strength and Conditioning Association Journal*, **5**(5), 12-19, 62-68.

4. Altug, Z., Altug, T., & Altug, A. (1987). A test selection guide for assessing and evaluating athletes. *National Strength and Conditioning Association Journal*, **9**(3), 62-66.

5. Amusa, L.O., & Obajuluwa, V.A. (1986). Static versus dynamic training programs for muscular strength using the knee-extensors in healthy young men. *Journal of Orthopedic Sport, Medicine and Physical Therapy*, **8**(5), 243-247.

6. Anderson, T., & Kearney, J.T. (1982). Effects of three resistance training programs on muscular strength and absolute and relative endurance. *Research Quarterly*, **53**(1), 1-7.

7. Appen, L., & Duncan, P.W. (1986). Strength relationship of the knee musculature: Effect of gravity and sport. *Journal of Orthopedic Sport, Medicine and Physical Therapy*, **7**(5), 232-235.

8. Armstrong, L.E. (1988). The impact of hyperthermia and hypohydration on circulation, strength, endurance and health. *Journal of Applied Sport Science Research*, **2**(4), 60-65.

9. Åstrand, P.O., & Rodahl, K. (1986). *Textbook of work physiology*. New York: McGraw-Hill.

10. Atha, J. (1981). Strengthening muscle. In D.I. Miller (Ed.), *Exercise and sport science reviews* (pp. 1-74). Philadelphia: Franklin.

11. Austin, D., Roll, F., Kreis, E.J., Palmieri, J., & Lander, J. (1987). Roundtable: Breathing during weight training. *National Strength and Conditioning Association Journal*, **9**(5), 17-25.

12. Axtell, R.S., Gravenstein, R.O., & Lanese, R.R. (1986). The relationship between peak and mean torque in isokinetic exercise. *Medicine and Science in Sports and Exercise*, **18**(Suppl. 2), 278.

13. Banister, E.W., & MeKjavic, I.B. (1986). *Experiments in human performance*. Toronto, Canada: Holt, Rinehart, and Winston.

14. Baumgartner, T.A., & Jackson, A.S. (1982). *Measurements for evaluation in physical education*. Dubuque, IA: Brown.

15. Belanger, A.Y., & McComas, A.J. (1989). Contractile properties of human skeletal muscle in childhood and adolescence. *European Journal of Applied Physiology*, **58**, 563-567.

16. Bemben, M.G., Clasey, J.L., & Massey, B.H. (1990). The effect of the rate of muscle contraction on the force time curve parameters of male and female subjects. *Research Quarterly*, **61**(1), 96-99.

17. Berger, R. (1962). Effect of varied weight training programs on strength. *Research Quarterly*, **33**, 168-181.

18. Berger, R.A. (1967). Determination of a method to predict 1-RM chin and dip from repetitive chins and dips. *Research Quarterly*, **38**(3), 330-335.

19. Biddle, S.J. (1986). Personal beliefs and mental preparation in strength and muscular endurance tasks: A review. *Physical Education Review*, **8**(2), 90-103.

20. Bishop, P., Cureton, K., & Collins, M. (1987). Sex difference in muscular strength in equally-trained men and women. *Ergonomics*, **30**(4), 675-687.

21. Brazell-Roberts, J.V., & Thomas, L.E. (1989). Effects of weight training frequency on the self-concept of college females. *Journal of Applied Sport Science Research*, **3**(2), 40-43.

22. Brown, E.W., & Kimball, R.G. (1983). Medical history associated with adolescent powerlifting. *Pediatrics*, **72**, 630-644.

23. Brown, R.D., & Harrison, J.M. (1986). The effects of a strength training program on the strength and self-concept of two female age groups. *Research Quarterly*, **57**(4), 315-320.

24. Brownstein, B.A., Lamb, R.L., & Mangine, R.E. (1985). Quadriceps torque and integrated electromyography. *Journal of Orthopedic Sport, Medicine and Physical Therapy*, **6**(6), 309-314.

25. Burkett, L.N. (1970). Causative factors in hamstring strains. *Medicine and Science in Sports and Exercise*, **2**, 39-42.

26. Caiozzo, V.J., Perrine, J.J., & Edgerton, V.R. (1981). Training induced alterations of the invivo force velocity relationship of human muscle. *Journal of Applied Physiology*, **51**(3), 750-754.

27. Chmelar, R.D., Shultz, B.B., Ruhling, R.O., Fitt, S.S., & Johnson, M.B. (1988). Isokinetic characteristics of the knee in female, professional and university ballet and modern dancers. *Journal of Orthopedic Sport, Medicine and Physical Therapy*, **9**(12), 410-418.

28. Christensen, C.S. (1975). Relative strength in males and females. *Athletic Training*, **10**, 189-192.

29. Cisar, C.J., Johnson, G.O., Fry, A.C., Housh, T.J., Hughes, R.A., Ryan, A.J., & Thorland, W.G. (1987). Preseason body composition, build and strength as predictors of high school wrestling success. *Journal of Applied Sport Science Research*, **1**(4), 66-70.

30. Cisar, C.J., Johnson, G.O., Fry, A.C., & Ryan, A.J. (1987). Assessment of preseason muscular strength as a basis for specific conditioning. *Journal of Applied Sport Science Research*, **1**(3), 60.

31. Clark, H.M. (1967). *Application of measurement to health and physical education.* Englewood Cliffs, NJ: Prentice Hall.

32. Clarke, D.M. (1986). Sex differences in strength and fatigability. *Research Quarterly*, **57**(2), 144-149.

33. Conroy, B., Stanley, D., Fry, A., & Kraemer, W.J. (1984). A comparison of isokinetic protocols. *Journal of Applied Sport Science Research*, **3**(3), 72.

34. Conroy, B.P., Kraemer, W.J., Maresh, C.M., & Dalsky, G.P. (1992). Adaptive responses of bone to physical activity. *Medicine, Exercise, Nutrition and Health*, **1**(2), 64-74.

35. Cook, E.E., Gray, V.L., Savinar-Nogue, E., & Medeiros, J. (1987). Shoulder antagonistic strength ratios: A comparison between college-level baseball pitchers and non-pitchers. *Journal of Orthopedic Sport, Medicine and Physical Therapy*, **8**(9), 451-461.

36. DiBrezzo, R., & Fort, I.L. (1987). Strength norms for the knee in women 25 years and older. *Journal of Applied Sport Science Research*, **1**(3), 45-47.

37. DiBrezzo, R., Gench, B.E., Hinson, M.M., & King, J. (1985). Peak torque values of the knee extensor and flexor muscles of females. *Journal of Orthopedic Sport, Medicine and Physical Therapy*, **7**(2), 65-68.

38. Dudley, G.A., & Djamil, R. (1985). Incompatibility of endurance and strength training modes of exercise. *Journal of Applied Physiology*, **59**, 1446-1451.

39. Dudley, G.A., Tesch, P.A., Miller, B.J., & Buchanan, P. (1991). Importance of eccentric actions in performance adaptations to resistance training. *Aviation Space and Environmental Medicine*, **62**, 543-550.

40. Edgerton, V.R., & Perrine, J.J. (1978). Muscle force-velocity and power-velocity relationships under isokinetic loading. *Medicine and Science in Sports and Exercise*, **10**(3), 159-166.

41. Enoka, R.M. (1988). Muscle strength and its development—New perspectives. *Sports Medicine*, **6**, 146-168.

42. Epler, M., Nawoczenski, D., & Englehardt, T. (1988). Comparison of the Cybex II standard shin adaptor versus the Johnson anti-sheer device in torque generation. *Journal of Orthopedic Sport, Medicine and Physical Therapy*, **9**(8), 284-286.

43. Faigenbaum, A.D., Skrinar, G.S., Cesare, W.F., Kraemer, W.J., & Thomas, H.E. (1990). Physiologic and symptomatic responses of cardiac patients to resistance exercise. *Archives of Physical Medicine and Rehabilitation*, **71**, 395-398.

44. Fleck, S.J., & Kraemer, W.J. (1987). *Designing resistance training programs.* Champaign, IL: Human Kinetics.

45. Fleck, S.J., & Kraemer, W.J. (1988). Resistance training: Basic principles. *The Physician and Sportsmedicine*, **16**(3), 160-171.

46. Fleming, L.K. (1985). Accommodation capabilities of Nautilus weight machines to human strength curves. *National Strength and Conditioning Association Journal*, **7**(4), 68.

47. Francis, K., & Hoobler, T. (1987). Comparison of peak torque values of the knee flexor and extensor muscle groups using the Cybex II and Lido 2.0 isokinetic dynamometers. *Journal of Orthopedic Sport, Medicine and Physical Therapy*, **8**(10), 480-483.

48. Frontera, W.R., Meredith, C.N., O'Reilly, K.P., Knuttgen, H.G., & Evans, W.J. (1988). Strength conditioning in older men: Skeletal muscle hypertrophy and improved function. *Journal of Applied Physiology*, **64**(3), 1038-1044.

49. Fry, A. (1985). Weight room safety. *National Strength and Conditioning Association Journal*, **7**(4), 32-33.

50. Fry, A.C., Bibi, K.W., Eyford, T., & Kraemer, W.J. (1990). Stature variables as discriminators of foot contact during the squat exercise in untrained females. *Journal of Applied Sport Science Research*, **9**, 23-32.

51. Fry, A.C., & Kraemer, W.J. (1991). Physical performance characteristics of American collegiate football players. *Journal of Applied Sport Science Research*, **5**(3), 126-138.

52. Fry, A.C., Kraemer, W.J., Weseman, C.A., Conroy, B.P., Gordon, S.E., Hoffman, J.R., & Maresh, C.M. (1991). The effects of an off-season strength and conditioning program on starters and non-starters in women's intercollegiate volleyball. *Journal of Applied Sport Science Research*, **5**(4), 174-181.

53. Fry, A.C., & Powell, D.R. (1987). A comparison of isokinetic and isometric muscle balance characteristics. *Journal of Applied Sport Science Research*, **1**(3), 59.

54. Fry, A.C., & Powell, D.R. (1987). Hamstring/quadricep parity with three different modes of weight training. *Journal of Sports Medicine and Physical Fitness*, **27**, 362-367.

55. Fry, A.C., Powell, D.R., & Kraemer, W.J. (1992). Validity of isokinetic and isometric testing modalities for assessing short-term resistance exercise strength gains. *Journal of Sport Rehabilitation*, **1**(4), 275-283.

56. Fry, A.C., Schmidt, R.J., Johnson, G.O., Tharp, G.D., & Kraemer, W.J. (1993). Recovery heart

rate and blood pressure responses to a graded exercise test and heavy resistance exercise. *Isokinetics and Exercise Science*, **3**(2), 74-84.

57. Gettman, L.R., & Pollock, M.L. (1981). Circuit weight training: A critical review of its physiological benefits. *The Physician and Sportsmedicine*, **9**(1), 44-60.

58. Going, S.B., Massey, B.H., Hoshizaki, T.B., & Lohman, T.G. (1987). Maximal voluntary static force production characteristics of skeletal muscle in children 8-11 years of age. *Research Quarterly*, **58**(2), 115-123.

59. Grace, T., Sweetser, E.R., Nelson, M.A., Ydens, L.R., & Skipper, B.J. (1984). Isokinetic muscle imbalance and knee joint injuries. *Journal of Bone and Joint Surgery*, **66A**, 734.

60. Graves, J.E., & James, R.J. (1990). Concurrent augmented feedback and isometric force generation during familiar and unfamiliar muscle movements. *Research Quarterly*, **61**(1), 75-79.

61. Gregor, R.J., Edgerton, V.R., Perrine, J.J., Capion, D.S., & DeBus, C. (1979). Torque-velocity relationships and muscle fiber composition in elite female athletes. *Journal of Applied Physiology*, **47**(2), 388-392.

62. Hageman, P.A., Gillaspie, D.M., & Hill, L.D. (1988). Effects of speed and limb dominance on eccentric and concentric isokinetic testing of the knee. *Journal of Orthopedic Sport, Medicine and Physical Therapy*, **10**(2), 59.

63. Häkkinen, K. (1989). Neuromuscular and hormonal adaptations during strength and power training. *Journal of Sports Medicine and Physical Fitness*, **29**, 9-26.

64. Häkkinen, K., Kauhanen, H., & Komi, P.V. (1987). Aerobic, anaerobic, assistant exercise, and weightlifting performance capacities in elite weightlifters. *Journal of Sports Medicine and Physical Fitness*, **27**, 240-246.

65. Harman, E.A. (1984). *A biomechanical analysis of the bench press exercise*. Unpublished doctoral dissertation, University of Massachusetts, Amherst.

66. Harman, E., Sharp, M., Manikowski, R., Frykman, P., & Rosenstein, R. (1987). Analysis of a muscle strength data base. *Journal of Applied Sport Science Research*, **2**(3), 54.

67. Harman, E.A., Frykman, P.N., Clagett, E.R., & Kraemer, W.J. (1988). Intra-abdominal and intra-thoracic pressures during lifting and jumping. *Medicine and Science in Sports and Exercise*, **20**(2), 195-201.

68. Hemba, G. (1985). Hamstring parity. *National Strength and Conditioning Association Journal*, **7**(3), 30-31.

69. Heyward, V.H., Johannes-Ellis, S.M., & Romer, J.F. (1986). Gender differences in strength. *Research Quarterly*, **57**(2), 154-159.

70. Hill, D.W., Collins, M.A., Curenton, K.J., & De-Mello, J.J. (1989). Blood pressure response after weight training exercise. *Journal of Applied Sport Science Research*, **3**(2), 44-47.

71. Hoeger, W.K., Barette, S.L., Hale, D.F., & Hopkins, D.R. (1987). Relationship between repetitions and selected percentages of one repetition maximum. *Journal of Applied Sport Science Research*, **1**(1), 11-13.

72. Hoffman, J.R., Fry, A.C., Howard, R., Maresh, C.M., & Kraemer, W.J. (1991). Strength, speed, and endurance changes during the course of a Division I basketball season. *Journal of Applied Sport Science Research*, **5**(3), 144-149.

73. Hoffman, J.R., Maresh, C.M., & Armstrong, L.E. (1992). Isokinetic and dynamic constant resistance strength testing: Implications for sport. *Physical Therapy Practice*, **2**(1), 42-53.

74. Hortobagyi, T., & Katch, F.I. (1990). Role of concentric force in limiting improvement in muscular strength. *Journal of Applied Physiology*, **68**, 650-680.

75. Hortobagyi, T.T., LaChance, P.F., & Katch, F.I. (1987). Prediction of maximum isokinetic force, power and isotonic velocity and power from maximum force and power measured during hydraulic bench press exercise. *Journal of Applied Sport Science Research*, **1**(3), 58.

76. Housh, T.J., Johnson, G.O., Hughes, R.A., Cisar, C.J., & Thorland, W.G. (1988). Yearly changes in the body composition and muscular strength of high school wrestlers. *Research Quarterly*, **59**(3), 240-243.

77. Housh, T.J., Johnson, G.O., Hughes, R.A., Housh, D.J., Hughes, R.J., Fry, A.C., Kenney, K.B., & Cisar, C.J. (1989). Isokinetic strength and body composition of high school wrestlers across age. *Medicine and Science in Sports and Exercise*, **21**(1), 105-109.

78. Housh, T.J., Johnson, G.O., Marty, L., Eischen, G., Eischen, C., & Housh, D.J. (1988). Isokinetic leg extension and extension strength of university football players. *Journal of Orthopedic Sport, Medicine and Physical Therarpy*, **9**(11), 365-369.

79. Huegli, R., Richardson, T., Graffis, K., Kroll, B., & Epley, B. (1989). Roundtable: Safe facility design and standards for safe equipment. *National Strength and Conditioning Association Journal*, **11**(5), 14-27.

80. Hunter, G.R., & Culpepper, M.I. (1988). Knee extension torque joint position relationships following isotonic fixed resistance and hydraulic resistance training. *Athletic Training*, **23**(1), 16-20.

81. Hunter, G.R., McGuirk, J., Mitrano, N., Pearman, P., Thomas, B., & Arrington, R. (1984). The effects of a weight training belt on blood pressure during exercise. *Journal of Applied Sport Science Research*, **3**(1), 13-18.

82. Hurley, B.F., Hagberg, J.M., Goldberg, A.P., Seals, D.R., Ehsani, A.A., Brennan, R.E., & Holloszy, J.O. (1988). Resistive training can reduce coronary risk factors without altering V̇O₂max or percent body fat. *Medicine and Science in Sports and Exercise*, **20**(2), 150-154.

83. Ikai, M., & Steinhaus, A.H. (1961). Some factors modifying the expression of human strength. *Journal of Applied Physiology*, **16**(1), 157-163.

84. Jenkins, W.L., Thackaberry, M., & Killian, C. (1984). Speed-specific isokinetic testing. *Journal of Orthopedic Sport, Medicine and Physical Therarpy*, **6**(3), 181-183.

85. Keleman, M.A., Stewart, K.J., Gillilan, R.E., Valenti, S.A., Manley, J.D., Keleman, M.D., & Ewart, C.K. (1984). Circuit weight training in a cardiac rehabilitation program. *Medicine and Science in Sports and Exercise*, **16**(2), 128.

86. Kindig, L.E., Soares, P.L., Wisenbaker, J.M., & Mrvos, S.R. (1984). Standard scores for women's weight training. *The Physician and Sportsmedicine*, **12**(10), 67-74.

87. Klopfer, D.A., & Greij, S.D. (1988). Examining quadriceps/hamstrings performance at high velocity isokinetics in untrained subjects. *Journal of Orthopedic Sport, Medicine and Physical Therarpy*, **10**(1), 18-22.

88. Knuttgen, H.G., & Kraemer, W.J. (1987). Terminology and measurement in exercise performance. *Journal of Applied Sport Science Research*, **1**(1), 1-10.

89. Kraemer, W.J. (1983). Measurement of strength. In A. Weltman & C.G. Spain (Eds.), *Proceedings of the White House Symposium on physical fitness and sports medicine* (pp. 35-36). Washington, DC: President's Council on Physical Fitness and Sports.

90. Kraemer, W.J. (1990). Physiological and cellular effects of exercise training. In W.B. Leadbetter, J.A. Buckwalter, & S.L. Gordon (Eds.), *Sports-induced inflammation* (pp. 659-676). Park Ridge, IL: American Academy of Orthopedic Surgeons.

91. Kraemer, W.J., & Baechle, T.R. (1989). Development of a strength training program. In F.L. Allman & A.J. Ryan (Eds.), *Sports medicine* (2nd ed.) (pp. 113-127). Orlando, FL: Academic Press.

92. Kraemer, W.J., Deschenes, M.R., & Fleck, S.J. (1988). Physiological adaptations to resistance exercise: Implications for athletic conditioning. *Sports Medicine*, **6**, 246-256.

93. Kraemer, W.J., & Fleck, S.J. (1993). *Strength training for young athletes*. Champaign, IL: Human Kinetics.

94. Kraemer, W.J., Fleck, S.J., & Noble, B.J. (1991). Muscle strength and endurance following long distance treadmill running. *Journal of Human Muscle Performance*, **1**(3), 32-39.

95. Kraemer, W.J., Fry, A.C., Frykman, P.N., Conroy, B., & Hoffman, J. (1989). Resistance training and youth. *Pediatric Exercise Science*, **1**, 336-350.

96. Kraemer, W.J., Gordon, S.E., Fleck, S.J., Marchitelli, L.J., Mello, R., Dziados, J.E., Friedl, K., Harman, E., Maresh, C., & Fry, A.C. (1991). Endogenous anabolic hormonal and growth factor responses to heavy resistance exercise in males and females. *International Journal of Sports Medicine*, **12**(2), 228-235.

97. Kraemer, W.J., & Koziris, L.P. (1992). Muscle strength training: Techniques and considerations. *Physical Therapy Practice*, **2**(1), 54-68.

98. Kraemer, W.J., Marchitelli, L., McCurry, D., Mello, R., Dziados, J.E., Harman, E., Frykman, P., Gordon, S.E., & Fleck, S.J. (1990). Hormonal and growth factor responses to heavy resistance exercise. *Journal of Applied Physiology*, **69**(4), 1442-1450.

99. Kraemer, W.J., Noble, B.J., Clark, M.J., & Culver, B.W. (1987). Physiologic responses to heavy-resistance exercise with very short rest periods. *International Journal of Sports Medicine*, **8**, 247-252.

100. LaChance, P.F., Gabriel, D.A., Hortobagyi, T.T., & Katch, F.I. (1987). Muscular peak torque during fast and slow uni- and bi-directional concentric hydraulic resistance exercise. *Journal of Applied Sport Science Research*, **1**(3), 59.

101. LaChance, P.F., Katch, F.I., Mistry, D.J., & Hortobagyi, T.T. (1988). Day-to-day reliability during high and low resistance bi-directional hydraulic exercise. *Journal of Applied Sport Science Research*, **2**(3), 57.

102. Lander, L.B., Franklin, B.A., Wrisley, D., & Rubenfire, M. (1986). Acute cardiovascular responses to Nautilus exercise in cardiac patients: Implications for exercise training. *Annals Sports Medicine*, **2**, 165-169.

103. Landers, J. (1985). Maximum based on reps. *National Strength and Conditioning Association Journal*, **6**(6), 60-61.

104. Legg, S.J., & Pateman, C.M. (1984). A physiological study of the repetitive lifting capabilities of healthy young males. *Ergonomics*, **27**(3), 259-272.

105. Lewis, C.L., & Spitler, D.L. (1989). Effect of tibial rotation on measures of strength and endurance

of the knee. *Journal of Applied Sport Science Research*, **3**(1), 19-22.

106. MacDougall, J.D., Tuxen, D., Sale, D.G., Moroz, J.R., & Sutton, J.R. (1985). Arterial blood pressure response to heavy resistance exercise. *Journal of Applied Physiology*, **58**(3), 785-790.

107. Meese, G.B., Schiefer, R.E., Kustner, P., Kok, R., & Lewis, M.I. (1986). Subjective comfort vote and air temperature as predictors of performance in factory workers. *European Journal of Applied Physiology*, **55**, 195-197.

108. Morrissey, M.C. (1987). The relationship between peak torque and work of the quadriceps and hamstrings after meniscectomy. *Journal of Orthopedic Sport, Medicine and Physical Therarpy*, **8**(8), 405-408.

109. Morrissey, M.C., & Brewster, C.E. (1986). Hamstring weakness after surgery for anterior cruciate injury. *Journal of Orthopedic Sport, Medicine and Physical Therapy*, **7**(7), 310-312.

110. Nagle, F.J., Seals, D.R., & Hanson, P. (1988). Time to fatigue during isometric exercise using different muscle masses. *International Journal of Sports Medicine*, **9**, 313-315.

111. National Strength and Conditioning Association. (1985). Position paper on prepubescent strength training. *National Strength and Conditioing Association Journal*, **7**(4), 27-31.

112. Nosse, L.J. (1982). Assessment of selected reports on the strength relationship of the knee musculature. *Journal of Orthopedic Sport, Medicine and Physical Therapy*, **4**(2), 78-85.

113. Nosse, L.J., & Hunter, G.R. (1985, Fall). Free weights: A review supporting their use in training and rehabilitation. *Athletic Training*, **20**(3), 206-209.

114. Nunn, K.D., & Mayhew, J.L. (1988). Comparison of three methods of assessing strength imbalances at the knee. *Journal of Orthopedic Sport, Medicine and Physical Therapy*, **10**(4), 134-138.

115. Osternig, L.R. (1986). Isokinetic dynamometry: Implications for muscle testing and rehabilitation. In K.B. Pandolf (Ed.), *Exercise and sport science reviews* (Vol. 14) (pp. 45-104). New York: MacMillan Publishing.

116. Osternig, L.R., Sawhill, J.A., Bates, B.J., & Hamill, J. (1983). Function of limb speed on torque patterns of antagonistic muscles. In H. Matsui & K. Kobayashi (Eds.), *Biomechanics VIII-A* (pp. 251-257). Champaign, IL: Human Kinetics.

117. Patteson, M.E., Nelson, S.G., & Duncan, P.W. (1984). Effects of stabilizing the non-tested lower extremity during isokinetic evaluation of the quadriceps and hamstrings. *Journal of Orthopedic Sport, Medicine and Physical Therapy*, **6**(1), 18-20.

118. Patton, J.F., Kraemer, W.J., Knuttgen, H.G., & Harman, E.A. (1990). Factors in maximal power production and in exercise endurance relative to maximal power. *European Journal of Applied Physiology*, **60**, 222-227.

119. Poulmedis, P. (1985). Isokinetics maximal torque power of Greek elite soccer players. *Journal of Orthopedic Sport, Medicine and Physical Therapy*, **6**(5), 293-295.

120. Rankin, J.M., & Thompson, C.B. (1983). Isokinetic evaluation of quadriceps and hamstring function: Normative data concerning body weight and sport. *Athletic Training*, **18**, 110-113.

121. Rizzardo, M., Bay, G., & Wessel, J. (1988). Eccentric and concentric torque and power of the knee extensors. *Canadian Journal of Sport Sciences*, **13**(2), 166-169.

122. Rose, K., & Ball, T.E. (1992). A field test for predicting maximum bench press lift of college women. *Journal of Applied Sport Science Research*, **6**(2), 103-106.

123. Rutherford, O.M., Greig, C.A., Sargeant, A.J., & Jones, D.A. (1986). Strength training and power output transference effects in the human quadriceps muscle. *Journal of Sports Sciences*, **4**, 101-107.

124. Rutherford, O.M., & Jones, D.A. (1986). The role of learning and coordination in strength training. *European Journal of Applied Physiology*, **55**, 100-105.

125. Safran, M.R., Garrett, W.E., Seaber, A.V., Glisson, R.R., & Ribbeck, B.M. (1988). The role of warm-up in muscular injury prevention. *American Journal of Sports Medicine*, **16**(2), 123.

126. Sailors, M., & Berg, K. (1987). Comparison of responses to weight training in pubescent boys and men. *Journal of Sports Medicine and Physical Fitness*, **27**, 30-38.

127. Sale D., & Delman, A. (1983). Fatigability in young men and women during weight lifting exercise. *Medicine and Science in Sports and Exercise*, **15**, 146.

128. Sale, D.G. (1988). Neural adaptation to resistance training. *Medicine and Science in Sports and Exercise*, **20**(5) (Suppl.), S135-S145.

129. Sale, D.G., & MacDougall, J.D. (1979). Effect of strength training upon motoneuron excitability of man. *Medicine and Science in Sports*, **11**(1), 77.

130. Sale, D.G., & Norman, R.W. (1982). Testing strength and power. In J.D. MacDaugall, H.A. Wenger, & H.J. Green (Eds.), *Physiological testing of the elite athlete* (pp. 7-37). Ithaca, NY: Mouvement Publications.

131. Sapega, A.A., Nicholas, J.A., Sokolow, D., & Saraniti, A. (1982). The nature of torque overshoot

in Cybex isokinetic dynamometry. *Medicine and Science in Sports and Exercise*, **14**, 368-375.

132. Seger, J.Y., Westing, S.H., Hanson, M., Karlson, E., & Ekblom, B. (1988). A new dynamometer measuring concentric and eccentric muscle strength in accelerated, decelerated, or isokinetic movements. *Journal of Applied Physiology*, **57**, 526-550.

133. Shankman, G.A. (1984). Training related injuries in progressive resistance exercise programs. *National Strength and Conditioning Association Journal*, **6**(4), 36-37.

134. Sharp, M.A., Harman, E., Vogel, J.A., Knapik, J.J., & Legg, S.J. (1988). Maximal aerobic capacity for repetitive lifting: Comparison with three standard exercise testing modes. *European Journal of Applied Physiology*, **57**, 753-760.

135. Smidt, G.L., Albright, J.P., & Densingerm, R.H. (1984). Pre- and postoperative functional changes in total knee patients. *Journal of Orthopedic Sport, Medicine and Physical Therapy*, **6**(1), 25-29.

136. Smith, T.K. (1984). Preadolescent strength training: Some considerations. *Journal of Physical Education, Recreation and Dance*, **80**, 43-44.

137. Stone, M., & O'Bryant, H. (1987). *Weight training: A scientific approach*. Minneapolis: Bellwether Press.

138. Thomas, L. (1984). Isokinetic torque levels for adult females: Effects of age and body size. *Journal of Orthopedic Sport, Medicine and Physical Therapy*, **6**, 21-24.

139. Thomeé, R., Renström, P., Grimby, G., & Peterson, L. (1987). Slow or fast isokinetic training after knee ligament surgery. *Journal of Orthopedic Sport, Medicine and Physical Therapy*, **8**(10), 495-499.

140. Thomson, D.B., & Chapman, A.E. (1988). The mechanical response of active human muscle during and after stretch. *European Journal of Applied Physiology*, **57**, 691-697.

141. Thomson, R., Fix, B., White, P., Moran, R., Longo, P., Van Haianger, D., & Rhode, B. (1989). Roundtable: Safe facility design and standards for safe equipment. *National Strength and Conditioning Association Journal*, **11**(3), 14-22.

142. Thorstensson, A., Grimby, G., & Karlsson, J. (1976). Force-velocity relations and fiber composition in human knee extensor muscles. *Journal of Applied Physiology*, **40**, 12-16.

143. Viitasalo, J.T., Era, P., Leskinen, A.L., & Häkkinen K. (1985). Muscular strength profiles and anthropometry in random samples of men aged 31-35, 51-55 and 71-75 years. *Ergonomics*, **28**(11), 1563-1574.

144. Walmsley, R.P., & Szybbo, C. (1987). A comparative study of the torque generated by the shoulder internal and external rotator muscles in different positions and by varying speeds. *Journal of Orthopedic Sport, Medicine and Physical Therapy*, **9**(6), 217-222.

145. Wathen, D., Borden, R., Dunn, B., Everson, J., Gieck, J., Hill, B., Klein, K., O'Shea, J.P., & Stone, M. (1983). Prevention of athletic injuries through strength training and conditioning. *National Strength and Conditioning Association Journal*, **5**(2), 14-19.

146. Weltman, R., Tippett, S., Janney, C., Strand, K., Rians, C., Cahill, B.R., & Katch, F.I. (1988). Measurement of isokinetic strength in prepubertal males. *Journal of Orthopedic Sport, Medicine and Physical Therapy*, **9**(10), 345-351.

147. Westing, S.H., Seager, J.Y., Karlson, E., & Ekblom, B. (1988). Eccentric and concentric torque-velocity characteristics of the quadriceps femoris in man. *European Journal of Applied Physiology*, **58**, 100-104.

148. Winter, D.A., Wells, R.P., & Orr, G.W. (1981). Errors in the use of isokinetic dynamometers. *European Journal of Applied Physiology*, **46**, 397-408.

149. Zemper, E.D. (1990). Weightroom safety: Four year study of weightroom injuries in a national sample of college football teams. *National Strength and Conditioning Association Journal*, **12**(3), 32-34.

CHAPTER 9

Skeletal Muscle Structure and Function

William J. Fink, MA
David L. Costill, PhD

Ball State University

One of the critical steps in the development of exercise physiology was the development of the percutaneous needle biopsy technique of Duchenne, which was adopted by Bergstrom in 1962 (1). This technique allowed the direct study of human skeletal muscle metabolism with a relatively easy (and surprisingly nontraumatic) method. Early studies with this technique focused on muscle glycogen metabolism and on the fundamental structure of human skeletal muscle. The range and depth of studies possible with this technique are summarized in the text *Muscle Metabolism During Exercise* edited by Bengt Pernow and Bengt Saltin in 1971 (2). Beginning in the early 1970s, following a sabbatical visit to Scandinavia, we have had a significant interest in the study of human skeletal muscle metabolism. The laboratory techniques that we have accumulated, modified, or developed are detailed at some length in our own laboratory manual *Analytical Methods for the Measurement of Human Performance* (22). This chapter includes edited versions of some of these techniques, which may serve as a convenient starting point for investigators interested in skeletal muscle physiology.

MUSCLE BIOPSY PROCEDURE

The following account is intended to provide a verbal description of the needle biopsy technique. Because this procedure requires some minor surgery, it should be performed by a physician or under medical supervision. With care and proper direction to the subject, there is little distress associated with this procedure. Nevertheless, it is important to develop good rapport with the subject and to describe the procedure in enough detail that the subject can anticipate moments of discomfort.

Generally, samples are obtained from muscles that have few large blood vessels or nerves.

Equipment and Reagents:
Biopsy needles, 4 to 5 mm, catalog numbers 6625-14 and 6625-18 (DuPuy Manufacturing, PO Box 988, Warsaw, IN 46580; telephone (219) 267-8143)
Xylocaine with epinephrine, 1%
Surgical prep (e.g., Betadine)
3-cc sterile syringes
25-gauge, 0.5 to 0.75-in. (or finer) sterile needles
No. 11 sterile scalpel blades

4 in. × 4 in. sterile gauze
Adhesive bandages
Clippers
Razor

The muscles most frequently sampled are the gastrocnemius, vastus lateralis, and third deltoid. To locate the site for each incision, we ask the subject to contract the muscle so that we define the thickest portion of the muscle and identify the proper site for entry into the muscle.

After all of the hair from the skin over the proposed incision is removed, the skin is cleaned with surgical prep. A local anesthetic (xylocaine) is injected into a small area about 3 cm in diameter through three or four punctures. The total amount of xylocaine required should not exceed 1.5 cc. Portions of the xylocaine should be injected under the fascia and into the superficial layers of the skin (not deep into the muscle). The epinephrine in the xylocaine will reduce bleeding in the skin. The procedure causes some burning and mild stinging, so forewarn the subject.

The scalpel blade is used to make a 1-cm incision through the skin and fascia. Pressure is immediately applied to the area with sterile gauze until all bleeding is stopped. Prior to the taking of the biopsy, the subject is instructed to keep the muscle as relaxed as possible and to be aware that he or she will feel an unusual pressure in the muscle and a slight tendency for the muscle to cramp.

With the needle notch closed (cutting blade closed), the biopsy needle is inserted into the incision and the tip pressed lightly against the fascia. The needle point is moved across the fascia until the incision in the fascia is located. The needle is inserted about 0.5 cm into the muscle, then the needle's shaft is inclined so that the needle can be fully introduced into the belly of the muscle. The angle of entry should be perpendicular to the length of the muscle fibers, with the needle notch oriented upward so that the muscle fibers can fill the notch. The needle is inserted deep enough to insure that the *entire notch* is inside the muscle. The needle should enter with little resistance and without discomfort to the subject. The needle should not be inserted into a contracted muscle. If the subject tenses up, talk him or her into relaxing the muscle before the procedure continues.

Once the needle is in position, the blade is drawn back to open the notch and then closed sharply. Often two cuts are made. After the second cut, the blade is held down (notch closed) and the needle withdrawn quickly. The time required to insert the needle, cut the sample, and withdraw the needle is generally 5 to 10 s. Better samples are obtained, however, if suction is applied to the needle as the muscle is cut (3). This is done by fitting a large syringe (≥ 20 cc) with a rubber tube and a tip that will insert into the end of the biopsy needle. Once the needle is positioned in the muscle and the notch opened, an assistant pulls suction on the syringe while the physician makes the cut. Once the cut is made, the suction is relaxed and the needle withdrawn. This method can increase four- or fivefold the size of the muscle piece obtained.

When the needle is withdrawn, pressure is applied directly over the incision with a sterile gauze. We have found that if the pressure is maintained for 10 to 20 min, all bleeding can be stopped. The degree of soreness experienced by the subject following this procedure is related to the amount of bleeding into the biopsy site.

If multiple biopsies are to be taken from the same muscle (e.g., before and after exercise), the needle may be inserted in the same incision but angled away from the previous biopsy. For biopsies from the same muscle taken hours or days after the first, a new incision should be made about 3 cm away from the original site. When it is necessary to biopsy the muscle immediately after an exercise bout on a cycle ergometer, the leg must be prepped and the incision made before the bout begins. At the end of exercise, the subject immediately puts the leg up on a stool or similar support and leans back into the arms of an assistant. Another assistant quickly removes the pressure bandage over the incision, and the physician takes the biopsy, immediately putting the muscle sample into a container of liquid nitrogen.

Biopsies taken at rest should be taken from a position where the muscle is under the least stretch. This is important because a smooth biopsy depends on a relaxed muscle. For the vastus lateralis this might be a seated position with the foot on the floor. But because it is not a good idea to have the subject sitting up and watching the procedure, this biopsy is usually done with the subject lying down with the leg out straight. With some subjects it is helpful to lightly brace the foot if it wants to fall over. For the gastrocnemius muscle, the subject lies prone with the lower leg and foot elevated on a cushion. For the deltoid, the subject is seated and usually extends the arm laterally and horizontally, resting it on a support.

After the biopsy, the incision is pulled closed with adhesive bandages and the subject is instructed not to remove them for 3 days. If exercise is to be performed after a biopsy, a gauze/tape pressure bandage should be applied over the adhesive bandages. In any case, a pressure bandage is kept over the band-aids for the first day. In our experience, adhesive bandages work better than steristrips for closing the incision, because steristrips are more likely to pull the skin loose, creating a very sore skin burn.

HANDLING AND WEIGHING OF TISSUE

Tissue samples can be handled and weighed at room temperature. Start a watch when the sample is removed from the needle and weigh the sample for 1-min intervals (30 s is adequate, times 2 to make a minute). Because the tissue evaporates water at a constant rate, these repeated weights can be used to compute the muscle's weight at the time it was removed from the needle. This calculation is as follows:

$$W_0 = [(W_1 - W_2) \times T_1] + W_1$$

where W_1 is the first weight recorded, W_2 is the second weight recorded (1 min after W_1), T_1 is the time of the first weight measurement (min) at W_1, and W_0 is the muscle weight at zero time. Subtract pan weight if one was used.

Having been weighed, the samples are frozen in liquid nitrogen and stored at −80 °C or directly in the liquid nitrogen. Samples that must be analyzed fresh are immediately homogenized as described in the specific method.

For many assays the slight weight loss to evaporation while the muscle sample is removed from the needle, cleaned, and sectioned is insignificant, and the muscle may more conveniently be frozen immediately in liquid nitrogen for later weighing in a freezer.

Muscle stored in liquid nitrogen should be put in vials that are vented in order to avoid the vials' exploding, when they are removed from storage, because of the rapid warming of any liquid nitrogen trapped inside. Cryotubes (Vangard International, Neptune, NJ) are self-venting and work very well. Other vials will need to be vented with a small hole before use. If the muscle is kept on dry ice or in a freezer at −80 °C, the vials should be airtight.

CONVENIENT FORMULAS: MIXING AND DILUTING

For simplicity, most muscle tissue studies are conducted with convenient dilutions to produce volumes that are easy to work with and provide results in the range of conventional laboratory instrumentation. Because basic laboratory methods for mixing chemicals are not otherwise reviewed in this book, we have included some formulas and methods we find useful.

Mixing a Solution of Molarity and Volume From a Solid

To mix a solution of a given *molarity* and *volume* from a solid, use this equation:

molecular weight × desired molarity
× volume in liters = grams of substance
to be weighed out and dissolved in chosen volume

For example, to mix 50 ml of a 0.05-M Tris base,

consider that Tris base has a molecular weight of 121.1. Fifty milliliters is the same as 0.05 L. Therefore, 121.1 × 0.05 M × 0.05 L = 0.30275 g. Weigh out this amount and dissolve it in the total *final* volume of 50 ml.

Note that other definitions and formulas should be apparent.

Molarity (M) = moles/liter
mM = mmol × L^{-1}
mol = g/M.W. or M × L
mmol = mg/M.W. or mM × L

Examples: 1 mol of Tris base = 121.1 g.
1 mmol of Tris base = 0.121 g or 121.1 mg.

One milliliter (0.001 L) of a 1-M solution contains 0.001 mol, which is the same as 1 mmol.

It should be noted, therefore, that

ml × M = mmoles
ml × mM = μmoles
mmol/ml = M
μmol/ml = mM

Mixing a Solution of Molarity and Volume From Liquid

To mix a solution of a given *molarity* and *volume* from liquid stock, use this equation:

(desired molarity/stock molarity)
× desired volume = volume of stock to be
diluted to desired volume

For example, to mix 50 ml of a 0.05-M Tris base from a 1-M stock, (0.05 M/1 M) × 50 ml = 2.5 ml of stock brought to a total volume of 50 ml.

The terms of expression in this formula must be uniform. If we express the desired concentration in molarity, we must express the stock concentration in molarity. If we wish to measure the volume in milliliters, we must read the calculated amount of stock to be diluted in milliliters. If we choose to calculate a desired concentration of 50 mM, then a 1-M stock concentration must be expressed as 1,000 mM.

Dilutions

The previous formula is a simple dilution formula. It is useful in setting up recipes for reagent cocktails (solutions containing several active ingredients of known concentrations) so that stocks, final concentrations, and volumes are clear and easily adaptable to the needs of an assay and the capabilities of the laboratory. Thus, many biochemical assays are set up as shown in Table 9.1.

Table 9.1 Example of a Biochemical Assay

Reagent	Stock concentration	Final concentration	Volume of stock to make: 25 ml	Volume of stock to make: 50 ml
ATP	100 mM	0.3 mM	0.075 ml	0.15 ml
HK	1000 U/ml	1 U/ml	0.025 ml	0.05 ml

It is always best to begin mixing the reagent cocktail by adding the ingredients to a volume of water a little less than the desired final volume, and to begin by adding the buffer ingredients (e.g., the Tris base and the HCl).

Dilution Factors

It is often very helpful to derive the dilution factor involved in the preparation of a sample. If, for example, 25 μL of stock is diluted in 10 ml of cocktail, this gives a dilution factor of 400. That is, 10 ml/0.025 ml = 400. The volume of stock constitutes 1/400th of the total volume. The final concentration of the ingredient in the cocktail is also 1/400th of the stock concentration: 100 mM/400 = 0.25 mM.

Likewise, we are often required to dilute biological materials one or more times in the course of an analysis. If we are asked to dilute a sample 20 times, for example, that means we must make the sample 1/20th of some chosen convenient volume. To do that in 1 ml (1 ml/20 = 0.05 ml), 50 μL of sample would be brought to a total volume of 1 ml.

In practice, however, it is usually much more convenient to add 50 μL to 1 ml. In this case, the dilution is actually 21 (1.05 ml/0.05 ml = 21). As can be seen, what is more important than pipetting numerically even dilutions is to keep track of them. It should be noted, then, that the dilution factor is figured by dividing the total volume by the sample volume.

dilution factor = total volume/sample volume

It is this dilution factor that is so often needed to calculate back to original concentrations or activities in biological material. If 0.5 ml of serum is extracted with 1 ml of 1-M acid, it is diluted three times: 1.5 ml total volume/0.5 ml sample volume.

If 1 ml of this is drawn off and neutralized with 0.5 ml of 2-M base, it is diluted another 1.5 times: 1.5 ml total volume/1 ml sample volume.

The total dilution factor would be the product of these: $(1.5/0.5) \times (1.5/1) = 4.5$.

Thus, the extract of serum to be used in various analyses, which may call for further dilutions, is 4.5 times more dilute than the serum itself.

Dilutions of muscle tissue are made on the *assumption* that 1 g by weight is equivalent to 1 ml by volume. Thus, a 20-fold dilution of muscle means there is 1 part muscle and 19 parts homogenizing buffer. One gram of tissue would be diluted and homogenized in 19 ml of buffer. A 1:100 dilution of 15 mg of human muscle would be 0.015 grams × 99 = 1.485 ml.

In other assays, it is important to know the actual weight of muscle contained in a small volume of muscle homogenate. This is simply a matter of dividing the weight of the muscle by the volume in which it is homogenized. In this regard, it is helpful to remember that:

a 1:1,000 dilution = 1 μg/μL
a 1:100 dilution = 10 μg/μL
a 1:50 dilution = 20 μg/μL

MIXING SIMPLE BUFFERS

A buffer is most easily described as a solution that resists a change in pH. Its importance in biochemistry is its ability to maintain an optimal acid–base condition for a given procedure. It does this by exerting a moderating control on the free hydrogen ion concentration, $[H^+]$ (actually H_3O), in the solution, for it is the free hydrogen ion concentraiton (measured in molarity) that determines the pH. pH by definition is the negative log of this hydrogen ion concentration—a *negative* log because it is the common logarithm of a number less than 1.

The log of 10 is 1.
The log of 1 is 0.
The log of 0.5 is −.301.
The log of 0.00005 is −4.301.

(A calculator comes in handy here.)

Thus, a solution that has a free hydrogen concentration of 1×10^{-7} M has a log of −7 and a pH of 7. Because the *p* in the expression means "negative log," the minus sign is omitted when stating a pH value. It should be apparent, then, that pH values are usually applied to rather dilute solutions, because a solution whose free hydrogen concentration is 1 M would have a pH of zero. It should also be kept in mind that in order to convert the pH back into a hydrogen ion concentration, one must take the antilog of the *negative* number. For example, the hydrogen ion concentration of a solution whose pH is 7.4 is not 2.51×10^7, but 3.98×10^{-8} M.

Let us return to buffers. To understand how a buffer exerts a moderating control on the free hydrogen concentration, it is necessary to take a look at how free hydrogen is produced in certain systems. What is basic to this notion is to understand that various compounds in a water solution have a characteristic ionization or dissociation, where all or part of certain hydrogens will separate from their conjugate groups and form H_3O, or what is called free hydrogen.

If a chemical compound dissociates completely, it is called a strong acid (or strong base).

$$HCl \rightarrow H^+ + Cl^-$$
$$NaOH \rightarrow Na^+ + OH^-$$

If the chemical compound does not dissociate completely, it is called a weak acid (or weak base), and the extent of the dissociation is expressed by a constant ratio of products to reactants (K). Thus, acetic acid dissociates partially and is described as

$$K = [H^+][Oac^-]/[HOac] = 1.8 \times 10^{-5}$$

Each acid has its characteristic constant, which is determined experimentally and can be found in various chemical handbooks. By rearranging the previous equation, we see that

$$[H^+] = [HOac]/[Oac^-] \times K$$

If this solution had equal concentrations of acid and base, the hydrogen ion concentration would equal the constant ($[H^+] = 1 \times K$), and the pH would be the negative log of that number. With the pure acid (HOac), however, the concentration of conjugate base (Oac^-) nowhere equals the concentration of acid (but it does equal the concentration of free hydrogen). If we have a 0.1-M acetic acid, the concentrations of free hydrogen and conjugate base can be easily determined from the dissociation constant. The acid dissociates into equal molar concentrations of hydrogen and conjugate base, an amount that must be subtracted from the original concentration of acid.

$$[HOac] \rightarrow [H^+] [Oac^-]/[HOac] = K = 1.8 \times 10^{-5}$$

The free hydrogen = x; the conjugate base = x; HOac = $0.1 - x$.

$(x)(x)/(0.1 - x) = 1.8 \times 10^{-5}$
(Ignore the x in the denominator.)
$x^2/0.1 = 1.8 \times 10^{-5}$
$x^2 = 1.8 \times 10^{-6}$
(Take the square root.)
$x = 1.34 \times 10^{-3}$
(This equals the free hydrogen and conjugate base molar concentrations.)

If we take the log of that number, pH = 2.87.

Note that an accurate solution to this problem would require solving a quadratic equation, but a workable approximation can be had by ignoring the x in the denominator; its value, compared to the concentration of acid, is insignificant. This can be done whenever the difference between the concentration of the acid and the value of K is at least 10^3. On the other hand, the dissociation characteristics are most ideal when the acid is most dilute.

Salt Buffers

At any rate, to create a buffer, more conjugate base must be added to the acid. This is often done by adding the salt of the acid—sodium acetate (NaOac), for example. Because most salts dissociate completely, the amount of conjugate base added would be the same as the concentration of salt added. Now it is possible to mix a solution that has a concentration of conjugate base (Oac^-) approching that of the acid (HOac). This provides a system that exerts a moderating control of pH by being able to form more conjugated acid from any hydrogen (e.g., HCl) that is added. These buffer systems follow precise characteristics, which are best described by the Henderson-Hasselbalch equation, developed by taking the log of both sides of the equation $[H^+] = \dfrac{[Acid]}{[Base]} \times K$:

$$pH = pK + \log [Base]/[Acid]$$

The pK is the log of the dissociation constant. As we indicated indirectly in the previous section, when the acid and conjugate base are equal molar concentrations, the free hydrogen concentration equals the dissociation constant. Thus, the pH also equals the pK. It is at this value that a given buffer is most effective.

What is said here of "salt" buffers (acetic acid–sodium acetate, NaH_2PO_4–Na_2HPO_4) is also true of the more modern synthetic buffers like Tris, MOPS, HEPES, and TES. Here HCl or NaOH, a strong acid or base, is added to the buffer until the proper ratio of base form and acid form is produced. In fact, acetic acid (HOac) and sodium hydroxide (NaOH) will create a proper salt buffer, too, because the strong base has the effect of producing more conjugate base (Oac^-) from the acid. Table 9.2 provides some convenient pK values for frequently used buffers, as well as the molar concentrations of some common concentrated acids.

Let's look at two examples: A phosphate buffer is made by mixing acid phosphate, NaH_2PO_4, and basic phosphate, Na_2HPO_4. The equilibrium that is most active, and the one we are interested in, is

Table 9.2 PK Values and Concentrations for Frequently Used Buffers and Acids

Useful pK's (approx.) for buffers

Acetate	4.76
2-amino-2-methyl-1-propanol	9.90
Carbonate	10.36
Glycine, K_2	9.74
Glycylglycine	8.21
HEPES	7.48
Hydrazine	8.23
Imidazole	7.07
MOPS	7.01
Phosphate, K_2	7.12
TEA	7.80
TES	7.44
Tris	8.10

Normality of concentrated acids

Acetic	17.0
Hydrochloric	12.0
Nitric, 68%	15.0
Perchloric, 70%	11.6
Sulfuric	36.0

$$H_2PO_4 \rightarrow H^+ + HPO_4$$

The pK of a 0.1-M phosphate solution is 6.8. If we want a buffer with a pH of 7.4, we simply apply the Henderson-Hasselbalch equation.

$$pH = pK + \log [base]/[acid]$$
$$7.4 = 6.8 + \log [base]/[acid]$$
$$0.6 = \log [base]/[acid]$$

The antilog of 0.6 = 4 (approximately). The ratio of base to acid is then 4:1, which means there is a total of 5 parts. If the desired concentration of buffer is 0.1 M, then

$$4/5 \times 0.1 M = 0.08\text{-M base}$$
$$1/5 \times 0.1 M = 0.02\text{-M acid}$$

Now a particular volume of this could be mixed in various ways. An appropriate amount of each salt could be weighed out to mix a certain volume of buffer with these concentrations of base and acid, or 0.1-M solutions of each salt could be mixed and added in volumes 4 parts base to 1 part acid. To make 100 ml,

$$4/5 \times 100 \text{ ml} = 80 \text{ ml Na}_2\text{HPO}_4$$
$$1/5 \times 100 \text{ ml} = 20 \text{ ml Na}_2\text{HPO}_4$$

This last method is the most convenient and allows the buffer to be adjusted easily with a pH meter to an exact pH.

Tris Buffer

Tris has a pK of 8.1. This buffer can be purchased in the pure base form and several acid forms. Each, then, could be weighed out, or mixed and added together by volume as we have described. But it is much more convenient to add HCl to Tris base, thus forcing Tris into whatever ratio of acid to base is desired.

To mix a Tris buffer with a pH of 8.5,

$$pH = pK + \log [base]/[acid]$$
$$8.5 = 8.1 + \log [base]/[acid]$$
$$0.4 = \log [base]/[acid]$$
$$\text{antilog of } 0.4 = 2.5$$

Therefore, the ratio of base to acid is 2.5:1, and there is a total of 3.5 parts.

To make a 0.1-M Tris buffer,

$$2.5/3.5 \times 0.1 M = 0.07\text{-M base}$$
$$1/3.5 \times 0.1 M = 0.03\text{-M acid}$$

To make 100 ml of this buffer, we would most conveniently mix a 0.1-M Tris base and add enough HCl to make the same volume 0.03 M in acid. This kind of mixing is best done from previously mixed stock solutions so that mixing the buffer is simply a matter of making the appropriate dilutions. If we used 1-M stocks,

$$0.1 M/1 M \times 100 \text{ ml} = 10 \text{ ml Tris base}$$
$$0.03 M/1 M \times 100 \text{ ml} = 3 \text{ ml HCl}$$

These volumes are added to water and adjusted to a final volume of 100 ml.

Note that this 0.1-M Tris is 0.1 M in *total* Tris but only 0.07 M in Tris base. Any acid that may be added, as in perchloric acid (PCA) extract, contributes to a concentration that must be subtracted from 0.07 M, *not* from 0.1 M, and added to the 0.03 M to establish the new ratio of base to acid.

If, for example, we were working with 1 ml of the buffer described, 0.1-M Tris with a pH of 8.5, and add to it 10 μL of a 1-M PCA extract, what happens to the pH? Originally, we have a base to acid ratio of 0.07-M base/0.03-M acid.

Ten μL of 1-M PCA added to this 1 ml of Tris buffer (ignoring the slight change in volume) effectively makes this another 0.01 M in acid. The new ratio would be $(0.07 - 0.01)/(0.03 + 0.01) = 0.06/0.04 = 1.5$.

The new pH would be:

$$pH = pK + \log [base]/[acid]$$
$$pH = 8.1 + \log 1.5$$
$$pH = 8.1 + 0.176$$
$$pH = 8.276$$

It should be noted, then, that adding 25 μL of a 1-M PCA extract to 1 mL of a 0.05-M Tris buffer with a pH of 8.1 would destroy the buffer. At that pH the pH equals the pK, and the 0.05-M Tris is actually 0.025 M in both acid and base. Adding 25 μL of 1-M acid would make the 1-ml volume another 0.025 M in acid—in other words, converting all of the 0.05-M Tris into its acid form.

CALIBRATION OF THE FLUOROMETER

Because the coenzymes NAD-NADH and NADP-NADPH participate in many biochemical reactions or can be linked to them through a sequence of enzymatic steps, their measurement provides an easy and flexible means of determining both substrate concentrations and enzyme activities.

Spectrophotometer Measures of NAD-NADH (NADP-NADPH)

NADH or NADPH can be measured on both the spectrophotometer and the fluorometer because they absorb light at 340 nm (where NAD and NADP do not) and fluorescent light at about 460 nm (where NAD and NADP do not). The fluorometer, however, is much more sensitive than the spectrophotometer because the absorbance of light is dependent upon the concentration of NADH or NADPH, whereas the fluorescence of light depends far more on the intensity of the exciting light.

Because of the Lambert-Beer law, we can determine the concentration of NADH/NADPH directly on the spectrophotometer. All we need to know is the molar extinction coefficient of NADH/NADPH at a wavelength of 340 nm in a light path of 1 cm. This has been determined experimentally in several laboratories and is taken to be 6,270, 6,220, or 6,200, depending on whom you read. What this means is that a 1-M concentration of NADH or NADPH would have an absorbance of 6,270 at a wavelength of 340 nm. Such a high absorbance is impossible to read on a spectrophotometer, however. Nevertheless, this number serves as a standard in calculating the concentration of more dilute samples. Consequently, the absorbance of any sample of NADH or NADPH will reveal its concentration.

For example, if absorbance = 0.500, then concentration = 0.500/6220 = 0.0000804 M, or 0.0804 mM.

This method is used in calculating the concentration of an NADH/NADPH solution because it is far more accurate than weighing out and dissolving NADH/NADPH. (The purity and stability of a given package of NADH/NADPH is never accurately known.)

Fluorometer Measures

To use the fluorometer to measure the concentration of NADH/NADPH, the instrument must first be calibrated with a known concentration (or a dilution thereof) determined on the spectrophotometer. (Remember that the fluorometer does not read concentration directly, as a spectrophotometer does, but only under set conditions of light intensity, temperature, sample volume, etc.) Therefore, follow these steps:

1. Dissolve a small pinch of NADH (2 to 3 mg) in about 1 ml of alkaline buffer, pH 7.5 to 9.0. Shield from the light.
2. Zero and span the spectrophotometer at 340 nm with the buffer alone.
3. Add a precise amount of NADH solution (e.g., 100 μL) to a precise volume of buffer (e.g., 3 ml).
4. Read absorbance.
5. Calculate the concentration (see the following example):

$$absorbance = 0.500$$
$$concentration\ in\ the\ cuvette = 0.500/6.22$$
$$= 0.804\ mM$$
$$concentration\ of\ your\ stock = (0.500/6.22) \times$$
$$(total\ vol.\ in\ ml)/$$
$$(sample\ vol.\ in\ ml)$$
$$= (0.500/6.22) \times$$
$$(3.1/0.1)$$
$$= 2.49\ mM$$

6. Read the initial fluorescence of a known volume (e.g., 1 ml) of your buffer under your chosen conditions. That is, adjust the fluorometer for the aperture and range settings you are going to work with. For most standard work this would probably be the smallest aperture with a range setting of 0.1. (Not all fluorometers have range settings.)
7. Add a precise quantity of NADH solution, or a known dilution thereof, to the tube with the buffer. Mix.
8. Read the fluorescence.
9. Perform the calculations: Subtract the initial fluorescence from the final fluorescence, or blank the initial fluorescence of the buffer to zero. Then determine the μM concentration, or the number of micromoles that this fluorescence corresponds to. This fluorescence becomes your standard fluorescence. For example, 25 μL (0.025 ml) of a 0.080-mM NADH solution equals 0.002 μmol. (Note that ml times mM equals μmol.) If this gives a fluorescence of 10, your standard is 10 for that amount of NADH. On a more sensitive range or with more light, it may give a fluorescence of 100.

Notes on Fluorometers

When choosing a filter, remember that although the absorption maximum for NADH/NADPH is 340 nm, the usual excitation line chosen for the fluorometer is ≈ 360 nm. The primary filter used to work in this range (355-365 nm) is either glass number 5840 (filter 7-60) or glass number 5860 (filter 7-37). The fluorescence emission is ≈ 460 nm, and the secondary filters chosen for this line are usually the combination of glass number 3387 (yellow filter 3-72) and glass number 4303 (blue-green filter 4-72). The yellow filter is slightly fluorescent and is placed closest to the photocell. Some will use glass number 4308 (filter 4-70) instead of filter 4-72. The Turner fluorometer numbers for the secondary filters are 2A (yellow) and 48 (blue-green).

Most of the biochemical assays to be done on the fluorometer are most conveniently done in 1-ml volumes. This means that your fluorometer should be equipped to read 10 × 75 mm tubes. These tubes must be made of borosilicate glass. Soda lime glass tubes have a high fluorescence of their own that makes them unsuitable for use.

The fluorescence of NADH/NADPH is greatly affected by temperature, decreasing as the solutions warm up. For kinetic assays that require the sample to be in the fluorometer for some minutes, it is necessary to have some kind of temperature control system on the instrument. Assays that call for only quick readings can be done quickly, but do not leave the tube in the instrument long enough for the temperature to start rising.

HISTOCHEMICAL PREPARATION

The sectioning of frozen tissue is much quicker than the preparation of paraffin sections, and it leaves alive those enzymes that are the basis of some of the metabolic stains of interest. The principal concern in the freeze mounting of tissue is to avoid freeze artifact, which is the disruption of the tissue caused by the formation of ice crystals during freezing.

To avoid freeze artifact, the tissue must be frozen evenly without the formation of ice crystals. Although this can be done without liquid nitrogen (-190 °C), there are other reasons why it is advisable to freeze the small muscle mount as quickly as possible, not the least of which is the practical problem of freezing a cross-section of muscle before it falls over. This is usually done with liquid nitrogen, but if the muscle mount is plunged directly into liquid nitorgen, the gas evolved from the boiling nitrogen will form an insulating layer

around the tissue that will produce artifact. To overcome this problem, an organic compound with a low freezing point is cooled over the liquid nitrogen to the point where it begins to freeze. Freon (CCl_2F_2) or isopentane (2-methylbutane) are most often used for this, Freon having a freezing point of -150 °C and isopentane one of -160 °C. Both of these will drop to their freezing points without becoming very viscous, and when the warm piece of muscle is introduced into the nearly frozen organic fluid, its heat is drawn out rapidly without any boiling of the liquid.

Freon has the disadvantage of being more expensive than isopentane and of being a chlorofluorocarbon (a matter of concern for environmentalists), but isopentane carries the risk of being very flammable, having a flash point at room temperature. In our experience this has never been a problem, but we take the precaution of storing it in the freezer.

Equipment and Reagents:
Tragacanth gum (Sigma G-1128) or some form of cryoprotectant such as Ames Tissue-Tek (O.C.T.)
The top half of a size "0" cork
A scalpel with a no. 11 blade, or some such pencil-like instrument with a point that can hold the cork
Liquid nitrogen
A styrofoam container that will hold a moderate amount of liquid nitrogen
A small beaker (~125 ml), preferably metal, that will fit into the stryofoam container on top of the liquid nitrogen
Isopentane
Assorted blades and forceps for cutting the muscle
Cryotubes (Vangard International Inc., 2 ml, no. MS-4503)
A cryostat/microtome
Glass cover slips, 22 × 22 mm
Columbia (cover slip) jars (Thomas Scientific, no. 8542-C32)

Procedure

Once the biopsy is taken, or the muscle is ready to be mounted, pour some liquid nitrogen into the styrofoam container and about 0.5 in. or so of isopentane into the metal beaker. Place the beaker on the liquid nitrogen and allow the isopentane to begin to freeze. As it freezes, it will turn into a white solid. Ideally, it is ready to use when a small puddle of unfrozen isopentane remains at the center of its frozen surroundings.

In preparation for mounting the muscle, a small amount of the tragacanth gum is mixed with water until it forms a workable paste, not so thin that it runs and not so thick that the piece of muscle cannot be stuck into it. The wider end of the cork is affixed to the scalpel and a bit of tragacanth gum is put on the cork.

The muscle is carefully cut and oriented so that the direction of the fibers is clearly visible. Sometimes a magnifying light will help the technician to see this. Then, with a fine forceps, wetted in the tragacanth paste (or other cryoprotectant), the piece of muscle is placed vertically into the mounting medium on the cork and adjusted so that it sits well. There is no need to bury the muscle in the mounting medium. In fact, better sections are obtained if the muscle stands above the paste. Once the muscle is on the cork, it is frozen by being immersed upside-down into the isopentane. This is done rather quickly so that the muscle does not begin to fall over, and it is kept in the isopentane until it is thoroughly frozen. The cork with the mount on it is then removed to liquid nitrogen, placed in a labeled airtight vial (Cryotube), and stored either in liquid nitrogen or at −80 °C. *At no time should the muscle mount be allowed to thaw.*

Sectioning

Not much will be said about the actual sectioning of the muscle sample, because every cryostat/microtome needs to be learned for its own idiosyncrasies. In general, the cork-mounted muscle is affixed to a specimen mount with some mounting medium, the blade of the microtome aligned, and sections cut at 8 to 10 μm. The temperature of the cryostat is about −20 °C. Once the antiroll plate is adjusted, serial sections are picked up on glass cover slips simply by touching them to the muscle section as it lies on the blade. The sections are allowed to air dry at room temperature, then stained according to the procedures for each stain.

A good, sharp, solid blade (knife) is essential. Although this is the age of the disposable blade and automatic knife sharpeners, we have found that the easiest, least expensive, and most successful way to keep a good blade is to sharpen it before each use on an old-fashioned block strop (Baxter Scientific, M-7445). All that is needed is a knife back (Baxter M7225-2), a knife handle (Baxter M7320-1), and the block strop. The sharpening can be done in a matter of minutes, and the results are excellent.

The glass cover slips are placed in a Columbia jar for staining. This is a staining jar made for cover slips that holds only 10 to 12 ml of solution. In the absence of a Columbia jar, the cover slips can be stained in a petri dish.

FIBER TYPING— MYOFIBRILLAR ACTOMYOSIN ATPase

The enzyme ATPase is responsible for catalyzing the breakdown of ATP to ADP and inorganic phosphate (P_i). The histochemical staining for this reaction depends on a series of sequential substitutions that end in a visible product. The tissue section is incubated in a solution continaing ATP and calcium. The ATPase splits off the terminal phosphate from ATP, which reacts immediately with the calcium in the solution to form calcium phosphate. At an alkaline pH the calcium phosphate is insoluble and is deposited at the site of the enzyme activity. The section is then exposed to cobalt chloride, and the cobalt is exchanged for the calcium where the calcium was previously present. Finally, the section is exposed to ammonium sulphide, which results in the formation of a black, insoluble cobaltous sulphide. Thus, the site of the enzyme originally present is demonstrated, and nothing is visible until this last step.

Nomenclature of Fiber Types

Muscle may be clasified into four systems based on different approaches of investigation, and thus the descriptive characteristics of muscle are limited by the approach used by the investigator. Muscle may be classified by

- anatomical appearance, including red vs. white, high vs. low granularity, dark vs. light;
- physiological behavior, including slow vs. fast, high vs. low resistance to fatigue;
- biochemical properties, including high vs. low respiratory capacity, high vs. low enzyme constituents; and
- histochemical features, including high vs. low enzyme content, or the enzyme "profile" of the fiber.

It is obvious that each system of classification overlaps the others. A physiologist examining the twitch characteristics of a muscle can say it is slow or fast, not red or white. A histochemist does not state that a muscle is slow or fast but that the fibers are type I or type II. In fact, however, the fiber in question may be all of these. Statements concerning muscle classification must be examined carefully so as not to conclude more than was actually indicated by the analysis.

Histochemical Manipulation for Fiber Typing: Altering pH

The routine reaction for ATPase is one in which both the preincubation and incubation are carried out at pH 9.4 or, more usually, with the preincubation at pH 10.3. The ATPase of type II fibers is alkaline stable and that of type I fibers is alkaline labile. As a result, type II fibers stain dark and type I fibers remain unstained, leaving a black and white pattern.

This staining pattern is reversed if the preincubation is carried out at a pH of 4.30 to 4.35. In this instance, the type I fibers stain black and type II fibers remain unstained. Occasionally, some type II fibers retain a moderate degree of reactivity at this pH; these are designated type IIC fiber subtypes.

A 5-min preincubation at pH 4.6 elicits a different staining pattern. In this case, the type I fibers stain black as before, but the type II fibers do not stain as a uniform group. The type II fibers that stain white as before are designated type IIA, but there are those that stain dark as the type I fibers do, and these are called type IIB fibers. To distinguish the type I fibers from the type IIB fibers, it is necessary to compare serial sections preincubated at pH 4.3 with those preincubated at pH 4.6.

This staining pattern is sometimes confusing to those who are accustomed to thinking in terms of metabolic stains such as succinate dehydrogenase (SDH) or NADH tetrazolium reductase, where the type I fibers, which are high in respiratory enzymes, stain dark. According to this logic, one would expect the type IIA fibers to stain dark because they are higher in aerobic capacity than type IIB fibers, and the type IIB fibers to stain light. But this is not the case. As it is usually used, the ATPase stain is not a gradient measure of an amount of ATPase present, but an all-or-nothing sort of stain that depends on the activation or inactivation of a type of myofibrillar actomyosin ATPase that is very pH sensitive to the acid or alkaline preincubation.

Occasionally, depending on the muscle, all three types can be differentiated in one stain with a preincubation at a pH of about 4.54. In this case, type I fibers stain dark, type IIA fibers remain unstained, and type IIB fibers stain intermediately with a moderately dark stain. The problem with this is that the pH must be just right for the type of muscle being stained. Sometimes it does not work, and just because no type IIB fibers are visible does not mean they are not there. In practice, it is usually necessary to run preincubations at pH 4.3, 4.54, and 4.6 to see if the stain worked. If it did, the three types will be visible in the pH 4.54 stain. If it did not, the pH 4.54 preincubation will be the same as the pH 4.6 preincubation.

When fiber typing is used to characterize a subject, it is often sufficient to report just the type I (slow twitch) and type II (fast twitch) fiber percentages. In such cases, one stain with a preincubation at either pH 10.3 or pH 4.3 would be sufficient. In human muscle, the type II fibers are normally equally divided between type IIA and type IIB fibers *in untrained muscle*. However, even in moderately trained individuals, we find that all but about 2% of the type II fibers are type IIA.

One will find several variations of this stain in the literature, all trying to simplify the procedure to identify all the fiber types in one stain, or trying to manipulate the preincubation time, pH, or temperature to identify a variety of fiber subtypes. It is important to appreciate how sensitive this staining procedure is to even slight changes in pH, preincubation time, and temperature. The method given here makes use of pH as the principal determinant of the staining pattern. Given a precise pH, muscle preincubated for about 5 min at a standard room temperature (~22 °C) will generally give a consistent staining pattern.

This said, however, it is important to note that a 5-min preincubation at pH 4.3 is enough time to complete the reversal of the staining pattern seen at pH 10.3 and to inactivate some fiber subtypes that might have developed with a much shorter preincubation. Gollnick et al. (4), for instance, have demonstrated three subtypes of type II fibers in rat plantaris muscle early in the acid preincubation as the intensity of the stain moves toward the reversal of the staining pattern seen at pH 10.3. They see this happening when the muscle is preincubated at pH 4.34 for 2 to 3 min at 15 °C, and the time course for this change is much faster and more unpredictable at room temperature. Even so, these three subtypes are not synonymous with the type IIA, IIB, and IIC fibers identified after preincubations at pHs of 10.3, 4.6, and 4.3. All of this points up the importance of identifying fiber types only after the consistent application of a well-defined procedure.

Reagent Preparation

Follow this procedure to prepare the reagent.

1. Prepare the alkaline stock solution by mixing together the following ingredients in about 300 ml of distilled water.

Glycine	2.25 g
Calcium chloride	2.40 g
Sodium chloride	1.76 g
Sodium hydroxide	1.10 g (or ~25 ml of 1-N NaOH)

   Adjust the pH to 9.4 and bring to a final volume of 400 ml. Store in the refrigerator. Freezing will produce an unwanted precipitate.
2. Prepare the alkaline preincubation solution by removing the needed volume of alkaline stock solution and adjusting its pH to 10.3 using 1-N NaOH or 1-N HCl as needed.
3. Prepare the acid preincubation stock solution by mixing together 1.94 g of sodium acetate and 2.94 g of sodium barbital in 100 ml of distilled water. Store in the freezer.
4. To prepare the working acid preincubation solution, for each Columbia jar (~12 ml), mix 2.5 ml

of barbital/acetate stock, 5.0 ml of 0.1-N HCl, and 4.0 ml of H_2O.

Adjust the pH to 4.30, 4.54, or 4.60 with 1-M NCl as necessary. This is easily done by mixing a relatively large volume, adjusting all of it to pH 4.6, pouring off what is needed, and continuing to adjust the next pH, and so on. This should be done with continuous mixing and with a pH meter sensitive to at least 0.01 pH units, preferably to 0.001 pH units. All solutions must be adjusted at the temperature at which they will be used.

5. To prepare the incubation solution, for each Columbia jar (~12 ml), add 17 mg of ATP (e.g., Sigma A 5394) to the alkaline stock and adjust the pH to 9.4. Make enough for all Columbia jars.
6. Mix 500 ml of a 1% calcium chloride solution (1 g/100 ml H_2O). Store at room temperature.
7. Mix 500 ml of a 2% cobalt chloride solution (2 g/100 ml H_2O). Store at room temperature.
8. Right before using, mix a 1% ammonium sulphide solution (0.5 ml concentrated ammonium sulphide to 50 ml H_2O).

Procedure

During preincubation, add the appropriate *acid* pH pre-incubation solution to the sections in their Columbia jar and incubate at room temperature for 5 min. Agitate the jars occasionally. If staining single fibers that have been separated from freeze-dried muscle, increase the preincubation time to 15 min.

Add the *alkaline* preincubation solution to the appropriate jar, agitate slightly, and incubate for 10 to 15 min at room temperature.

Follow these steps during the incubation stage:

1. Pour off the preincubation solution and rinse the sections well with distilled water.
2. Add the incubation ATP solution to each jar and incubate for 45 min at 37 °C.
3. Pour off the incubation solution and rinse well with distilled water.
4. Incubate in the 1% calcium chloride solution for 3 min.
5. Pour off the calcium solution and rinse well with distilled water.
6. Incubate in the 2% cobalt chloride solution for 3 min.
7. Pour off the cobalt solution and rinse well with distilled water.
8. Incubate in the 1% ammonium sulphide solution for 1 min.
9. Pour off the ammonium sulphide solution and rinse well in distilled water.
10. Allow the sections to air dry or dehydrate in ascending alcohols, and clear in xylene. Mount

as usual in Permount or some similar mounting medium. The sections will tend to fade in time, especially if exposed to light.

NADH TETRAZOLIUM REDUCTASE

This stain is a measure of the respiratory capacity of muscle, producing a blue stain proportional to the muscle's ability to process NADH. Because this is done principally in the electron transport chain of the mitochondria, the stain is taken to be a measure of the aerobic capacity of muscle. Besides the mitochondria, it also stains the sarcoplasmic reticulum and transverse tubules, thus defining an intermyofibrillar reticular pattern in cross-sections of muscle fibers, which makes the stain very useful in demonstrating a variety of disruptions of fiber architecture. The indicator reaction of the method is the reduction of a tetrazolium salt (nitro blue tetrazolium, NBT) by NADH. In its oxidized form, NBT is light yellow or colorless in solution, but blue in its reduced form.

$$NBT_{colorless} + NADH \xrightarrow{cytochromes} NBTH_{blue}$$

Reagents
NBT (Sigma N-6876)
NADH (Sigma N-8129)
Tris (Sigma T-1503)
HCl

To stain the fiber, prepare a stock of Tris buffer, 0.2 M, pH 7.4. For every 10 ml of reagent, mix together 2 mg NBT, 8 mg NADH, and 10 ml of Tris buffer.

Incubate for 30 min at 37 °C. Rinse with water, dehydrate in ascending alcohols to xylene, and mount.

This stain is often used together with an ATPase fiber-typing stain to classify fibers. In human muscle, type I fibers will stain dark blue and type II fibers will generally stain light blue. In rodent muscle, the stain is used to help identify the type IIA highly oxidative, fast-twitch fiber (FOG). Because of the effect of aerobic training on the stain and because of the natural gradation in the intensity of the color, it is impossible to use this stain for fiber typing. It is a useful stain, however, for visualizing a number of muscle disorders.

ALPHA-GLYCEROPHOSPHATE DEHYDROGENASE (GLYCEROL-3-PHOSPHATE DEHYDROGENASE)

This stain, like NADH tetrazolium reductase, makes use of nitro blue tetrazolium (NBT), mediated by menodione, as the hydrogen acceptor in the reaction:

$$\text{Glycerol-3-phosphate} + \text{NBT}_{colorless}$$
$$\xrightarrow{\alpha\ GPDH} \text{DHAP} + \text{NBTH}_{blue}$$

It is characteristic of this stain that it produces a staining pattern opposite to that produced by NADH tetrazolium reductase. In other words, the type II fibers tend to stain dark and the type I fibers light. Nevertheless, the gradation of color is somewhat gradual, so this stain is not very useful for fiber typing. It is useful, however, for measuring fiber size, because the fibers are less subject to distortion than they are in ATPase stains.

Reagents
NBT (Sigma N-6876)
Menadione (Sigma M-5625)
Glycerol-3-phosphate (Sigma G-2138)
Tris buffer, 0.2 M, pH 7.4

Prepare a stock of Tris buffer, 0.2 M, pH 7.4, and store in the refrigerator. For every 10 ml of reagent, mix together 30 mg glycerol-3-phosphate, 2 mg NBT, 2 mg menadione, and 10 ml Tris buffer.

The menadione will not dissolve in water, but it is enough that it is broken up and dispersed in solution with a small spatula. Alternatively, it can be dissolved in a small amount (~0.2 ml) of acetone.

Incubate the sections for 45 min in a water bath at 37 °C.

Rinse in distilled water, dehydrate in ascending alcohols to xylene, and mount in Permount.

PERIODIC ACID–SCHIFF STAIN (PAS)

This stain is used to visualize glycols (carbohydrate/glycogen) in cellular material. The glycols are first oxidized in periodic acid to dialdehydes and then reacted in Schiff's reagent (pararosaniline and sodium metabisulfite) to produce a magenta-colored adduct to the dialdehydes. In a cross-section of muscle, the darker the stain, the more glycogen in the fiber. The glycogen content can be assessed qualitatively by grouping the fibers as light, medium, or dark; or it can be measured quantitatively by determining the absorbance of each fiber (23). The average absorbance of each section can then be compared to the glycogen content of that muscle measured biochemically. Once glycogen values are correlated with absorbance values, then, by matching fibers with those in an ATPase stain, glycogen content can be determined for each fiber type.

The PAS stain is a standard histochemical stain that is conveniently available in a kit (Sigma 395). Schiff's reagent is somewhat unstable and unpredictable (not to mention messy), so it is probably wise to purchase the kit rather than make the Schiff's reagent in the laboratory. Nevertheless, it can be made as follows.

Schiff's Reagent

Dissolve 1 g of basic fuschsin (pararosaniline, Sigma 7632) in 200 ml of boiling distilled water. Cool to 50 °C and filter. Add 20 ml 1-N HCl. Cool to room temperature and add 1 g sodium metabisulfite (Sigma 1516) and leave in the dark overnight. Add 2 g of decolorizing charcoal (Sigma 5260), shake for 2 min, filter, and store in a dark bottle in the refrigerator.

Fixatives

Several traditional fixatives can be used, such as formalin-ethanol, formal saline, acetic ethanol, formalin-acetone, and picric ethanol. For glycogen, an alcoholic fixative is usually recommended; Carnoy's fixative seems to work well. Carnoy's is composed of 6 parts ethanol, 3 parts chloroform, and 1 part glacial acetic acid. Store either in the refrigerator or at room temperature.

Oxidizing Reagent

Mix a 0.5% to 1% periodic acid solution in distilled water (0.5 to 1.0 g periodic acid is dissolved in 100 ml of distilled water). Store in the refrigerator, but bring to room temperature before using.

Procedure

Take the following steps to prepare the PAS stain:

1. Fix sections in Carnoy's fixative for 5 to 10 min. This should be done fairly promptly after sectioning and can be done at refrigerator temperature (4 °C). This may enhance glycogen preservation and help prevent streaming artifact.
2. Wash in distilled water with several rinses.
3. Add 1% periodic acid solution for 5 min.
4. Rinse with distilled water.
5. Add Schiff's reagent for 15 min. Be sure that the Schiff's reagent has had enough time to warm to room temperature. This reagent will develop a precipitate over time. Do not mix this, but carefully pour the clear reagent off the top. Return the Schiff's reagent to the refrigerator as soon as possible.
6. Wash in running *tap water* for 10 min. Do not rinse with distilled water.
7. Dehydrate in ascending alcohols (80%, 90%, 100%).
8. Mount in a toluene-based mounting medium such as Permount.

Capillary Density

The stain for capillary density is the same as that for glycogen, but in order to visualize the capillaries, the glycogen in the fibers must first be removed with an amylase digestion. Then the mucopolysaccharides in the capillary walls can be oxidized in periodic acid and stained in Schiff's reagent.

1. Prepare a 1% amylase solution (1 g/dl) (Sigma 2771). This is a crude amylase suspension.
2. After the fixation and rinse, incubate the sections in the amylase solution for 30 min at 37 °C.
3. Rinse well in distilled water and continue with the periodic acid step as previously mentioned.

Notes on Procedure

There are several things in this method that will affect the intensity and consistency of the stain, such as the freshness of the reagents, incubation times, and temperatures. For this reason, it is imperative that tissue sections that are going to be compared (e.g., pre- vs. post-exercise) be stained in the same batch. If absorbance readings are going to be taken on the sections and correlated with total glycogen content, it is also necessary to make one's calculations from sections done together in the same jar. To ensure the uniform staining of all the tissue sections in the jar, it is good to agitate the jars periodically in all the incubation steps and to rinse the sections well.

FIBER CROSS-SECTIONAL AREA

In this age of the computer, some very sophisticated methods have been devised for measuring muscle fiber area. A number of programs are available for digitizing areas, and even complete systems that will make measurements and calculations from a videotape of the muscle section. In lieu of these, however, there are some old methods that work fairly well. All of these methods require some sort of image magnification and projection, such as a drawing tube or a ground-glass viewing screen for the microscope, a microscope slide projector, or a photograph. In our laboratory, before the day of the microscope video camera and printer, we usually made use of a microscope slide projector, where the muscle section was projected downward to a piece of white paper and the fibers traced with a pencil. Assuming this was done, we can take one of three approaches for determining the cross-sectional area of the fibers.

Tracing

One of the oldest methods that needs the least special equipment is to trace the fibers on a piece of uniform standard-weight paper, cut out the shapes with scissors, and weigh the pieces on an analytical balance. The area of a standard circle or square, *the approximate size of the fibers*, is used for the calculations. This is drawn with a compass or ruler from a stage micrometer slide projected from the same height as the muscle fibers. The circle or square is cut out and weighed, and that weight *and the area it represents* are used as the standard against which the areas of the unknown fibers are determined.

For example, if the calculated area that the standard piece of paper represents is 3,600 μm^2, the weight of the standard piece is 23.0 mg, and the weight of the sample fiber piece of paper is 25.1 mg, then the area of the muscle fiber = $(25.1/23.0) \times 3,600 \ \mu m^2 = 3,939 \ \mu m^2$.

This method is obviously an approximation and rests on certain assumptions about the areas of similar shapes, as well as the uniform weight of the paper, and the proportionality of paper weight to paper size. In essence, however, the method tries to measure the area of the fiber shape as it appears in the muscle section. A second method for doing this, and perhaps the one most used in recent years, is planimetry.

Planimetry

A planimeter is an instrument that measures the area of a figure by tracing its perimeter. As the tracer point of the planimeter moves along the periphery of the figure, arbitrary planimeter units are accumulated on the planimeter wheel. These units are then converted to an area by measuring the perimeter of a circle whose area is known.

Measuring the Fibers

Place the slide containing the muscle section on the stage of the microscope projector and project it downward onto a piece of white paper. Adjust the height and focus of the projector to give a fiber size that is large enough to work with conveniently.

Trace the outline of the fibers with a pencil. This can be done one fiber at a time, or a group of about 20 fibers of one fiber type can be fitted together like the pieces of a jigsaw puzzle by maneuvering the paper to produce a tight fit.

Trace the periphery of the fibers with the planimeter, moving the tracer point clockwise, and record the number of wheel units displayed. Repeat this at least three times to ensure accuracy and average the results.

Calibration of the Planimeter

Place a stage micrometer slide (Baxter Scientific 400 BF or 311690 BX) in the microscope slide projector at the same height as that chosen to project the muscle section.

From the image of the micrometer, select a radius (e.g., 0.5 mm) and draw a circle using a compass. Try to make the size of this circle similar to the size of the fibers you wish to measure, if you are going to measure each fiber one at a time. If you wish to group fibers into a larger area, draw a circle similar to that area. In fact, it will reduce the error of the measurement if you first determine the average number of planimeter units for the periphery of the grouped fibers and then draw a circle that has a circumference equal to that number of units.

Calculate the area of this circle using the formula $A = \pi r^2$.

Trace the circle several times with the planimeter, moving the tracer point clockwise, and average the results. This number of planimeter units now represents the area of the standard circle.

Calculations

Using the planimeter values obtained in measuring the muscle fibers and the values obtained for the standard circle, calculate the area of the unknown in the usual way. For example, if the radius represented by the standard circle is 500 µm, the area of the standard circle is 785,400 µm^2, the planimeter units for the circumference of the standard circle are 1,204, and the planimeter units for the circumference of a group of 20 fibers are 154, then you calculate the fiber cross-sectional area this way: $(154/1,204) \times 785,400$ µm^2 ÷ 20 = 5,022 µm^2 per fiber.

The problem with both of these methods, even with due care given to minimizing the error of the measurement, is that they attempt to determine the cross-sectional area of fibers by their shapes as they appear in the muscle sections. This is probably based on a false assumption. Seldom do fibers appear as round as we assume them to be *in vivo*. Rather, they appear in a variety of oval and flattened shapes that are the result of oblique cuts and fiber kinking typical of less than perfect mounts. The result is a fiber shape that often overestimates the cross-sectional surface of the fiber. To avoid this difficulty, *the preferred method of determining fiber area today is the method of the least fiber diameter*.

Least Fiber Diameter

This method is as simple as they come. The least fiber diameter is the maximum diameter across the lesser aspect of the muscle fiber. That is, it is the diameter drawn through the center of the fiber at its smallest width. This diameter will be the same for a round cut, an oblong cut, or any variety of irregular shapes. With this method, the area will be neither overestimated nor underestimated, but values may well be somewhat less than those presented in the literature for which planimetry was used or, indeed, any method that is based on measuring the area of the surface as seen in the section.

The diameter of the average human muscle fiber is usually between 50 to 70 µm, becoming smaller with atrophy and larger with hypertrophy. The physiological assumption on which this method rests is that the muscle fiber is most like a cylinder, and its cross-sectional area is best described as the area of a circle ($A = \pi r^2$). If this is true, then the cross-sectional area of a fiber with a diameter of 70 µm would be 3,838 µm^2 (3.1416×35^2).

To use this method, one would have to project the muscle fibers and trace them with a pencil as before, and the micrometer slide would also have to be projected and marked out with a rule to indicate the length of 0.5 to 1.0 mm. Then with a fine ruler the lesser diameter of each fiber is measured and the area calculated as previously mentioned.

It is important to note that, however it is done, fiber areas are probably valid only for making comparisons within the same section. There, relative sizes of type I and type II fibers can be compared. It is much more difficult to make comparisons in longitudinal studies, or even in cross-sectional studies, unless the number of observations is large. The primary reason for this is that one never knows the true state of the fibers in this particular muscle mount or what has happened to them in this particular stain. One can only assume that if every procedure is done in the same way, then the distortions should be similar. Nevertheless, it is worth noting that studies looking at muscle hypertrophy with training have advanced beyond fiber area measurements to CAT scans and other imaging techniques.

MUSCLE GLYCOGEN

Glycogen is the storage form of carbohydrate in the body. It is a macromolecule of glucose residues linked together at the alpha 1-4 or 1-6 carbons. In this procedure, the glycogen in a small piece of muscle is hydrolyzed in HCl to its constituent glucose residues and measured enzymatically. The method is the hexokinase/glucose-6-phosphate dehydrogenase reaction for measuring glucose.

$$\text{Glucose} + \text{ATP} \xrightarrow{HK} \text{glucose-6-phosphate} + \text{ADP}$$

$$\text{G-6-P} + \text{NADP} \xrightarrow{G\text{-}6\text{-}PDH} \text{6-phosphogluconic acid} + \text{NADPH}$$

The NADPH produced can be read on a spectrophotometer at 340 nm if the concentration of glucose is high enough, or on a fluorometer even at very low concentrations. The following procedure is designed for the fluorometer.

A reagent cocktail is mixed from stock reagents that are kept frozen. Once thawed, the reagents are mixed gently before pipetting. The cocktail is mixed in a flask containing a volume of H_2O somewhat less than the final volume, and begun by adding the buffer ingredients first. Table 9.3 shows the ingredients, concentrations, and volumes of the reagent cocktail.

A shortcut for making this cocktail is to purchase it in a kit for measuring serum glucose (e.g., Sigma No. 16-UV) and dilute it in half with 0.05-M Tris buffer. Background fluorescence, however, may be higher than desired. If no fluorometer is available, enough extract can be used with this cocktail to use a spectrophotometer.

Preparation of the Muscle Sample

Once the muscle is attained, it is frozen in liquid nitrogen and stored either in a liquid nitrogen refrigerator (Dewar) or in some airtight container at −80 °C. (Cryotubes from Vangard International, Inc., Neptune, NJ, are good. The small 1.2-ml tube, no. 4501, is suitable.)

When it is time to do the assay, label at least in duplicate 12 × 75 mm glass culture tubes for each muscle sample to be measured, and pipet into these tubes 0.5 ml 2-M HCl. The muscle samples are placed in a freezer or cold room and allowed to come up to about −15 °C. The muscle is then cut into pieces of about 5 to 15 mg and weighed frozen to at least 0.1 mg, and the weight is recorded. As each piece of muscle is cut and weighed, it is placed in the corresponding tube of acid. At this point, the tube can be handled at room temperature.

When all of the muscle is cut and placed in the tubes, each tube is weighed on an analytical balance and the weight recorded to the nearest milligram. The

tubes are then covered with marbles and heated in an oven at 100 °C for 2 hours. (The marbles allow the tubes to vent without undue evaporation.) The tubes should be agitated occasionally during the incubation. Do not allow the oven to get so hot that the muscle begins to burn. After the 2 hours, the tubes are allowed to cool to room temperature and then reweighed so that their original weight can be reconstituted by adding distilled water. This replaces the volume evaporated during the incubation. The water can be added with an adjustable microliter pipet on the basis of 1 mg/μL. If the tube lost 200 mg of water during the incubation, it would be reconstituted with 200 μL of distilled water. Alternatively, water can be added directly to the tube on the balance (a 100-μL constriction pipet is useful) until the original weight is reached.

After the original volume of HCl has been reconstituted to 0.5 ml, it is neutralized with NaOH. A convenient volume is 1.5 ml of 0.67-M NaOH. This gives 2 ml of muscle extract that is theoretically pH neutral. In all likelihood all the glucose from the muscle is in solution, but it would be prudent to shake each tube against a piece of parafilm until the muscle is dissolved. This sometimes takes hard shaking. Vortexing will not work.

Assay Procedure

Use the following procedure to measure muscle glycogen:

1. Pipet 1 ml of reagent cocktail into 10 × 75 mm borosilicate glass culture tubes.
2. For very precise work it is necessary to read and record the initial fluorescence of each tube. For the most part, however, you will find that the initial fluorescence is quite uniform and a look at a couple of blanks is sufficient.
3. Pipet 10 to 20 μL of muscle extract, or standard, or distilled water into the reagent cocktail for the samples, standards, and blanks, respectively. Run duplicates. Mix. A convenient standard concentration is 0.5 mM.
4. Let the reaction proceed to its endpoint (5-10 min).
5. Read and record the final fluorescence of all tubes at the range and aperture settings you have chosen. Usually, for 10 mg of muscle, the number 1 or 0.1 setting is sufficient.
6. Subtract the initial fluorescence (or blank) from the final fluorescence of samples and standards.
7. Calculate the values:

$$(\Delta F_{sample} / F_{std}) \times (mM\ conc_{std} \times ml\ Vol_{std}) \times dilution_{muscle} / mg\ wt_{muscle} \times 1,000 =$$

Table 9.3 Reagent Cocktail for Measuring Glycogen

Reagent (pH 8.1)	Stock	Final	Volume to make 25 ml
Tris base	1 M	50 mM	1.25 ml
HCl	1 M	25 mM	0.625 ml
MgCl$_2$	1 M	1 mM	0.025 ml (25 μL)
DTT (dithiothreitol)	0.5 M	0.5 mM	0.025 ml (25 μL)
ATP	0.1 M	0.3 mM	0.075 ml (75 μL)
NADP	0.05 M	0.05 mM	0.025 ml (25 μL)
HK	1000 U/ml	1 U/ml	0.025 ml (25 μL)
G-6-PDH	1000 U/ml	0.1 U/ml	0.0025 ml (2.5 μL)
Glucose std.	0.5 M		25 μL in 25 ml H$_2$O

μmoles glucosyl units/gram wet weight

(Use these example values to practice the calculation.)

Fluorescence of the sample = 70
Fluorescence of the standard = 50
Concentration of the standard = 0.5 mM
Volume of samples and standards = 0.02 ml (20 μL)
Weight of muscle = 10 mg
Total volume of muscle extract = 2 ml

$$(70/50) \times (0.5 \text{ mM} \times 0.02 \text{ ml}) \times$$
$$(2 \text{ ml}/0.02 \text{ ml}) / 10 \text{ mg} \times 1,000 =$$
140 μmol glycosyl units of glycogen per
gram of wet muscle, or 140 mmol/kg wet weight

Because the molecular weight of glucose is 180, this would also be 25.2 g per kilogram of muscle, or 2.5 g per 100 g of muscle. Both of these usages are found in the literature. (One gram of glycogen per 100 g of muscle is the same as 55.5 mmol/kg.) The procedure remains the same for freeze-dried musle, except that now 10 mg of wet muscle becomes about 2 mg, and the final value, per kilogram, is about 4 times what it would be for wet muscle.

This method measures the free glucose and glucose-6-phosphate in the muscle as well as the glycogen, but these concentrations are usually so small that they can be ignored. This is certainly true of muscle taken at rest. Immediately after intense exercise, approximately 5 to 6 mmol/kg of the glycogen value may be G-6-P. If this is of interest, it can be measured first in a reagent cocktail without the enzymes added. After an initial fluorescence is taken on the cocktail with the sample in it, the reaction is started by adding the G-6-PDH. When the reaction is completed, a final fluorescence is taken and the change in fluorescence is the measure of the G-6-P. G-6-P is present in much lower concentrations than the glucose liberated from glycogen, so these fluorescences will need to be read on a more sensitive range. Corresponding working standards of G-6-P of around 10 to 100 μM, made from a stock standard of about 100 mM, should be run. After this reaction is completed, the hexokinase can be added to start the glycogen measurement, and that can then be read at a less sensitive setting on the fluorometer. Be sure to use the same settings for both the initial and the final fluorescence of each substrate of interest. The enzymes can be added separately in convenient 25-μL aliquots by mixing appropriate enzyme stocks. For example, to add 1 unit of hexokinase to the sample tube in a 25-μL aliquot, add 0.040 ml (40 μL) of the 1,000-U/ml HK stock to 1 ml of reagent (or buffer). This will provide 1 unit of HK in every 25 μL. To provide 0.1 U of G-6-PDH in every 25 μL, add 4 μL to 1 ml of reagent.

It would be better to measure G-6-P in a separate assay on a different piece of muscle extracted as it would be for the measurement of ATP, CP, and so on.

Free glucose in muscle is also very low (~1 mmol/kg even after intense exercise) and can be ignored. But if it is necessary for some reason to isolate only the glycogen from a piece of muscle or from a muscle homogenate, a glycogen pellet can be precipitated from ice-cold ethanol after the muscle is dissolved in hot potassium hydroxide (KOH). In this case, 50 to 100 μL of a 1:10 muscle homogenate, or 5 to 10 mg of muscle, can be placed in a tube of 1 ml 30% KOH saturated in sodium sulfate (NA_2SO_4), sealed, and boiled for 20 to 30 min until all the muscle is dissolved. The tubes are then cooled and 1.2 ml of pure, ice-cold ethanol is added. They are then centrifuged hard for about 20 min and decanted. The glycogen pellet is then resuspended in ethanol and the precipitation repeated. Finally, the pellet is dissolved in 0.5 ml of 1-M HCl, heated at 100 °C for 2 hours, and neutralized in NaOH as before.

Expected Values

The concentration of glycogen in human muscle depends on the level of carbohydrate nutrition and training. Normally fed, untrained persons will have muscle glycogens about 55 to 85 mmol/kg. Normally fed, trained individuals will be around 110 to 135 mmol/kg, and, if they are well rested, their values may rise to 180 mmol/kg. If carbohydrate loaded, they may be as high as 220 to 240 mmol/kg.

MUSCLE LACTATE

The assay for muscle lactate is basically the same enzymatic analysis used for blood lactate, with two further considerations. The amount of lactate in a small piece of muscle is small, so a fluorometer is used for the analysis instead of a spectrophotometer. Muscle enzymes are active at room temperature, so the lactate must be extracted from the tissue while it is still frozen.

Preparation of the Muscle

The muscle is obtained, presumably with a biopsy needle, and frozen immediately in liquid nitrogen. Experience has shown, however, that it does no harm (at least to the lactate) to take a few seconds to open the needle and remove the muscle with a pair of fine forceps to put it into the liquid nitrogen. This avoids the somewhat cumbersome task of trying to remove tissue that is frozen in the barrel of the needle without partially thawing it or breaking it to pieces. The muscle is placed in an appropriately labeled tube and kept in a freezer at −80 °C. If the muscle is stored in a freezer, care should be taken to have it in an airtight tube to keep it from drying out before it is weighed.

At the time of the assay, the muscle is placed in the dissecting and weighing freezer or in the cold room and allowed to come up to −20 to −15 °C. The muscle is cleaned of any visible blood or connective tissue, cut into pieces of about 5 to 10 mg, and weighed frozen. The weight is recorded for later calculations.

At this time it is necessary to have on hand appropriately labeled 10 × 75 mm glass culture tubes. Into each tube is placed 0.25 ml 3-M perchloric acid (PCA), which is frozen with liquid nitrogen or dry ice. The frozen, weighed muscle is placed on the frozen PCA and allowed to come to a temperature of −8 to −10 °C for 15 min (or longer). This allows the PCA to thaw and begin to penetrate the still-frozen muscle. This can be accomplished by placing the tubes into an alcohol or dry ice bath adjusted to this temperature, or by placing the tubes into a refrigerator freezer adjusted to this slightly warmer temperature.

When you are ready to proceed, bring the temperature of the tubes up to +5 °C (refrigerator temperature) for 5 min to allow the muscle to completely thaw in the PCA. This can be done either in a refrigerator or by placing the tubes in a bath of that temperature. At this point the tubes can be sealed and refrozen for later processing, the PCA extract can be used as is, or the PCA extract can be neutralized for storage or for the analysis of various substrates other than lactate. If muscle lactate is the only item of interest, the PCA extract can be used without further processing, and that is the procedure that will be presented here.

Procedure

The fluorometric procedure is similar to that given for blood lactate except that the buffer is considerably stronger. If you choose to neutralize an aliquot of the 3-M PCA extract, the reagent cocktail can be mixed the same as in the fluorometric method for blood lactate. Table 9.4 shows the mixing of the reagent cocktail. The ingredients are brought to their final volume with distilled water.

If a 1-M glycine/hydrazine stock has been prepared, only one pipetting will be necessary. The pH of the cocktail is adjusted to 9.8 to 10. This may be more conveniently done by dissolving a pellet of NaOH in the buffer and watching it in the pH meter. A little practice will give you a feel for this. It is best to do this before adding the NAD. The LDH will be added in aliquots after an initial fluorescence is taken on each tube.

Table 9.4 Reagent Cocktail for Muscle Lactate

Reagent (pH 9.8)	Stock	Final	Volume to make 25 ml
Glycine	1 M	0.33 M	8.25 ml
Hydrazine (hydrate, 100%)	20 M	0.33 M	0.41 ml
NAD	0.1 M	0.20 mM	0.05 ml
LDH	5000 U/ml	8 U/ml	See step 4 in the procedure

1. Pipet 1 ml of the reagent cocktail into 10 × 75 borosilicate glass culture tubes.
2. Pipet 0.025 ml (25 μL) of PCA extract into the corresponding tubes for the samples. Pipet 0.025 ml (25 μL) 3-M PCA into triplicate tubes for the blanks and standards. Pipet 0.002 ml (2 μL) of the Sigma lactate standard (Sigma 826-10, 4.44 mM) into the standard tubes.
3. Read and record the initial fluorescence of each tube.
4. Add 8 units LDH to each tube. To do this in 0.025-ml (25-μL) aliquots, add approximately 0.064 ml (64 μL) of the stock LDH given previously to 1 ml of reagent cocktail or buffer. Vortex. Add the 0.025 ml of the LDH mix to each tube. Vortex.
5. Let stand at room temperature for 45 to 60 min.
6. Read and record the final fluorescence. Subtract the initial fluorescence from the final fluorescence for all tubes, samples, standards, and blanks. Subtract the change in the blank fluorescence from the change in fluorescence of the samples and standards.
7. Calculate the muscle lactate values.

$$(\Delta F_{sample} / F_{std}) \times (mM\ conc_{std} \times ml\ vol_{std}) \times dilution_{sample} / mg\ wt_{muscle} \times 1{,}000 = mmol/kg\ wet\ wt.$$

(Use these example values to practice the calculation.)

Initial fluorescence of sample = 7
Initial fluorescence of standard = 6
Initial fluorescence of blank = 6
Final fluorescence of sample = 98
Final fluorescence of standard = 83
Final fluorescence of blank = 14
Volume of sample and blank = 0.025 ml
Volume of muscle PCA extract = 0.25 ml
Volume of standard = 0.002 ml
Concentration of standard (Sigma 826-10) = 4.44 mM
Wet weight of the muscle = 6.0 mg

$$(83/69) \times (4.44\ mM \times 0.0002\ ml) \times (0.25\ ml/0.025\ ml) / 6.0\ mg \times 1{,}000 = 17.8\ \mu mol/g\ or\ mmol/kg\ wet\ wt.$$

Normal Values

Resting values of approximately 1 mmol/kg or less; highs of approximately 25 to 30 mmol/kg.

INTRODUCTION TO ENZYME ASSAYS

Enzyme activities are measured on muscle tissue that has been homogenized in a buffer designed to maintain an appropriate pH for the assay (usually a physiological pH between 7.0 and 7.4). Such a buffer will also contain a variety of stabilizers or activators whose purpose it is to keep the enzymes alive. The buffer from M. Chi et al. (10) shown in Table 9.5 is a good example of such a homogenizing medium.

The muscle is homogenized to a workable dilution on the assumption that 1 g of muscle is equivalent to 1 ml of homogenizing buffer. A 1:100 dilution would have 1 part muscle and 99 parts buffer. Such a dilution for 20 mg of muscle would be 0.020 g $\times$ 99 = 1.98 ml. The piece of muscle would be homogenized, on ice, in that amount of buffer. Whether this is done with a handheld tissue homogenizer or a motor-driven model, the muscle is gently coaxed into solution, taking care to be as quick as possible without generating a lot of frictional heat in the process.

PHOSPHOFRUCTOKINASE (PFK)

Phosphofructokinase (PFK) is usually considered to be the key regulatory enzyme in glycolysis. For this reason, it is often measured as an index of a muscle's glycolytic capacity, as succinate dehydrogenase or citrate synthase may be measured as an index of a muscle's aerobic capacity. PFK catalyzes the phosphorylation of fructose-6-phosphate to fructose-1,6-diphosphate and is under the control of a complex interplay of stimulants and inhibitors. Principal among the stimulants are phosphagens other than ATP (AMP, ADP, P_i) and substrates (F6P, F2,6P). PFK is inhibited by rising levels of ATP, H^+, and feedback from citrate. *In vivo* regulation, however, remains very complex and fleeting, and may be beyond our ability to measure. *In vitro* measurement can be manipulated to give a wide range of activities.

Presented here are two fluorometer methods, a direct, kinetic method and an indirect, two-step method. PFK, much like its aerobic counterpart SDH, is a fragile enzyme that very quickly becomes inactive. To prevent this, the muscle is homogenized on ice in a special buffer. The following is an example of such a buffer (from Baldwin [5]). Table 9.6 shows the ingredients, concentrations, and volumes for mixing the homogenizing buffer for PFK.

Homogenizing Buffer

Potassium phosphate, pH 8.2	100 mM
Gluthathione (reduced)	10 mM
ATP	0.5 mM
$MgSO_4$	5 mM
NaF	30 mM

Kinetic Method

The kinetic method is a direct method that follows the decrease in NADH over a set period of time. This can be done with pencil and paper and stopwatch, but it is more conveniently followed if the fluorometer is connected to a chart recorder or some such integrator. The reaction is as follows:

$$\text{Fructose-6-phosphate + ATP} \xrightarrow{\text{PFK}} \text{Fructose 1,6-diphosphate}$$

$$\text{F-1,6-P}_2 \xrightarrow{\text{Aldolase}} \text{Dihydroxyacetonephosphate + Glyceraldehyde-3-phosphate}$$

$$\text{G-3-P} \xrightarrow{\text{Triosphosphate isomerase}} \text{DHAP}$$

$$\text{DHAP + NADH} \xrightarrow{\text{Glycerophosphate DH}} \text{Glycerol-3-phosphate + NAD}$$

Table 9.5 Homogenizing Buffer

Reagent (pH 7.4)	Stock	Final	Volume to make 25 ml
Glycerol	100%	50%	12.5 ml
K_2HPO_4	1 M	0.02 M	0.5 ml
2-Mercaptoethanol	1 M	0.005 M	0.125 ml
EDTA	0.1 M	0.05 mM	0.125 ml
BSA	10%	0.02%	0.05 ml

Table 9.6 Homogenizing Buffer Ingredients for PFK

Reagent (pH 8.2)	Stock	Final	Volume to make 25 ml
K_2HPO_4	1 M	0.10 M	2.500 ml
Glutathione	powder	0.01 M	77 mg
ATP	0.1 M	0.50 mM	0.125 ml
$MgSO_4$	1 M	5.00 mM	0.125 ml
NaF	1 M	30.00 mM	0.750 ml

For every mole of fructose-1,6-diphosphate produced, 2 mol of NADH are converted to NAD. Consequently, the activity of PFK is half the turnover of NADH.

Mix the cocktail shown in Table 9.7 in the usual way from reagent stocks kept in the freezer (substrates) or refrigerator (enzyme suspensions).

Some methods in the literature give enzyme concentrations in terms of micrograms per milliliter, and others in terms of units per milliliter, and the same is true of commercial preparations of enzymes. Because the number of units per microgram can vary depending on the source of the enzyme and the purity of the preparation, the amount of enzyme in the assay cocktail can also vary. It is also the case that different recipes call for different concentrations. Although these are based on calculations of K_m (the Michaelis-Menten constant) and V_{max} (maximal velocity), there is no hard-and-fast requirement for exact concentrations of reagents in order for an assay to work. A balance is often struck between too little and too much. Obviously, the auxiliary enzymes will have to be present in enough activity, and the substrates in enough concentration, as to not limit the speed of the reaction. But putting in too much will often introduce unwanted side reactions that would otherwise be insignifiant. Each cocktail should be tested when first mixed by running a few different dilutions or volumes of muscle homogenate to see where maximal activity is attained and whether doubling the sample enzyme will double its velocity.

Direct assays that follow the formation of NADH are more convenient than those, like this one, that follow its disappearance, because the sensitivity of the fluorometer limits the amount of NADH that can be put into an assay without its going off the scale. On the typical fluorometer, the most NADH that can be read at the least sensitive settings without blanking is about 10 to 20 µM. This can become a problem when NADH should be maintained at saturating levels in order to produce a linear maximal velocity over a reasonable period of time. Fortunately, the K_m for NADH in this reaction is low, about 2 µM, so that a 10 to 20 µM concentration should provide enough NADH to produce a sensitive reaction that is linear for about 3 to 4 min.

Procedure

1. Homogenize the muscle on ice in the usual way in PFK homogenizing buffer. A dilution of 1:100 is sufficient, although it can be more dilute. Centrifuge briefly to settle the cell debris.
2. Adjust the NADH content of the cocktail until it reaches a satisfactory point up scale on the fluorometer about 80 to 100. It is usually more convenient to use preweighed vials of NADH (Sigma 340-5, 101) in mixing this. It takes only about 0.4 mg of NADH to make 25 ml of a 20-µM concentration. Further fine-tuning can be made with the adjustments on the fluorometer. *It is important to remember, however, that with every adjustment of the fluorometer it will be necessary to recalibrate it to a known concentration of NADH.*
3. Pipet 1 ml of cocktail into a 10 × 75 mm borosilicate glass culture tube.
4. Add 3 to 5 µL of a 1:100 dilution of muscle. Mix.
5. Follow the disappearance of NADH for about 3 min. The reaction should remain linear during this period after a short lag time or give sufficient indication where it departs from linearity. A tissue blank may be run in some reagent cocktail prepared without F-6-P to check on the extent of any nonspecific decrease in NADH over the same period of time. If this activity is significant, it can be subtracted from the measurement of PFK activity.
6. Calculate the results from the change in fluorescence per minute from the linear part of the curve or from the initial velocity if that can be clearly distinguished. (The initial velocity is sometimes masked by irregularities at the very beginning of the reaction. Sometimes the lag time seems to be exaggerated, and sometimes there is an overshoot of fluorescence that rapidly declines to a more regular pattern. Some of these things should be examined at the start to determine if a more or less dilute sample should be used.)

$$(F/min_{sample} / F_{NADH\ std}) \times \mu mol_{NADH\ std} \times dilutions_{muscle} / 2 = \mu mol/g/min$$

(Use these example values to practice the calculation).

Table 9.7   Cocktail Ingredients for PFK (Kinetic Method)

Reagent (pH 8.2)	Stock	Final	Volume to make 25 ml
Glycylglycine	0.5 M	0.05 M	2.5 ml
MgCl$_2$	1 M	1 mM	0.025 ml
ATP	0.1 M	1 mM	0.25 ml
F-6-P	0.1 M	1 mM	0.25 ml
BSA	10%	0.1%	0.025 ml
L-Cysteine	fresh	14 mM	55 mg
NADH	fresh	≈20 µM	up scale
Aldolase (Sigma A-7145)	100 U/ml	0.4 U/ml	≈0.1 ml
Triosphosphate isomerase/a-Glycerophosphate DH (Sigma G-6755)	100 U/ml	0.08 U/ml	0.02 ml

Dilution of muscle in the homogenate = 100
Volume of cocktail in assay = 1 ml
Volume of homogenate in assay = 3 μL
Dilution of muscle in the cocktail = 1:334
Total dilution of muscle = 1:33,400
Change in fluorescence per minute = 15 units
Calibration of fluorometer: 20 μM = 100 units
(that is, 0.02 μmol/ml = 100 units)

$$(15/100) \times 0.02 \ \mu mol \times 33,400 \ / \ 2$$
$$= 50.1 \ \mu mol/g/min$$

Expected Values

As in all enzyme procedures, the temperature of the assay will make a considerable difference if we assume a Q_{10} effect (the rate of an enzyme mediated reaction doubling with an increase in temperature of 10 °C). Most assays, however, are done at room temperature or at 25 °C. Sometimes these are adjusted to reflect an activity at 30 °C or 37 °C. Consequently, a wide range of activities are often reported in the literature. (If one attempts to measure the reaction in the fluorometer at 30 °C or 37 °C, it is important to remember that the NADH calibration of the instrument will also have to be made at that temperature, because the fluorescence of NADH decreases rapidly with rising temperatures.) The enzyme is also fiber-type dependent, being higher in type II fibers than in type I. Samples from mixed human muscle may often reflect the error in the muscle fiber sampling. Overall, however, PFK seems to change little with training, perhaps decreasing slightly with aerobic training and increasing slightly with detraining, and this might reflect only the volume change of mitochondria in the muscle fiber. Values can range from 15 to 80 μmol/g/min.

Indirect Method

The indirect method is often more convenient because it allows one to batch a number of muscle samples and do them in duplicate or triplicate in a relatively short time. In this assay, it also allows for ample NADH to be put into the reaction, because the excess is destroyed before the final step. The NAD produced in the reaction is then changed to a fluorescent product in NaOH and read on the fluorometer as an increase in fluorescence.

Procedure

The muscle can be homogenized as in the previous method, but the final dilution should be 1:1,500. This is more conveniently done by making a first homogenate of a 1:100 dilution and then further diluting another 15 times. This can be accomplished by adding 0.1 ml of

the 100 dilution to 1.4 ml of homogenizing buffer. If the muscle is homogenized in the buffer given at the beginning of this section, it should be immediately diluted in a PFK buffer. In addition to the buffer described previously, the following has also been used.

Tris buffer	50.0 mM
K_2HPO_4	10.0 mM
2-Mercaptoethanol	5.0 mM
EDTA	0.5 mM
BSA	0.02%

Table 9.8 shows *how* a muscle homogenizing buffer can be mixed.

Mix the cocktail shown in Table 9.9 in the usual way from stock reagents kept in the refrigerator or freezer.

Add the cocktail to the 1-mg vial of NADH to rinse it into the solution. The triosphosphate isomerase and the a-glycerophosphate dehydrogenase can be added separately

Table 9.8   Muscle Homogenizing Buffer

Reagent (pH 8.2)	Stock	Final	Volume to make 25 ml
Tris base	1 M	.05 M	12.500 ml
HCl	1 M	0.025 N	0.625 ml
K_2HPO_4	1 M	10 mM	0.250 ml
EDTA	100 mM	0.5 mM	0.125 ml
2-Mercaptoethanol	1 M	5 mM	0.125 ml
BSA	10%	0.02%	0.050 ml

Table 9.9   Cocktail Ingredients for PFK (Indirect Method)

Reagent (pH 8.1)	Stock	Final	Volume to make 10 ml
Tris base	1 M	0.05 M	0.500 ml
HCl	1 M	0025 M	0.025 ml
F-6-P	0.1 M	1 mM	0.100 ml
ATP	0.1 M	1 mM	0.100 ml
K_2HPO_4	1 M	10 mM	0.100 ml
$MgCl_2$	1 M	2 mM	0.020 ml
2-Mercaptoethanol	1 M	1 mM	0.010 ml
BSA	10%	0.05%	0.050 ml
Adolase (Sigma A-7145)	100 U/ml	0.1 U/ml	0.010 ml
TPI/a-GPDH (Sigma G-6755)	≈1000 U/ml / ≈100 U/ml	10 U/ml / 1 U/ml	0.100 ml
NADH (Sigma 340-101)	1 mg vial	0.124 mM	Pour reagent cocktail into vial
F-1,6-P_2(std)	0.1 M	0.5 mM	0.050 ml

if desired. The enzyme preparations given here are sulfate free to avoid sulfate inhibition in the reaction.

1. Pipet 0.1 ml of cocktail into 10 × 75 mm borosilicate glass culture tubes for samples, standards, and blanks. Run duplicates or triplicates.
2. For each sample tube, add 2 µL of the 1,500 dilution of muscle. Mix gently. Incubate at room temperature for 1 hour. Standards can be prepared by adding 2 to 5 µL of 0.5-mM F-1,6-P$_2$ to the cocktail in the standard tubes. Nothing need be added to the blanks, because 2 to 5 µL is an insignificant volume in this assay.
3. After the hour's incubation, add 10 µL of a 0.75-M HCl to each tube. Mix and let stand for 10 min. This acidification destroys the excess NADH.
4. To each tube add 1 ml of a 6-M NaOH/10-mM imidazole solution. (This should be prepared ahead of time and stored in a dark bottle. One hundred milliliters can be made by dissolving 24 g of NaOH in distilled water and adding to it 1 ml of a 1-M imidazole.) Vortex each tube immediately and vigorously when the solution is added.
5. When all the tubes are pipetted, place the rack into a water bath at 60 °C for 20 min.
6. After the 20 min, remove the rack to a room-temperature water bath for a few minutes. Then remove the rack from the bath, blot, and let the tubes stabilize at room temperature before reading. Gently dry each tube with a Kimwipe before placing it in the fluorometer.
7. Read the blanks and standards and a couple of samples to set the fluorometer to an appropriate range and sensitivity. Then read and record the fluorescence of all tubes, samples, standards, and blanks.
8. Subtract the average fluorescence of the blanks from the samples and standards and calculate the results in the usual way.

$$(F_{sample}/F_{std}) \times (mM\ conc_{std} \times ml\ vol_{std})\ /$$
$$g\ wt_{muscle}\ /\ time = µmol/g/hr\ or\ min$$

See this example:

$$Dilution\ of\ muscle = 1,500$$
$$Volume\ of\ muscle$$
$$homogenate\ in\ assay = 2\ µL$$
$$Weight\ of\ muscle\ in\ assay = 1.33\ µg\ wet\ wt.$$
$$Concentration\ of\ standard = 0.5\ mM$$
$$Volume\ of\ standard\ in\ assay = 0.005\ ml$$
$$Fluorescence\ of\ sample = 70$$
$$Fluorescence\ of\ standards = 65$$
$$Fluorescence\ of\ blanks = 10$$

$$(60/55) \times (0.5\ mM \times 0.005\ ml)\ /\ 1.33^{-6}$$
$$/\ 60\ min = 34.2\ µmol/g/min$$

Expected Values

Values can range from 15 to 80 µmol/g/min. (This is the same as for the direct method.)

HEXOKINASE

Hexokinase is the enzyme responsible for introducing glucose into the glycolytic pathway by phosphorylating it to glucose-6-phosphate. Although it is considered a glycolytic enzyme, it is higher in type I fibers than in type II by about twofold, and it increases its activity with endurance training in a manner similar to that of the oxidative enzymes. Even so, its activity is low compared to other enzymes and usually ranges from about 1 to 5 µmol/g/min.

Direct Method

The direct assay measures the rate of production of NADPH in the following reaction:

$$Glucose + ATP \xrightarrow{Hexokinase}$$
$$Glucose\text{-}6\text{-}phosphate + ADP$$
$$G\text{-}6\text{-}P + NADP \xrightarrow{G\text{-}6\text{-}PDH}$$
$$6\text{-}phosphogluconolactone + NADPH$$

Mixing the Cocktail

Muscle is homogenized in an appropriate buffer such as that given in Table 9.5. A 2% Lubrol can be added to free the enzyme from membranes. Care should be taken in mixing in the Lubrol to avoid foaming. Other detergents such as Triton X-100 could also be used. Alternatively, a 0.5% Triton X-100 could be added to the cocktail.

Mix the cocktail in Table 9.10 in the usual way from stock reagents kept in the freezer. Adjust the pH to 8.1.

Table 9.10 Cocktail Ingredients for Hexokinase

Reagent (pH 8.1)	Stock	Final	Volume to make 25 ml
Tris base	1 M	0.05 M	1.25 ml
HCl	1 M	0.025 N	0.625 ml
Glucose	0.1 M	1 mM	0.25 ml
ATP	0.1 M	2 mM	0.5 ml
MgCl$_2$	1 M	5 mM	0.125 ml
NADP	0.5 M	0.1 mM	0.05 ml
BSA	10%	0.02%	0.05 ml
G6PDH	1000 U/ml	≈0.1 U/ml	2.5 µL

Procedure

1. Homogenize the muscle in a 1:100 dilution.
2. Pipet 1 ml of cocktail into a 10 × 75 mm borosilicate glass culture tube.
3. Pipet into the cocktail 10 to 25 µL of muscle homogenate. Mix gently and follow the change in fluorescence for about 5 min. As with other assays, the amount of muscle to be added might vary depending on the activity of the enzyme. Some preliminary troubleshooting may be necessary to find the right dilution or volume of homogenate to use. Ideally, one would use the most dilute preparation that would give a satisfactory linear response.
4. Calculate the results from the change in fluorescence per minute and from the dilutions of the muscle in the homogenate and the assay. A standard NADH (or NADPH) is used to calibrate the fluorometer.

$$(\Delta F/min_{sample} /F_{std} \; NADH) \times$$
$$\mu mol_{std} \; NADH \times dilutions_{muscle} = \mu mol/g/min$$

See this example:

Dilution of muscle in the homogenate = 100
Volume of muscle homogenate in assay = 0.025 ml
Dilution of muscle in the assay tube = 41
Change in fluorescence per
minute of assay = 2
NADH calibration of the
fluorometer: 0.002 µmol = 10 units

$(2/10) \times 0.002 \; \mu mol \times 100 \times 41 = 1.64 \; \mu mol/g/min$

Indirect Method

As with other indirect methods, this one separates the enzymatic reactions into two distinct steps.

Step 1 Glucose + ATP $\xrightarrow{\text{Hexokinase}}$
Glucose-6-phosphate + ADP
Step 2 G6P + NADP $\xrightarrow{\text{G-6-PDH}}$
6-P-gluconolactone + NADPH

The advantages of doing this are the convenience of doing a large number of samples in duplicate in a relatively short time and the avoidance of possible side reactions that might oxidize the NADPH if the two steps were not separated in a long incubation.

Procedure

1. Mix the reagent in Table 9.11 (Reagent #1) in the usual way, adjusting the pH to 8.1.
2. Homogenize the muscle in a 1:50 dilution using the buffer as described for the direct method of measuring hexokinase (Table 9.5). Keep the homogenate in an ice bath.
3. Pipet 0.1 ml of Reagent #1 into 10 × 75 mm borosilicate glass culture tubes for samples, standards, and blanks. Run duplicates or triplicates.
4. Pipet about 4 µL of the muscle homogenate (~80 µg) into a corresponding tube of reagent cocktail. Standards of 5 to 20 µL of a 0.5-mM glucose-6-phosphate, and blanks with little or no H_2O, should be run along with the samples. Incubate at room temperature for 1 hour.
5. At the end of the hour, stop the reaction by adding 10 µL of a 1-N HCl to each tube. Mix and let stand for 10 min.
6. Mix, or have mixed, the reagent in Table 9.12 (Reagent #2), adjusting its pH to 8.1. The phosphoglucose isomerase is included in the cocktail to convert back to glucose-6-phosphate the fructose-6-phosphate that was produced by the muscle PGI during the long incubation.
7. Pipet 1 ml of Reagent #2 into each tube, mix, and let stand for about 10 min.
8. Use a few tubes of blanks, standards, and samples to adjust the fluorometer to convenient settings. Read and record the fluorescence of all tubes.
9. Calculate the results in the usual way. Subtract the average fluorescence of the blank from the average fluorescence of standards and samples.

Table 9.11 Reagent #1

Reagent (pH 8.1)	Stock	Final	Volume to make 10 ml
Tris base	1 M	50 mM	0.50 ml
HCl	1 M	25 mM	0.25 ml
Glucose	0.1 M	5 mM	0.50 ml
ATP	0.1 M	5 mM	0.50 ml
$MgCl_2$	1 M	2 mM	0.02 ml
Triton X-100	10%	0.5%	0.50 ml
BSA	10%	0.05%	0.05 ml

Table 9.12 Reagent #2

Reagent (pH 8.1)	Stock	Final	Volume to make 25 ml
Tris base	1 M	50 mM	1.25 ml
HCl	1 M	25 mM	0.625 ml
NADP	0.05 M	0.05 mM	0.025 ml
EDTA	0.1 M	1 mM	0.25 ml
PGI	1000 U/ml	0.5 U/ml	≈12.5 µL
G6PDH	1000 U/ml	0.1 U/ml	≈2.5 µL

$$(F_{sample}/F_{std}) \times (mM\ conc_{std} \times$$
$$ml\ vol_{std})/g\ wt_{muscle}/time = \mu mol/g/time$$

See the example:

Dilution of muscle
in the homogenate = 50
Volume of muscle homogenate
in assay = 4 μL
Weight of muscle in assay = 80 μg or 8^{-5} g
Concentration of the standard = 0.5 mM
Volume of standard in assay = 0.01 ml
Average fluorescence of the blank = 10
Fluorescence of the standard = 50
Fluorescence of the sample = 85
Incubation time = 60 min

$$(75/40) \times (0.5\ mM \times 0.01\ ml)\ /\ 8^{-5}$$
$$g\ /\ 60\ min = 1.95\ \mu mol/g/min$$

Another Procedure

A more sophisticated two-cocktail procedure, which will not be given here, is also available in the literature (24). It goes to extra lengths to avoid the possibility of underestimating hexokinase activity from the nonspecific oxidation of NADH (NADPH). It makes use of G-6-PDH from Leuconostoc mesenteroides, which reacts with NAD as well as with NADP, and ends by measuring the amount of 6-P-gluconate produced in the reaction instead of the NADH. It proceeds as follows:

Step 1 Glucose + ATP $\xrightarrow{Hexokinase}$
Glucose-6-phosphate
G6P + NAD $\xrightarrow{G-6-PDH}$
6-P-gluconate + NADH
Step 2 Acid and heat to destroy
the NADH and kill the enzymes
Step 3 6-P-gluconate + NADP
$\xrightarrow{G-6-PDH}$Ribulose-5-P + NADPH

A comparison of these two indirect methods illustrates the great flexibility available in enzymatic assays.

SUCCINATE DEHYDROGENASE (SDH)

Succinate dehydrogenase (SDH) and citrate synthase (CS) are two mitochondrial enzymes that are often used as an index of Krebs cycle activity and, inferentially, of the aerobic capacity of tissue. Because SDH is a membrane-bound enzyme, its measurement is also considered to be an index of mitochondrial protein.

SDH is the enzyme that catalyzes the oxidation of succinate to fumarate. When this is done *in vivo*, FAD serves as the hydrogen acceptor, being reduced to FADH, which carries the H^+ to the electron transport chain. The problem with this is that the reduction of FAD is not easily monitored in the laboratory. Consequently, the assay is carried out in two steps, where the second step reacts the fumarate produced by the SDH to a point where an equimolar amount of NADH is produced that can be read on a fluorometer.

Step 1 Succinate + electron acceptor
$\xrightarrow{SDH}$Fumarate
Step 2 Fumarate $\xrightarrow{fumarase}$Malate
Malate + NAD $\xrightarrow{MDH}$
Oxalacetate + NADH

Reagents
Homogenizing buffer:
Potassium phosphate, 0.17 M, pH 7.4
2-mercaptoethanol, 10 mM
Bovine serum albumin, 0.05%
Incubation medium:
Sodium succinate, 600 mM
Potassium ferricyanide, 8 mM
Prepare by dissolving 320 mg of sodium succinate and 5.2 mg of potassium ferricyanide in 2 ml of 0.17-M phosphate buffer, pH 7.4. Prepare fresh.
Deproteinizing and neutralizing reagents:
3-M PCA
3-M KOH
Fluorometric reaction medium:
Hydrazine-HCl buffer, 0.2 M, pH 9.2. (This is conveniently made from a 100% hydrazine hydrate [64% hydrazine], which is a 20-M hydrazine solution.)
NAD, 0.36 mM. (To make 25 ml of cocktail, add 90 μL of 0.1-M NAD stock to the above.)
Enzyme mix:
Fumarase, final concentration, 0.25 μg/ml (Sigma F4631)
MDH, final concentration, 5 μg/ml (Sigma M-9004)

Prepare a working stock enzyme mix in a phosphate buffer that would allow you to add 25 to 50-μL aliquots to each tube to produce the previously mentioned final concentrations. For example, 25-μL aliquots could be provided by making a working stock that is 10 μg/ml fumarase and 200 μg/ml MDH.

Procedure

The first step in measuring SDH is to cause it to produce fumarate. Follow these procedures:

1. Weigh and homogenize the tissue in the homogenizing buffer. Dilute 1:200 to 1:400 for heart or 1:50 to 1:100 for skeletal muscle (i.e., on the basis

of gram weight to milliliter volume). Homogenization is done as gently as possible, keeping the homogenizer in ice. Afterward, the homogenate can be transferred to another tube and kept in an ice bath. Do not centrifuge the homogenate for the SDH assay, but gently mix it before use.

2. For each homogenate, prepare three 12×75 mm glass culture tubes, two for duplicates and one for a blank, keeping them in the ice bath. Pipet 0.1 ml of the homogenate into each tube.

3. Place the succinate/ferricyanide incubation medium into a water bath at 37 °C and allow it enough time to come up to temperature.

4. Place the duplicate sample tubes into the water bath and allow them to come to temperature (~1 min).

5. Add 0.1 ml of the incubation medium to each sample tube, mix gently, and incubate for *exactly 5 min*. It is wise to figure out some workable timed sequence for this pipetting. If a number of tubes are being run, it may be necessary to have an assistant for this part of the procedure.

6. After the 5-min incubation, remove the tube from the bath and stop the reaction by adding 0.1 ml 3-M PCA. Mix and return the tube to the ice bath.

7. At this time, 0.1 ml 3-M PCA is also added to the tissue blank tube, and this is followed by adding 0.1 ml of incubation medium to each blank tube.

8. When all the tubes are back in the ice bath, 0.1 ml of 3-M KOH is added to each tube, including blanks. At this point, the total volume in each tube should be 0.4 ml.

9. Centrifuge all the tubes briefly to pellet the potassium perchlorate precipitate and return them to the ice bath.

The second step is to measure the fumarate produced in the first step. To do so, follow these procedures:

1. Pipet 1 ml of the hydrazine/NAD cocktail into 10 × 75 mm borosilicate glass culture tubes.

2. Pipet 20 to 50 µL of samples and tissue blank into a corresponding cocktail tube. A working standard of fumarate or malate (0.1-0.5 mM) can be run, or a standard NADH can be used.

3. Read and record the initial fluorescence of each tube.

4. Add a 25-µL aliquot of the enzyme mix to each tube. Mix. Let stand at room temperature for 1 hour.

5. Read and record the final fluorescence of all tubes. Subtract the initial fluorescence from the final fluorescence of all tubes, and the change in the tissue blank fluorescence from the change in the fluorescence of the sample. Calculate the results.

$$(dF_{sample}/dF_{std}) \times (mM\ conc_{std} \times ml\ vol_{std}) \times dilution_{sample} / tissue\ wt_{grams} / time_{min} = \mu mol/min/g$$

See this example:

Initial fluorescence of the cocktail = 3
Final fluorescence of the sample = 35
Final fluorescence of the
    tissue blank = 7
Final fluorescence of the standard = 98
Concentration of the standard = 0.5 mM
Volume of samples, blanks,
    and standard = 0.02 ml
Dilution factor of sample volume = 0.4 ml/
    0.02 ml = 20
Dilution of muscle in
    the homogenate = 1:100
Amount of muscle tissue
    in the reaction = 0.001 g
Incubation time = 5 min

$$(28/95) \times (0.5\ mM \times 0.02\ ml) \times (0.4\ ml/0.02\ ml) / 0.0001\ g / 5\ min = 11.8\ \mu mol/min/g$$

Notes

The measurement of malate is slow and labors under many of the problems we see with the lactate and glycerol assays. The reaction requires a large excess of NAD, but this should pose no problem in the method presented here. The use of buffers in addition to hydrazine, such as glycine or 2-amino-2-methylpropanol, help to stabilize pH, but they also contribute to higher blank values, which tend to increase with time. Hydrazine alone is not a very effective buffer, so some preliminary troubleshooting and adjusting of the pH may be warranted. The malate reaction, however, may be completed well short of an hour. To check on this, a fluorescence reading should be taken on the standard and a few samples at 30 min and then again a short time later. An alternative method of measuring malate with glutamate-oxalacetate transaminase is also available and avoids some of these problems, especially if very low levels of malate are to be measured (16).

If problems occur in the assay, however, they are most likely to happen in the first part of the procedure, not the second. The first item of concern is the fragile nature of the enzyme. SDH does not store well. Best results are achieved with fresh tissue. When tissue is frozen and stored, it should be kept in liquid nitrogen. Once the tissue is homogenized, SDH should be analyzed without delay, the first of any other enzymes to be measured in the homogenate. And, needless to say, the homogenate cannot be refrozen for later analysis without a great loss of activity.

It is also necessary to test the potency of the ferricyanide in the incubation medium. This reagent should remain yellow when it is added to the tissue homogenate. Occasionally, for unknown reasons, the homogenate will completely reduce the ferricyanide to a colorless state and effectively destroy its ability as an electron acceptor. Should this happen in a preliminary check, double the amount of potassium ferricyanide in the incubation medium.

Expected Values

SDH is expected to be present in these amounts in the following populations:

Rat muscle:	Heart	25 to 30 μmol/min/g
	White muscle	2 to 3 μmol/min/g
	Red muscle	5 to 7 μmol/min/g
Human muscle:	Untrained	2 to 6 μmol/min/g
	Trained	10 to 20 μmol/min/g

CITRATE SYNTHASE

Citrate synthase is the mitochondrial enzyme that catalyzes the synthesis of citrate from acetyl-CoA and oxalacetate to start a new turn of the citric acid cycle. It is neither rate limiting nor membrane bound, but it is still very useful in measuring the mitochondrial development of tissue and, inferentially, its aerobic capacity. One of the practical advantages of measuring citrate synthase instead of SDH (see that assay) is that it is a very hardy enzyme. It will take a lot of abuse, freezing and refreezing, and still repeat its activity.

The disadvantages of this assay are mainly matters of convenience, which are not insurmountable. The assay we describe here is a kinetic measurement, which requires the technician to follow the reaction for each sample in the spectrophotometer. If there are many samples, this will take a long time. Another disadvantage is that this assay works through the reduction of DTNB (5,5'-dithiobis-2-nitrobenzoate) by the CoA-SH released in the cleaving of acetyl-Co-A.

$$\text{Acetyl-Co-A} + \text{Oxalacetate} \xrightarrow{CS} \text{Citrate} + \text{CoA-SH}$$

$$\text{Co-A-SH} + \text{DTNB}_{\text{pale yellow}} \rightarrow \text{CoA} + \text{DTNB}_{\text{dark yellow}}$$

Unfortunately, there are many sulfhydryl (SH) compounds (glutathione, 2-mercaptoethanol, dithiothreitol, cysteine) that are put into homogenizing buffers to protect enzymes from oxidation that will reduce the DTNB in the assay. Consequently, the tissue used for this assay must be homogenized in a buffer without these stabilizers/activators needed for other enzymes. In practice, this means that a separate piece of tissue will have to be cut for this assay, if other enzymes are also to be measured, to avoid these problems. A two-step assay is available, but it is much more complex than the kinetic method of Srere given here.

The last disadvantage of this assay is that acetyl-CoA is very expensive and must be weighed out and prepared fresh with each use. Even so, the ease and reliability of this method make it very attractive.

Reagents

100-mM Tris buffer, pH 8.3. A quantity of this can be prepared and kept in the refrigerator.

1-mM DTNB (Sigma D-8130). About 4 mg is dissolved in 10 ml of 100-mM Tris buffer, pH 8.3. This can be kept in a dark bottle and stored in the refrigerator for a couple of days, but it slowly begins to turn a dark yellow over time. It is easy to mix this fresh each time.

10-mM Oxalacetate (Sigma O-4126). Dissolve 13.2 mg in 10 ml of 100-mM Tris buffer, pH 8.3. Prepare fresh daily.

3-mM acetyl-CoA (Sigma A-2897). Dissolve 3.1 mg in 1 ml of distilled water. Prepare fresh daily. This reagent is not stable in Tris.

Homogenizing medium, 0.175-M KCl/2-mM EDTA, pH 7.4. This can be prepared and stored in either the refrigerator or freezer.

Reagent Cocktail

Each assay tube is prepared individually in a 1-ml volume, preferably in the cuvette that will go into the spectrophotometer. Add the following to the cuvette:

0.70 ml Tris buffer
0.10 ml DTNB
0.15 ml Acetyl-CoA
0.05 ml Oxalacetate

Procedure

1. Weigh the tissue and homogenize it in the usual way in the 175-mM KCl medium. Homogenizing dilutions can range from 1:15 to 1:50 for muscle and 1:100 to 1:200 for heart. The homogenate should then be frozen and thawed a couple of times to ensure the freeze-fracture of the mitochondria. If the tissue was frozen beforehand when stored, this refreezing should be unnecessary.

2. Centrifuge the homogenate briefly (~5 min) to settle the cell debris and produce a clear supernatant. Keep the homogenate in an ice bath when not in use.

3. Set the spectrophotometer to 412 nm, zeroing as necessary on the reagent blank. As in all enzyme assays, the chosen temperature for the measurement should be controlled. If no special equipment is available, it is best to run the assay at a stable room temperature (~23 °C to 25 °C).

4. Pipet about 5 to 50 µL of tissue homogenate into the 1-ml cuvette of reagent cocktail. Mix by gentle inversion (e.g., on a piece of parafilm). Place the cuvette in the spectrophotometer and start a timer.

5. Follow the change in absorbance for about 2 to 4 min, recording the change every 15 to 30 s. (Some instruments will have an enzyme analysis mode that will do this automatically, or the reaction can be followed on a chart recorder.) After a short lag time, the enzyme will reach its maximal velocity and the change in absorbance will remain constant for a couple of minutes. It is this period of maximal steady activity that is used in the calculations. Some troubleshooting and adjusting of the sample volume may be necessary to find a velocity that is neither too slow nor too fast. If too little enzyme is put into the system, very little change will be detected and the change will probably be inconsistent. If too much enzyme is put into the system, the enzyme will overpower the system, producing a large change in absorbance at first and then dying off to ever smaller changes as the reaction proceeds. We usually look for absorbance changes of 0.02 to 0.04 units every 15 s.

6. Determine the average change in absorbance per minute after the reaction has reached its maximal steady state. Calculate the results on the basis of the molar extinction coefficient for DTNB at 412 nm (13,600) and the dilutions of the tissue, first in the homogenate and then in the assay volume.

$$\text{Abs/min} \div 13.6 \times \text{dilution factors}_{\text{muscle}} = \mu\text{mol/min/g}$$

Use these values for example:

Change in absorbance every 15 s = 0.03
Change in absorbance per minute = 0.12
Dilution in muscle homogenate = 1:20
Volume of muscle homogenate used = 5 µL
Dilution of muscle in assay volume = 201

$$0.12 \div 13.6 \times 20 \times 201 = 35.47 \ \mu\text{mol/min/g}$$

Expected Values

Citrate synthase is expected to be present in these amounts in the following populations:

Rat tissue:	Heart	~125 µmol/min/g
	Planataris	~10 to 30 µmol/min/g
	Soleus	~20 to 35 µmol/min/g
	White vastus	~10 to 15 µmol/min/g
Human muscle, mixed:		
	Untrained	~10 to 20 µmol/min/g
	Trained	~30 to 60 µmol/min/g

SUGGESTIONS FOR FURTHER READING

As we indicated at the start, this chapter represents a condensation of our own laboratory manual. For the scientist interested in working in this area, there are several works that should be carefully read and digested prior to visiting the laboratory. They represent, at the least, the backbone of analytic methods for muscle metabolism.

REFERENCES

1. Bergstrom, J. (1962). Muscle electrolytes in man. *Scandinavian Journal of Clinical Investigation*, **14**(Suppl. 68), 7-110.

2. Pernow, B., & Saltin, B. (Eds.). (1971). *Muscle metabolism during exercise*. New York: Plenum Press.

3. Evans, W.J., Phinney, S.K., & Young, V.R. (1982). Suction applied to a muscle biopsy maximizes sample size. *Medicine and Science in Sports and Exercise*, **14**, 101-102.

4. Gollnick, P.D., Parsons, D., & Oakley, C.R. (1983). Differentiation of fiber types in skeletal muscle from the sequential inactivation of myofibrillar actomyosin ATPase during acid preincubation. *Histochemistry*, **77**, 543-555.

5. Baldwin, K.M., Winder, W.W., Terjung, R.L., & Holloszy, J.O. (1973). Glycolytic enzymes in different types of skeletal muscle: Adaptation to exercise. *American Journal of Physiology*, **225**, 962-966.

6. Bancoft, J.D., & Stevens, A. (Eds.). (1982). *Theory and practice of histochemical techniques* (2nd ed.). Edinburgh, Scotland: Churchill Livingstone.

7. Bergmeyer, H.O. (Ed.). (1974). *Methods of enzymatic analysis* (2nd ed.) (Vols. 1-4). New York: Academic Press.

8. Bergmeyer, H.O. (Ed.). (1983). *Methods of enzymatic analysis* (3rd ed.) (Vols. 1-12). Deerfield Beach, FL: Verlag Chemie.

9. Brooke, M.H., & Kaiser, K.K. (1970). Three "myosin adenosine triphosphatase" systems: The nature of their pH lability and sulfhydryl dependence.

Journal of Histochemistry and Cytochemistry, **18** 670-672.

10. Chi, M.M.-Y., Hintz, C.S., Coyle, E.F., Martin, W.H., III, Ivy, J.L., Nemeth, P.M., Holloszy, J.O., & Lowry, O.H. (1983). Effects of detraining on enzymes of energy metabolism in individual human muscle fibers. *American Journal of Physiology*, **244**, C276-C287.

11. Costill, D.L., Pearson, D.R., & Fink, W.J. (1988). Impaired muscle glycogen storage after muscle biopsy. *Journal of Applied Physiology*, **64**(5), 2245-2248.

12. Dubowitz, V., Brooke, M.H., & Neville, H.E. (1973). *Major problems in neurology: Vol. 2. Muscle biopsy: A modern approach.* Philadelphia: W.B. Saunders.

13. Dubowitz, V., & Brooke, M.H. *Muscle biopsy: A practical approach* (2nd ed.). London: Baillière Tindall.

14. Estabrook, R.W., & Pullman, M.E. (Eds.). (1967). In S.P. Colowick & N.O. Kaplan (Eds.), *Methods in enzymology: Vol. X. Oxidation and phosphorylation.* New York: Academic Press.

15. Lowenstein, J.M. (Ed.). (1969). *Citric acid cycle.* In S.P. Colowick & N.O. Kaplan (Eds.), *Methods in enzymology: Vol. XIII. Citric acid cycle.* New York: Academic Press.

16. Lowry, O.H., & Passonneau, J.V. (1974). *A flexible system of enzymatic analysis.* New York: Academic Press.

17. Mattenheimer, H. (1970). *Micromethods for the clinical and biochemical laboratory.* Ann Arbor, MI: Ann Arbor Science.

18. Padykula, H.A., & Herman, E. (1955). The specificity of the histochemical method for adenosine triphosphatase. *Journal of Histochemistry and Cytochemistry*, **3**, 170-195.

19. Pesce, A.J., & Kaplan L.A. (Eds.). (1987). *Methods in clinical chemistry.* St. Louis: Mosby.

20. Srere, P.A. (1969). Citrate synthase. In S.P. Colowick & N.O. Kaplan (Eds.), *Methods in enzymology: Vol. XIII. Citric acid cycle.* New York: Academic Press.

21. Umbreit, W.W., Burris, R.H., & Stauffer, J.F. (1972). *Manometric and biochemical techniques: A manual describing methods applicable to the study of tissue metabolism.* Minneapolis: Borgess.

22. Costill, D.L. & Fink, W.J. (1990). *Analytical methods for the measurement of Human Performance.* Muncie, IN: Human Performance Laboratory, Ball State University.

23. Vollestad, N.K., Vaage, K.O., & Hermansen, L. (1984). Muscle glycogen depletion patterns in type I and subgroups of type II fibers during prolonged severe exercise in man. *Acta Physiologica Scandinavica*, **122**, 433-441.

24. Henriksson, J., Chi, M.M.-Y., Hintz, C.S., Young, D.A., Kaiser, K.K., Salmons, S., & Lowry, O.H. (1986). Chronic stimulation of mammalian muscle: Changes in enzymes of six metabolic pathways. *American Journal of Physiology*, **251** (Cell Physiology 20), C614-C632.

CHAPTER 10

The Measurement of Body Composition

Michael L. Pollock, PhD
Linda Garzarella, MS
University of Florida

James E. Graves, PhD
Syracuse University

The purpose of this chapter is to describe the more popular techniques that are used for the determination of body composition. The equipment used, methodology, pitfalls associated with the measurement technique, and accuracy (reliability) and validity of the various methods will be described. Where appropriate, controversial issues concerning the various protocols/procedures will be discussed.

Finally, normative data will be presented and inference as to the interpretation of body composition results for general health and fitness and athletic competition will be presented. The following techniques for measuring body composition will be reviewed: hydrostatic (underwater) weighing, anthropometry, bioelectrical impedance, ultrasound, and total body DEXA.

The measurement of body composition has become a popular and standard practice for many physicians, athletic trainers, and allied health professionals. Evidence supports the notion that being overweight (excess body fat) is related to musculoskeletal injury, nonadherence to exercise training, reduced athletic performance, and many health problems (1, 6). More specifically, excessive body fat has been shown to be associated with such health problems as hypertension, diabetes mellitus, depression, hyperlipidemia, and coronary heart disease

(CHD). In a 26-year follow-up of participants from the Framingham Heart Study, Hubert, Feinlab, McNamara, & Castelli (4) showed that obesity in itself is an independent risk factor for mortality from CHD. In most athletic events participants must move their body mass quickly and efficiently; thus, the accumulation of body fat can deter running speed and jumping ability as well as endurance performance.

The term *overweight* refers to an amount of total body weight (mass) above what is recommended based upon stature. The Metropolitan Life Insurance tables for height and weight have been used for years as a standard index for health professionals to determine appropriate body weight (7). More recently, the body mass index (BMI), which is the ratio of weight to height squared (BMI = wt/ht^2 expressed as kg/m²), became more popular for use in epidemiological research (8, 9). The problem with the term *overweight* and use of height–weight or BMI measures is their lack of specificity in describing leanness–fatness. Thus, the term *obesity* is used to depict specifically what proportion of the body composition is fat (i.e., being too fat).

When they evaluated football players, Wilmore and Haskell (10) demonstrated the problem with using the term *overweight* to describe body composition (leanness–fatness). Football players were shown to be overweight according to the BMI, but when body composition was determined by hydrostatic weighing they were not considered overfat; they were overweight as a result of having excessive amounts of fat-free mass (FFM), not fat weight. Thus, more recently, various techniques to measure body composition use models that differentiate fat from FFM.

The two-compartment model as proposed by Brozek et al. (11) and Siri (12) assumes that body composition is made up of fat and fat-free body compartments. The fat-free body (FFM) includes the muscle, bone, and other nonfatty tissues (see Figure 10.1). Although the two-compartment model is well accepted and used extensively in the research and clinical settings, it's not without problems. This system assumes that the composition of fat and FFM is constant for all individuals,

that is, that the density of fat is 0.900 g/cc and FFM is 1.100 g/cc. Clarys, Martin, and Drinkwater (13) studied dissection data from 25 cadavers and found a considerable variation among subjects in density for bone and muscle. The variation in FFM composition in this specific population was approximated at 0.006 g/cc by Lohman (14), which could cause an error of 2.5% in estimated percent fat. Lohman (15) has also pointed to the errors involved in determining body composition in children and youth prior to their age of "chemical maturity" (ages 15 to 18 years, for most). The FFM is not stable in growing children and youth because water content decreases and body solids (bone density) increase in concentration until maturity. At the opposite end of the age spectrum, FFM also changes composition in older adults. In particular, after menopause in females and 60 years of age in males, bone mineral density decreases significantly (16).

Lohman (15) has summarized the views of other investigators concerning two- to four-compartment systems used for body composition determination (Figure 10.1.). Because it is more time-consuming and technically difficult to measure bone mineral (density) and the chemical components of FFM and fat, the two-compartment system has continued to be used extensively. More recently, the availability of technology such as total-body dual-energy X-ray absorptiometry (DEXA), computerized tomography, and magnetic resonance imaging has made the *in vivo* estimation of the components of the four-compartment model more feasible. Even so, the cost of such technology limits the use of such techniques to a few researchers.

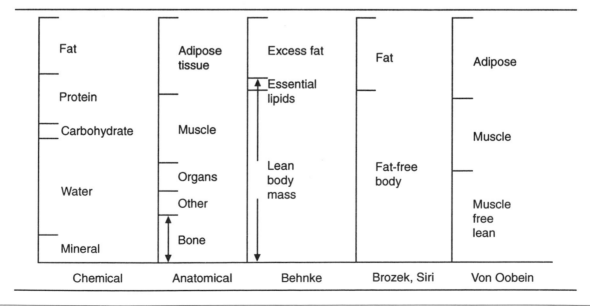

Figure 10.1 Models for determination of body composition by different investigators, from Lohman (15). Applicability of body composition techniques and constants for children and youth.

HYDROSTATIC WEIGHING

Hydrostatic or underwater weighing is the most widely used laboratory procedure for measuring body density (D_b) and often serves as a criterion method for other indirect techniques (17, 18). This method utilizes Archimedes' principle that a body immersed in a fluid is acted on by a buoyancy force that is evidenced by a loss of weight equal to the weight of the displaced fluid (18). Because the density of fat is less than that of water, fat contributes to the buoyancy force, as does any air in the lungs or trapped on the surface of the body. The density of bone and muscle tissue, however, is greater than that of water and will cause a person to sink. Therefore, a person having more bone and muscle mass and less fat will weigh more in the water and thus have a greater D_b—that is, a lower percent body fat and a greater percent FFM.

There are two basic methods of hydrostatic weighing used for determining D_b: underwater weighing and water displacement. Both techniques show similar high reliability and validity (19), but because underwater weighing tanks are more readily available, only this procedure will be described in detail.

Equipment and Methodology

Hydrostatic weighing can be performed in either a sitting or a supine position. For the seated position, which is used most commonly, necessary equipment includes a tank (recommended size $4 \times 4 \times 5$ ft) or pool of warm water, a chair or seat, an autopsy or similar type of scale (15- to 25-g increments) or load cell, a lift system (optional), and a weighted belt. Some subjects may also require a nose clip. The hydrostatic weighing tank can be made of stainless steel, fiberglass, ceramic tile, plexiglass, and so on. The chair, if suspended from a scale, can be made from PVC or a combination of PVC and webbing material. The lift system requires a 1/4-ton hoist or ratchet system that is mounted to the ceiling.

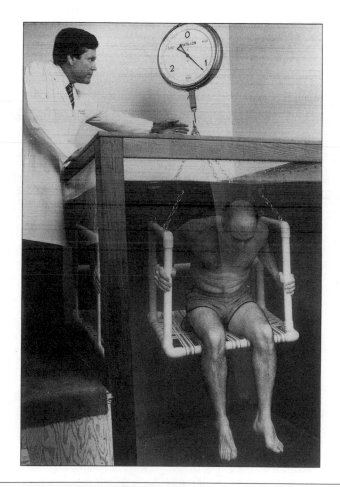

Figure 10.2 An underwater weighing tank used to determine body density. In this illustration the chair seat is attached to an autopsy scale. Residual volume is measured separately out of the water.
(Photographs by Wendy V. Watriss, 1985. Published with permission.)

The chair seat is suspended from the hoist or ratchet system (see Figure 10.2). The hoist is a luxury item; it assists in setting the chair height so that the chin is at water level. Scuba belts are the simplest weight devices to use. These can be adjusted easily and help keep fatter subjects firmly on the seat. If a swimming pool is used, special devices are commercially available that assist in suspending the scale and chair seat in the proper position in the water.

Figure 10.3 shows a modern alternative method of measuring underwater weight. Note that instead of being suspended from the ceiling, the chair seat rests on load cells that are directly connected to a recorder or a computer to provide near-instant analysis and feedback. Although a load cell system can make the measurement more objective and supply a permanent record of the procedure, it has not been shown to be more accurate with experienced technicians (20).

The advantages of a small tank over a swimming pool are numerous: privacy, no scheduling conflicts, less water turbulence, and greater control of water temperature. The water in a small tank must be treated with a disinfecting agent such as chlorine to avoid potential health hazards. If treating the water is not possible, the tank water should be changed between subjects. To avoid excessive shivering, and enhance subject comfort and cooperation, the water should be controlled at a comfortable temperature (32 °C to 35 °C). This can be accomplished with a commercial water heater and pump system or by periodically refilling the tank with warm water.

Subject instruction and preparation prior to underwater weighing are necessary for obtaining the best results. Pollock and Wilmore (17) recommend a normal diet, fluid intake, and exercise pattern the day prior to testing. Foods that cause excessive amounts of gas in the gastrointestinal (GI) tract should be avoided. Also, subjects should abstain from eating or smoking for a minimum of 2 hours prior to testing. Measuring subjects in the morning prior to breakfast is ideal. Females should not be hydrostatically weighed during menstruation or 3 days before or after. The underwater weighing measure is greatly affected by factors that influence hydration status, such as menstruation, drugs, physical activity, and saunas (21).

Minimal clothing should be worn during underwater weighing, to avoid trapping air. Ideally, men should be measured in a swimming brief and women should wear a bikini or similar type of two-piece swimsuit.

Before entering the tank, subjects should be asked to void their bladders and defecate if necessary. Next, the subject is weighed to determine dry weight or weight in air (W_a) to the nearest 100 g. After this, the subject climbs

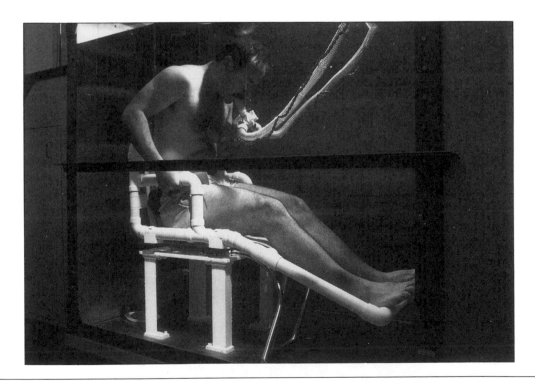

Figure 10.3   The tank shown in this figure is similar to the tank shown in Figure 10.2, but the chair seat is resting on three load cells that are directly connected to a computer and recorder. Residual volume is measured at the time of underwater weighing.
(Photograph from Harper Student Center, Medical University of South Carolina, Charleston, SC. Published with permission of Leslie W. Organ, MD.)

into the water tank, stands on the bottom if possible, gets completely wet, and rubs the hands over the entire body to remove any trapped air bubbles from skin, hair, and bathing suit. The subject then sits on the chair seat. If necessary, the subject will then put on the weight belt.

Once the subject is seated, the chair height is adjusted so that water level is just below the subject's chin. At this point, the test procedures are explained. The subject is instructed to hyperventilate four or five times after a deep breath, and start a full expiration while the head is still above the water.

When the subject feels like most of the air has been expelled, he or she bends forward slowly at the waist for complete submersion while continuing to exhale air. If the head is only partially submerged, the tester should tap the subject's head until it goes completely under. The subject's hands should be resting relaxed on top of the thighs, to safeguard against a rocking motion that can take place if subject is holding on to the knees or the chair. The rocking motion causes oscillation of the scale, making it difficult to read.

The tester should encourage the subject to continue to exhale underwater until no more air can be expelled. At this point, the subject sits as still and relaxed as possible. The underwater weight is then determined to the nearest 25 g. Once the underwater weight is obtained, the tester taps on the side of the tank to signal for the subject to surface.

The procedure should be repeated 6 to 10 times, or more if necessary, because there is a learning curve associated with the technique (22). It is important that the tester be patient and make the subject feel as comfortable as possible. The tester should also critique each trial, giving the subject feedback so that the next trial can be performed better.

Once the subject's weight levels off after repeated trials, the procedure is completed. The water temperature should be verified and recorded. In temperature-controlled tanks, usually only pre- and postprocedure values need to be recorded. The tare weight is determined after the subject gets out of the tank. Tare weight is the combined weight of the chair, chains, and, when applicable, the weighted belt, taken at the same level at which the underwater weight was observed. Tare weight is then subtracted from the underwater weight to derive the net underwater weight of the subject (W_w). Body density (D_b) is then calculated using the equation of Goldman and Buskirk (23):

$$D_b = \frac{W_a}{\frac{(W_a - W_w)}{D_w} - (RV + 100 \text{ cc})}$$

where D_b is body density (g/cc), W_a is body weight in air (kg), W_w is body weight in water (kg), D_w is density

of water (g/ml), and RV is residual lung volume (ml). One hundred cc is a correction factor that represents the approximate amount of air trapped in the gastrointestinal tract.

See Figure 10.4 for an example of a data collection form used for determining RV and D_b by underwater weighing. From the data found in Figure 10.4, Trials 5, 6, and 7 were used in the calculation of D_b. The subject in Figure 10.4 leveled off after Trial 4, but additional trials were taken to assure his best effort. The density of water (D_w) is temperature dependent (refer to Table 10.1).

Residual volume, the amount of air remaining in the lungs at the end of a maximal expiration, should be determined. However, if an estimation is used, the following equations developed by Goldman and Becklace (24) are recommended:

Men: RV = 0.017 (age in years) + 0.06858 (height in inches) − 3.477

Women: RV = 0.009 (age in years) + 0.08128 (height in inches) − 3.900.

Percent fat can then be calculated from D_b from one of the two following equations:

Brozek and colleagues (11):

$$\% \text{ fat} = [(4.57/D_b) - 4.142] \times 100$$

Siri (12):

$$\% \text{ fat} = [(4.95/D_b) - 4.500] \times 100$$

In the calculation of D_b in Figure 10.4, RV was measured twice and averaged. For verification, usually more than one RV measure is determined. Measures should be within the reported variation of the technique (usually 50-100 ml).

Table 10.1 Conversion Chart for Determining Water Density (D_w) at Various Water Temperatures (W Temp)

W Temp (°C)	D_w	W Temp (°C)	D_w
23	0.997569	31	0.995372
24	0.997327	32	0.995057
25	0.997075	33	0.994734
26	0.996814	34	0.994403
27	0.996544	35	0.994063
28	0.996264	36	0.993716
29	0.995976	37	0.993360
30	0.995678		

From Pollock & Willmore (17). Published with permission.

CENTER FOR EXERCISE SCIENCE
UNIVERSITY OF FLORIDA, GAINESVILLE, FL 32611
(904) 392-9575

BODY COMPOSITION ANALYSIS: DATA COLLECTION FORM

Name_____   Date_____02-07-90_____
Age_19_ Sex_F_ Tester_JEG_ SF_LMG_ UWW   Group_____
Weight___58.2__(kg)___128.2__(lb)   Height____168.1__(cm)___66.2__(in)

HYDROSTATIC WEIGHING

Trial	Wt(kg)	Trial	Wt(kg)
1	3.475	9	
2	3.500	10	
3	3.400	11	
4	3.450	12	
5	3.500	13	
6	3.500	14	
7	3.500	15	
8		16	

T_i(°C)_35.0_ T_f(°C)_35.0_

Average Weight = _3.500_ kg
Tare Weight   = _2.000_ kg
True UWW   = _1.500_ kg
Body Density   = _1.037_ g/ml

RESIDUAL VOLUME

Trial 1 _0.783_ L
Trial 2 _0.834_ L
Trial 3 _____ L

Average = _0.809_ L

SKINFOLDS (mm)

Chest	15.5
Axilla	14.0
Triceps	20.0
Subscapular	11.5
Abdominal	26.5
Suprailiac	18.5
Thigh	34.0
Sum of 7	140.0
Suprapatellar	27.0
Medial calf	19.5

SUMMARY

% Fat (SF)	=	26.1	%
% Fat (UWW)	=	27.4	%
Fat Wt.	=	35.1	lb
	=	15.9	kg
Fat Free Wt.	=	93.2	lb
	=	42.3	kg
Target % Fat	=	23.0	%
Target Wt.	=	121.0	lb
	=	54.9	kg

Figure 10.4 Body composition and pulmonary function form used in determining body density by underwater weighing. (Courtesy of the Center for Exercise Science, University of Florida, Gainesville, FL.)

Sources of Error

Although considered the criterion or "gold standard" when developing prediction equations for field methods, the hydrostatic technique is not free from measurement error. One potential source of error comes from the determination of total body volume. To calculate D_b (body mass/body volume) by the hydrostatic method, total body volume must be corrected for the RV and the volume of air trapped in the GI tract. Although GI gas volume can vary, Buskirk (25) proposed the use of the constant correction value of 100 ml. The error in the calculation of D_b associated with variation in GI gas is relatively small, so the constant of 100 ml has been used routinely. However, the error associated with RV can be large and can have a sizable effect on the final calculation of D_b (17, 26). Residual volume can be estimated from average population values based on age, sex, and height as shown earlier (24) or by an estimated percentage of the vital capacity (approximately 25% to 30%) (27, 28). Wilmore (26) compared the use of actual RV, and the two estimation techniques for measuring RV, in the assessment of body composition by underwater weighing for college-aged males and females. The results indicated a close agreement (< 0.001 g/cc) between measures of D_b, percent fat, and FFM, using the actual measurement of RV, and the two techniques used for estimating RV. Thus, estimated RVs can be used satisfactorily for screening purposes and when research is conducted on large populations. However, because of the variability of RV estimates based on age, height, and weight, or vital capacity, only actual measures are valid for use with individuals needing counseling or in research with small groups of subjects. Katch and Katch (27) showed that a 600-ml difference in RV could affect relative fat by 8% and FFM by 12 kg.

Should RV be measured before or after the underwater weighing procedure? Should RV be measured out of the water or in the water during the actual procedure (Figure 10.3)? Although 200- to 300-ml differences in RV have been reported in a subject's measurements taken in and out of the water (18), if care is taken to have the subject exhale fully and use similar body positions for the measurement of RV and underwater weight, the error is thought to be small (18, 29). For example, a 200-ml error in RV accounts for only a 1% error in percent body fat (Table 10.2). This is an acceptable amount of error for use in the clinical and research setting. The important factor is to replicate the technique consistently so that it will not affect serial analysis of D_b. In this case, the error in RV is constant in one direction. Although in most cases the difference between measuring RV in the water at the time of underwater weighing and measuring it out of the water is small, the number of trials needed to obtain an accurate D_b can be reduced when measuring RV in the water. This

is because it is not necessary for subjects to maximally exhale when RV is measured in the water. Another advantage of measuring RV in the water at the time of weighing is that many subjects can maximally exhale out of the water but feel uncomfortable doing so in the water.

In 1987, the authors and others had an unusual opportunity to evaluate the effect of measuring D_b while RV was determined out of or in the water during the underwater weighing procedure. As part of an eight-center research project, a subject visited each laboratory within a 2-week period for assessment of body composition. The purpose of the visit was to standardize testing procedures and determine interlaboratory variation among measures. All laboratories had experienced investigators and determined body density using the underwater weighing technique. Four of the laboratories measured RV while the subject was out of the water, and four measured it while he was in the water as part of the procedure. Among laboratories, body weight varied from 77.4 to 78.3 kg ($X = 77.9 \pm 0.35$ kg), D_b from 1.0717 to 1.0761 g/cc ($X = 1.0733 \pm 0.00136$ g/cc), RV from 1.00 to 1.44 L ($X = 1.22 \pm 0.13$ L), and percent fat from 10.0% to 11.9% ($X = 11.2\% \pm 0.6\%$). As can be seen, variation among laboratories was small, and there was no mean difference in D_b and percent fat between laboratories who measured RV in the water as compared with those who measured it out of the water (17; unpublished data from T. Lohman, University of Arizona, December 1987).

The determination of underwater weight is another source of error for the hydrostatic technique. How many trials are necessary to get valid results, and which trial(s) should be used for the calculation of D_b? Katch (22) conducted a study to determine the minimum number of trials necessary to establish "true" underwater weight during D_b measurements. He demonstrated that there is a learning curve associated with successive trials of underwater weighing. He concluded that 9 to 10 trials were necessary to obtain the most representative underwater weight for an individual and recommended that the average of the last 3 trials be used to calculate D_b. Behnke and Wilmore (18) also suggested performing 10 trials; however, they selected the true underwater weight as

1. the highest weight, if it is observed more than once;
2. the second-highest weight, if it is observed more than once and the first criterion is not met; or
3. the third-highest weight, if neither the first nor the second criterion is attained.

They chose this method of selection to reduce the possibility of underestimating the actual underwater weight

Table 10.2   The Effect of Errors in Residual Volume (RV), Scale Weight in the Water (W_1), and Body Weight Out of the Water (W_2) on Determination of Body Density (D_b) from Underwater Weighing

Measure	Actual*	Errors[†] 1	2	3
RV (L)	1.200	1.400	1.700	2.200
D_b (g/cc)	1.0605	1.0631	1.0669	1.0734
Fat (%)	16.74	15.63	13.95	11.16
W_1 (kg)	4.24	4.29	4.34	4.44
D_b (g/cc)	1.0605	1.0612	1.0618	1.0631
Fat (%)	16.74	16.46	16.18	15.62
W_2 (kg)	88.70	88.80	89.20	89.70
D_b (g/cc)	1.0605	1.0605	1.0601	1.0598
Fat (%)	16.74	16.78	16.91	17.09

*Actual values are from Figure 6-27, Pollock & Wilmore (17).

[†]Each error for D_b and percent fat is calculated with the other two variables from the actual values.

From Pollock & Wilmore (17). Published with permission.

on the subject who attained the highest value during the first 5 to 7 trials.

Thus, the measurement errors associated with the underwater weighing technique are mainly associated with errors in RV, body weight out of the water (W_a) and body weight in the water (W_w). For example, Table 10.2 shows the effect of errors in RV, W_a, and W_w on the determination of D_b from underwater weighing. The data for D_b are from our laboratory. The hypothetical errors of 200, 500, and 1,000 ml for RV; 50, 100, and 200 g for W_w; and 100, 500, and 1,000 g for W_a were added to the actual calculated D_b.

As shown in Table 10.2, errors in RV can have a dramatic effect on D_b (2% to 5.5% fat units). Errors of this magnitude are common when RV is estimated from age and height or vital capacity, and this is why estimations of RV are not recommended when D_b values are used for individual counseling. An error of 50 g or more in underwater scale weight (W_w) would be highly unusual, thus the error associated with an incorrect W_w should be less than 0.5% fat. Body weight (W_a) can be quite variable depending on time of day, dietary pattern, hydration status, and illness. As previously mentioned, excessive dehydration or hydration caused by such factors as exercise, sauna, diarrhea, medications, or menstruation cycle can have a significant effect on D_b (17, 21). For example, a 2- to 3-kg weight fluctuation could cause a 1.0% change in percent body fat.

A final consideration is the conversion of D_b to percent fat. The theoretical relationship between D_b and fatness can be derived if the fat and the FFM are assumed to have a constant density for all individuals (14). Percent fat is usually predicted from either the Siri (12) or the Brozek et al. (11) equation. The Siri formula avoids the assumption of a constant water content of the FFM and allows correction for abnormal hydration. However, it is still based on the assumption that fat density is 0.900 g/cc and FFM density is 1.100 g/cc (30). The equation of Brozek et al. (11) utilizes the concept of a reference man of a specified D_b and body composition (15.3% fat). Within D_b of 1.09 and 1.03 g/cc, the two formulas agree within 1% fat (14).

Although universally accepted, the Siri and Brozek equations are not without problems. Both are based on the results of direct compositional analysis of human cadavers, but only a few cadavers were used and they did not represent a distribution of the normal population (17, 18). As previously mentioned in this chapter, the density of FFM and fat are quite variable in humans (13) and can cause an error in estimating percent fat from D_b by 2.5% to 3.8% (14).

Reliability

Despite the potential sources of error, the hydrostatic technique has been shown to be highly reliable with

Pearson-product correlation coefficients greater than .95 when measurements were made over time intervals ranging from 30 min to a couple days (31-35). A small standard error of measurement (less than 0.002 g/cc) has also been observed (35, 36).

ANTHROPOMETRY

Anthropometry is the science that deals with the measurement of size, weight, and proportions of the human body. Anthropometric techniques (skinfold fat, circumference, and diameter measurements) are popular for predicting body composition in the field setting because they are inexpensive to attain, require little space, and are easy to perform (17, 18). Until recently, the techniques used to assess skinfold, circumference, and diameter measures varied and lacked standardization.

In 1985 at the Anthropometric Standardization Conference held in Airlie, VA, 50 professionals from the fields of epidemiology, exercise science, human biology, medicine, nutrition, physical anthropology, and physical education met to discuss how to standardize anthropometric procedures. The *Anthropometric Standardization Reference Manual* (ASRM) was a written consensus developed by the many experts attending this conference (37). The recommended procedures in the standardization manual will be described in this chapter. However, it is important that when body composition is predicted from anthropometric measures, the method employed to develop the prediction equation should be used to obtain the measures. Because of the popularity of the generalized equations for estimating D_b from skinfold and circumference measures developed by Jackson and Pollock for men (38) and Jackson, Pollock, and Ward for women (39), the differences of these techniques from those in the standardization manual will also be outlined.

This section will describe two of the popular techniques used for estimating body composition: skinfold fat and circumferences. Because diameter measures are more related to skeletal size than to body fat, they are not often used to predict body composition. See Lohman, Roche, and Martorell (37) and Pollock and Wilmore (17) for a more detailed description of diameter measures.

Skinfold Measurements

A skinfold thickness is actually two layers of skin and two layers of fat. To measure this thickness, a caliper that is accurately calibrated and has a constant pressure of 10 g/mm² is recommended (18). Although this is a general recommendation, some cheaper plastic calipers are acceptable for use in the nonresearch setting (40).

When measuring skinfold thicknesses, it is important to standardize site selection and location, because small differences in location can cause significant errors in measurement (37, 40). Depending on which caliper is used, measures are recorded to the nearest 0.1 cm or 0.5 cm. For standardization purposes, all measurements should be taken from the right side of the body.

Methodology

The following description of skinfold measurement technique is taken from the *Anthropometric Standardization Reference Manual* (37). When different, the techniques of Pollock and Wilmore (17) will also be presented.

General Technique

In the taking of skinfold measurements, the thumb and index finger of one hand are used to palpate the fat-muscle interface at about 1 cm proximal to the site at which the skinfold is to be measured (41). The thumb and index finger should be placed on the skin about 8 cm apart, on a line that is perpendicular to the long axis of the skinfold to be measured. The thicker the fat layer, the greater the distance needed between the thumb and index finger. The thumb and index finger are then drawn toward each other, and a fold is grasped firmly between them. The amount of subcutaneous tissue picked up should form a fold that has parallel sides, and the fold should be perpendicular to the surface of the body at the measurement site. With the other hand, pressure is exerted to separate the caliper jaws, and the caliper is placed over the skinfold so that the fixed arm of the caliper is positioned on one side of the fold approximately 1 cm adjacent to the first finger. The pressure on the caliper is then released gradually so that the caliper jaws come toward each other. It is best to line up one point of the caliper at one side of the fat fold first and then the other point as the caliper is released.

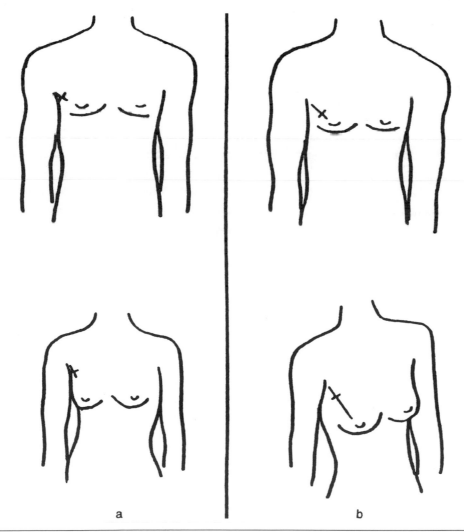

a   b

Figure 10.5   Measurement of the chest skinfold according to (a) Lohman, Roche, and Martorell (37) and (b) Pollock and Wilmore (17).

Measurement is made about 2 to 4 s after the pressure is released (18, 37). The measurement is repeated two or three times until a consistency is observed and the mean of the consistent measures is recorded. If the measure keeps getting smaller with each trial, stop and come back to that site later. The decrease in the fat fold is due to compression.

Pectoral (Chest) Skinfold

The ASRM recommends that the same chest skinfold site be used for both males and females (Figure 10.5a). Pectoral skinfold thickness is measured using a skinfold with its long axis directed to the nipple. The skinfold is picked up on the anterior axillary fold as high as possible; the thickness is measured 1 cm inferior to this. The measurement is taken while the subject stands with the arms hanging at the sides. According to Pollock and Wilmore (17), the chest skinfold is a diagonal fold one half of the distance between the anterior axillary line and the nipple, for men, and one third of the distance from the anterior axillary line and the equivalent position, for women (Figure 10.5b).

Midaxillary Skinfold

The subject stands erect with the right arm slightly abducted and flexed at the shoulder joint while the measurer stands facing the subject's right side. It may be more comfortable to have the subject rest the arm on the tester's shoulder. The ASRM recommends that the midaxillary skinfold be measured at the level of the xiphisternal junction in the midaxillary line, with the skinfold horizontal (Figure 10.6). According to Pollock and Wilmore (17), the location of the skinfold is the same, but a vertical fold is measured.

Triceps Skinfold

The ASRM recommends that "the triceps skinfold be measured 'vertically' in the midline of the posterior aspect of the arm, over the triceps muscle, at a point midway between the lateral projection of the acromion process of the scapula and the inferior margin of the olecranon process of the ulna" (Figure 10.7). The subject is measured standing with the arm hanging loosely and comfortably at the subject's side.

Subscapular Skinfold

The ASRM recommends that "the subscapula skinfold is picked up on a diagonal, inclined infero-laterally approximately 45° to the horizontal plane in the natural cleavage lines of the skin" (Figure 10.8a). "The site is just inferior to the inferior angle of the scapula. . . . The subject stands comfortably erect, with the upper extremities relaxed at the sides of the body. To locate the site, the measurer palpates the scapula, running the fingers inferiorly and laterally, along its vertebral border until the inferior angle is identified." For obese subjects, gently placing the right arm behind the back helps in locating the site. According to Pollock and Wilmore (17), the skinfold is taken on a diagonal line coming from the vertebral border, 1 to 2 cm from the inferior angle of the scapula (Figure 10.8b).

Abdominal Skinfold

The ASRM recommends that "the abdominal skinfold is taken horizontally at a site which is 3 cm lateral to the midpoint of the umbilicus and 1 cm inferior to it" (Figure 10.9a). The measure is taken with a horizontal fold. The subject stands and relaxes the abdominal wall musculature as much as possible and breathes normally. According to Pollock and Wilmore (17), a vertical fold is taken at a lateral distance of approximately 2 cm from the umbilicus (Figure 10.9b).

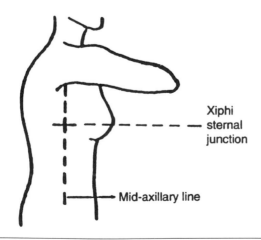

Figure 10.6 Illustration of the level of the xiphisternal junction at which the midaxillary skinfold is taken.

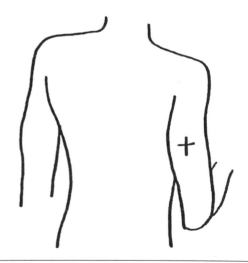

Figure 10.7 Landmark for the triceps skinfold. The elbow is bent to help locate the site, but the skinfold is measured with the arm hanging loosely at the subject's side.

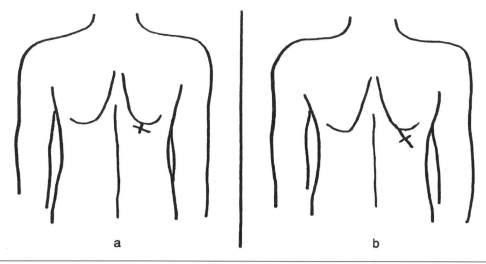

Figure 10.8   Landmark for the subscapular skinfold according to (a) Lohman, Roche, and Martorell (37) and (b) Pollock and Wilmore (17).

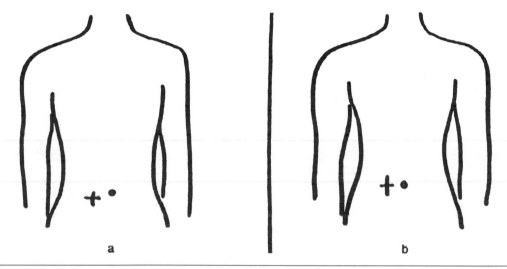

Figure 10.9   Landmark for the abdominal skinfold according to (a) Lohman, Roche, and Martorell (37) and (b) Pollock and Wilmore (17).

Suprailiac Skinfold

The ASRM recommends that "the suprailiac skinfold is measured in the midaxillary line immediately superior to the iliac crest. A diagonal skinfold is grasped just posterior to the midaxillary line following the natural cleavage lines of the skin" (Figure 10.10a). The subject stands erect with the arms hanging comfortably at the subject's sides. Sometimes the right arm or hand needs to be moved slightly posterior or be abducted to improve access to the site. According to Pollock and Wilmore (17), the suprailiac fold is measured as a diagonal fold above the crest of the ilium at the spot where an imaginary line would come down from the anterior axillary line (Figure 10.10b).

Anterior Thigh Skinfold

The ASRM recommends that "the thigh skinfold site is located in the midline of the anterior aspect of the thigh, midway between the inguinal crease and proximal border of the patella. The subject flexes the hip to assist location of the inguinal crease" (Figure 10.11). A vertical skinfold is measured while the subject stands with body weight shifted to the left leg and relaxes the right leg with the right knee slightly flexed.

Suprapatellar Skinfold

The ASRM recommends that "the suprapatellar skinfold site is located in the midsagittal plane on the anterior aspect of the thigh, 2 cm proximal to the proximal edge

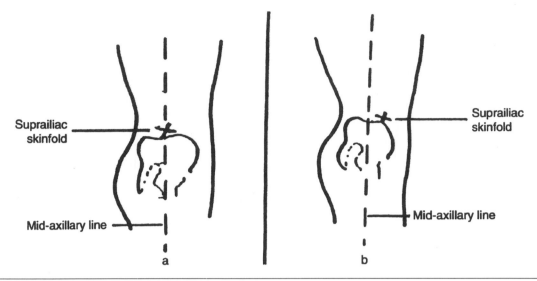

Figure 10.10   Landmark for the suprailiac skinfold according to (a) Lohman, Roche, and Martorell (37) and (b) Pollock and Wilmore (17).

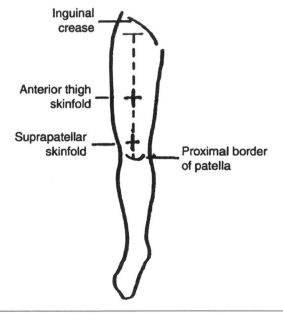

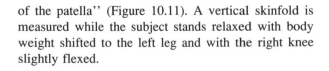

Figure 10.11   Location of the anterior thigh and suprapatellar skinfold sites.

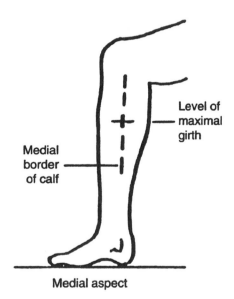

Figure 10.12   Medial calf skinfold site.

of the patella'' (Figure 10.11). A vertical skinfold is measured while the subject stands relaxed with body weight shifted to the left leg and with the right knee slightly flexed.

Medial Calf Skinfold

The ASRM recommends that the medial calf fold be measured with the subject standing and the right foot placed on a stool or bench so that the knee and hip are flexed to about a 90° angle (Figure 10.12). This fold can also be measured with the subject in the sitting

position. A vertical fold is measured on the medial aspect of the calf at the level of maximal girth.

Biceps Skinfold

The ASRM recommends that ''the biceps skinfold thickness is measured as the thickness of a vertical fold raised on the anterior aspect of the arm, over the belly of the biceps muscle'' (Figure 10.13). The subject stands with arms hanging relaxed at the sides with the right palm directed anteriorly.

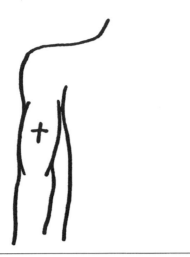

Figure 10.13 Location of the biceps skinfold site.

Sources of Error

Important potential sources of measurement error associated with skinfold measurements are caliper selection and tester reliability, including inter- and intraobserver measurement error and the variance associated with the selection of skinfold site (40). Differences in skinfold fat readings may result from the use of different calipers. According to Edwards et al. (42), the pressure exerted by the caliper has a significant effect on both the skinfold measurement and the consistency with which the measurement is repeated. Sloan and Shapiro (43) compared three calipers, the Harpenden, Lange, and MNL, and found that the Harpenden caliper yielded slightly better between-observer results. However, there were no systematic differences between measurements at any site among the calipers.

The results of Lohman and colleagues (44) were different—the Lange calipers consistently overestimated the results of the Harpenden calipers by approximately 1 to 2 mm per site. Gruber et al. (45) showed a high correlation between Harpenden and Lange skinfold fat calipers, but the Harpenden was 10% lower per skinfold site. This study demonstrated that using the Harpenden rather than the Lange caliper resulted in 10% difference in the sum of seven skinfolds, which caused a 10% underprediction of D_b. Thus, it is important that those estimating D_b/percent fat from skinfold fat equations use the same caliper that the investigator used to develop the equation. For example, if the Harpenden caliper is used and the generalized equations by Jackson and Pollock (38) and Jackson, Pollock, and Ward (39) are used in estimating D_b/percent fat, the 10% difference in the sum of skinfolds measured should be added.

Intratester reliability can be attained rapidly with practice and good instruction (40). Test-retest correlations well above .9 have been shown by Pollock et al. (46, 47) and Jackson et al. (48) for seven measures

(chest, axilla, triceps, subscapula, abdomen, suprailium, and anterior thigh). It has been suggested that approximately 50 to 100 persons need to be measured to attain a high level of competency in taking skinfolds (17, 27).

The best way to avoid interobserver variability is to have the same investigator take all the measurements. However, when others use published regression equations to estimate body composition, and in long-term epidemiological studies where several different investigators take skinfold measurements, the intertester source of measurement error cannot be avoided (44, 48). Lohman et al. (44) showed significant variation in skinfolds when experienced testers did not practice together or standardize procedures. One 30-min practice session minimized such errors. Jackson, Pollock, and Gettman (48) investigated intertester reliability of skinfold measurements and percent fat, and found that the variation among experienced testers who had practiced together was a relatively small source of measurement error (intertester reliability estimates exceeded .93). These results agree with findings reported by others (31, 49).

The most important factor associated with intertester error is variation in selection of skinfold site (40). In a study conducted by Lohman et al. (44), significant variation was found in the selection of sites with four experienced testers. Variation was greatest at the anterior thigh and suprailium. Size of the skinfold can also cause variation. Pollock, Jackson, and Graves (50) conducted a study to determine whether skinfold fat measurement error was related to the quantity of the skinfold measured rather than to site or sex. The results showed that, for trained testers, measurement error is more related to size of the skinfold than to site. The standard error among testers was approximately 1 mm for every 10 mm of skinfold fat—that is, 1 mm variation with a skinfold value of 10 mm; 2 mm with 20 mm; 3 mm with 30 mm; and so on.

Circumference Measurements

Circumference measurements, used either alone or in combination with skinfold measurements, provide information about body composition, growth, nutritional status, and fat patterning (18, 37, 51). Relatively accurate estimates of body composition (D_b/percent fat) have been found with circumference measures (52) using abdomen, right thigh, and right forearm circumferences for young women; abdomen, right thigh, and right calf for middle-aged women; right upper arm, abdomen, and right forearm for young men; and buttocks (hip), abdomen, and right forearm for middle-aged men. Refer to McArdle, Katch, and Katch (52a, pp. 813-819) for conversion charts to predict percent fat from the previously mentioned circumferences. Tracking by use of circumference measures before and after intervention programs for weight control or weight loss and exercise training makes the data important for use in the clinical setting.

Methodology

The following description of circumference measurement technique is taken from the *Anthropometric Standardization Reference Manual* (37). Where different, the techniques of Pollock and Wilmore (17) will also be presented.

General Technique

The tape measure should be flexible, nonstretchable (steel), approximately 0.7 cm wide, and easily retractable. Preferably, the tape should be in metric units on one side and inches on the other. Circumferences should be measured with the zero end of the tape held in the left hand (37). In the taking of circumference measurements, the tape is positioned in a horizontal plane or perpendicular to the length of the segment being measured. A mirror or assistant should be used to help ensure that the tape is horizontal or not accidentally hung up on a piece of clothing. Placement of the tape for each specific measurement is important because inconsistent positioning reduces validity and reliability. Tension on the tape should be snug around the body part but not so tight that it compresses the subcutaneous fat layer. For trunk circumferences (shoulder, chest, waist, and abdomen), measurements should be taken at the end of a normal expiration. According to Pollock and Wilmore (17), all trunk circumferences are taken during midtidal volume. Measures are recorded to the nearest 0.1 cm. Measures should be taken twice and agree within certain limits. The ASRM recommends that intra-intermeasure limits for circumferences should be within 1.0 cm for the shoulder, chest, abdomen, waist, and buttocks; 0.5 cm for the thigh; and 0.2 cm for the calf, ankle, wrist, arm, and forearm. If this standard is not met, the tester should repeat the measure two more times.

Shoulder Circumference

The subject stands upright with arms by the sides and weight evenly distributed. The tape is positioned horizontally at the maximal circumference of the shoulders at the level of the greatest protrusion of the deltoid muscles (Figure 10.14).

Chest Circumference

The subject stands erect and abducts the arms so the tape can be placed around the chest at the level of the

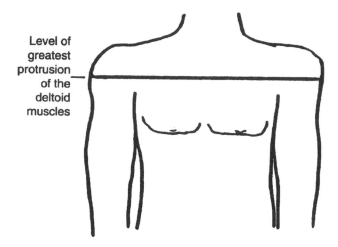

Figure 10.14   Tape placement for measurement of shoulder circumference.

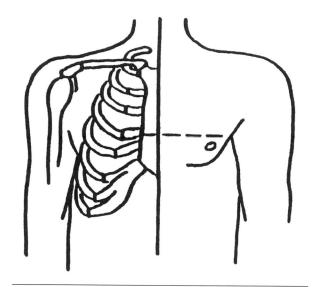

Figure 10.15   The level of the fourth costosternal joint for chest circumference measurements.

fourth costosternal joint. The measurement is taken in a horizontal plane at the end of a respiration. Once the tape is snugly in place, the arms are lowered to their natural position by the sides and the measurement is taken (Figure 10.15).

Waist Circumference

The waist circumference measurement should not be made over clothing. The subject stands erect with arms by the sides, feet together, and abdomen relaxed. The tape is placed in a horizontal plane at the level of the narrowest part of the torso as seen from the anterior (front) aspect. The measurement is taken after a normal expiration (Figure 10.16).

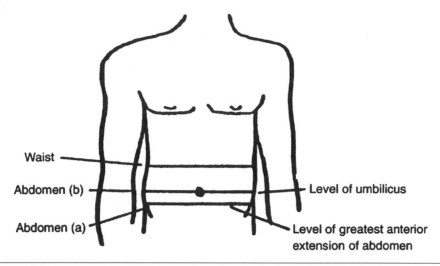

Waist

Abdomen (b)

Abdomen (a)

Level of umbilicus

Level of greatest anterior
extension of abdomen

Figure 10.16   Tape placement for measurement of waist circumference and abdominal circumference according to (a) Lohman, Roche, and Martorell (37) and (b) Pollock and Wilmore (17).

Abdomen Circumference

The abdomen circumference measurement should not be taken over clothing. The subject stands erect with arms by the sides, feet together, and abdomen relaxed. The tape is positioned horizontally at the level of the greatest anterior extension of the abdomen. This location is often but not always at the level of the umbilicus. Pollock and Wilmore (17) recommend that the tape be positioned at the level of the umbilicus (Figure 10.16). The measurement is taken at the end of a normal expiration.

Buttocks (Gluteal or Hip) Circumference

Ideally, the gluteal circumference measure is taken in a bikini (females) or supporter or swim brief (males). The subject stands erect with arms by the sides and feet together. The tape is placed in the horizontal plane at the level of maximum extension of the buttocks (Figure 10.17). Pollock and Wilmore (17) recommend that the gluteal circumference be measured while the buttock muscles are tensed.

Thigh Circumference (Proximal)

The subject stands erect with arms by the sides, feet approximately 10 cm apart, and weight evenly distributed. The tape is positioned horizontally immediately distal to the gluteal furrow (usually but not always the maximum circumference of the thigh) (Figure 10.18). Pollock and Wilmore (17) recommend that weight be shifted to the right leg and the thigh be tensed during

this measurement. Midthigh and distal thigh measures are not shown but are described by Lohman, Roche, and Martorell (37).

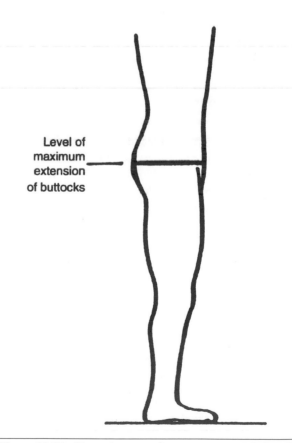

Level of
maximum
extension
of buttocks

Figure 10.17   Tape placement for measurement of gluteal circumference.

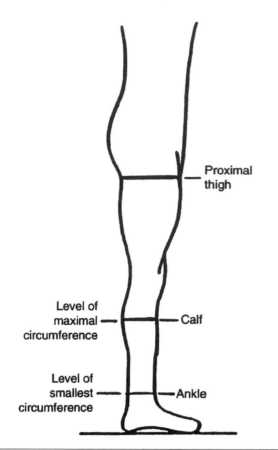

Figure 10.18 Lateral view of locations for thigh, calf, and ankle circumferences.

Calf Circumference

The subject either sits on a table so that the leg to be measured hangs freely or stands with the feet about 20 cm apart and weight evenly distributed. The tape is placed horizontally around the calf at the level of maximal circumference in a plane perpendicular to the long axis of the calf (Figure 10.18).

Ankle Circumference

The subject stands barefoot with feet slightly separated and weight distributed equally on both feet. The tape is placed at the smallest circumference of the lower leg just proximal to the malleoli in a plane perpendicular to the long axis of the calf (Figure 10.18).

Arm (Biceps) Circumference

The subject stands erect with the arms hanging freely at the sides with palms facing the thighs. The tape is positioned horizontally perpendicular to the long axis of the arm at the midpoint of the upper arm (Figure 10.19a). To locate the midpoint, the subject's elbow is flexed at 90° with the palm facing superiorly. The

measurer stands behind the subject and locates the lateral tip of the acromion by palpating laterally along the superior surface of the spinous process of the scapula. A small mark is made at the identified point. The most distal point of the acromial process is located and marked. A tape is placed so that it passes over the two marks, and the midpoint between them is marked. Pollock and Wilmore (17) recommend that the measurement be taken at maximal girth of the midarm when flexed to the greatest angle, with the underlying muscles fully contracted (Figure 10.19b).

Forearm Circumference

The subject stands erect with arms hanging downward but slightly away from the trunk, with the palms facing anteriorly. The tape is placed around the proximal part of the forearm, perpendicular to its long axis, at the level of maximum circumference (Figure 10.20a). Pollock and Wilmore (17) recommend that the measurement be taken at the largest circumference, with the forearm parallel to the floor, the elbow joint at a 90° angle, the hand clenched and in the supinated position, and the muscles flexed (Figure 10.20b).

Wrist Circumference

The subject stands erect and "flexes the arm at the elbow so that the palm is uppermost and the hand muscles relaxed. The tape is positioned perpendicular to the long axis of the forearm and in the same plane on the anterior and posterior aspects of the wrist. The tape must be no more than 0.7 cm wide, so that it can fit into the medial and lateral depressions at this level" (Figure 10.20).

Prediction Equations for Determining D_b From Anthropometric Measures

In 1951, Brozek and Keys (53) published the first regression equations predicting D_b using anthropometric techniques. Since then, more than 100 equations have been reported in the literature (54). Early equations were developed from various combinations of skinfold fat measurements (55, 56). In an attempt to produce more accurate prediction equations, researchers began adding body circumference and bone diameters as independent variables in the regression model (46, 47, 52, 57-60). These early equations were population-specific; that is, they were developed from relatively small, homogeneous samples. Application of these equations to different populations has shown that age, gender, and degree of fatness are important sources of D_b variation (14, 17, 54). Furthermore, these population-specific equations

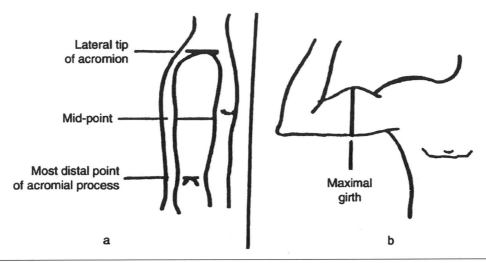

Figure 10.19 Tape placement for measurement of biceps circumference according to (a) Lohman, Roche, and Martorell (37) and (b) Pollock and Wilmore (17).

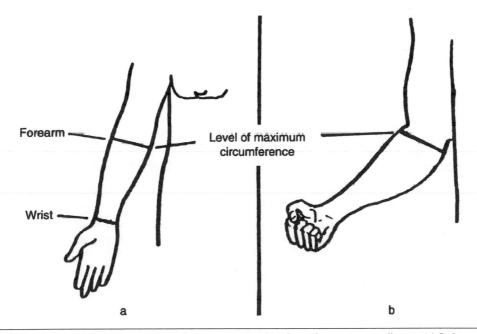

Figure 10.20 Tape placement for measurement of forearm and wrist circumferences according to (a) Lohman, Roche, and Martorell (37) and (b) Pollock and Wilmore (17).

were erroneously based on the assumption that the relationship between hydrostatically determined D_b and subcutaneous fat is linear. Figure 10.21 illustrates that this relationship is actually curvilinear. According to Pollock and Wilmore (17), population-specific equations predict most accurately at the mean of the population in which the data were collected and the equation developed. As subjects differ from the mean, the standard error of measurement increases significantly (54).

To avoid the limitations of population-specific equations, generalized equations were developed from larger, heterogeneous samples. Unlike population-specific equations, which can be applied only to samples having similar age and physical characteristics, generalized equations can be used with samples varying greatly in age and body fatness (54). The main advantage of the generalized approach is that one equation replaces several without a loss in prediction accuracy (17, 54).

Durnin and Womersley (61) were the first to use the generalized approach. They studied 272 women, ranging in age from 16 to 68 years, and developed five equations, one for each of the following age groups:

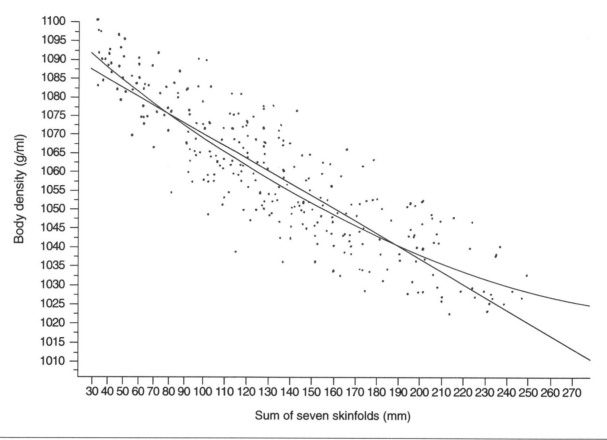

Figure 10.21 Scattergram of body density and the sum of seven skinfolds, with the linear and quadratic regression lines for adult men age 18 to 61 years.

From Jackson, A.S., and Pollock, M.L.: Generalized equations for predicting body density in men, *British Journal of Nutrition*, **40**, 497-504, 1978. Reprinted by permission of Cambridge University Press.

16-19, 20-29, 30-39, 40-49, and 50-68 years. All equations had a common slope, but the intercepts were adjusted to account for aging. The standard errors of the estimate for these equations ranged from 0.008 g/cc (for the 50- to 68-year-old group) to 0.013 g/cc (for the 30- to 39-year-old group). As an extension of the work of Durnin and Womersley, Jackson and Pollock also developed generalized equations for men (38) and women (39). To account for the potential changes in the ratio of internal to external fat and bone density with age, they added age to the prediction equation as an independent variable. Standard errors of the estimate for percent fat ranged from 3.4% to 3.9% for men and women, respectively.

The studies of Durnin and Womersley (61) and Jackson and Pollock (38, 39) realized the curvilinear nature of the data (Figure 10.21), and therefore used logarithmic transformations and quadratic forms of various sums of skinfold thicknesses as independent variables. See Table 10.3 for actual generalized equations for predicting D_b in women and men. For ease of determination of percentage of body fat, actual calculated percentages of body fat using age and the sum of chest, abdomen, and thigh skinfolds for men and the sum of triceps, suprailium, and thigh skinfolds for women are shown in Tables 10.4 and 10.5, respectively. Note that these skinfolds were taken with Lange calipers.

Pollock and Wilmore (17) note that the use of the quadratic component and age in generalized equations did not increase the correlation substantially over the linear version of the same equations. However, the value of the generalized equations over the linear equations is that they minimize large prediction errors that occur at the extremes of the D_b distribution. The equations of Jackson and Pollock have been cross-validated by several investigators (35, 62-67) and have been shown to accurately predict D_b for men and women up to 60 years of age and 40% fat.

Estimating body composition in the obese population has been difficult with most prediction equations and methods, which significantly underpredict the actual values of percent fat (17). Use of the BMI is generally recommended in the obese population.

Table 10.3   Generalized Regression Equations for Predicting Body Density (D$_b$) for Adult Women and Men

Variables	Regression equation	r	SE (D$_b$)	SE (% F)
	Adult Women			
Σ 7, Age	D$_b$ = 1.0970 − 0.00046971 (X$_1$) + 0.00000056 (X$_1$)^2 − 0.00012828 (X$_6$)	0.85	0.008	3.8
Σ 3, Age	D$_b$ = 1.0994921 − 0.0009929 (X$_2$) + 0.0000023 (X$_2$)^2 − 0.0001392 (X$_6$)	0.84	0.009	3.9
Σ 3, Age	D$_b$ = 1.0902369 − 0.0009379 (X$_5$) + 0.0000026 (X$_5$)^2 − 0.0001087 (X$_6$)	0.84	0.009	3.9
	Adult Men			
Σ 7, Age	D$_b$ = 1.11200000 − 0.00043499 (X$_1$) + 0.00000055 (X$_1$)^2 − 0.00028826 (X$_6$)	0.90	0.008	3.5
Σ 3, Age	D$_b$ = 1.1093800 − 0.0008267 (X$_3$) + 0.0000016 (X$_3$)^2 − 0.0002574 (X$_6$)	0.91	0.008	3.4
Σ 3, Age	D$_b$ = 1.1125025 − 0.0013125 (X$_4$) + 0.0000055 (X$_4$)2 − 0.0002440 (X$_6$)	0.89	0.008	3.6

Note. X$_1$ = Sum of seven skinfolds (mm); X$_2$ = sum of triceps, suprailium, and thigh skinfolds (mm); X$_3$ = sum of chest, abdomen, and thigh skinfolds (mm); X$_5$ = sum of chest, triceps, and subscapular skinfolds (mm); X$_5$ = sum of triceps, suprailium, and abdomen skinfolds (mm); X$_6$ = age in years.

From Pollock, M.L., Schmidt, D.H., and Jackson, A.S.: Measurement of cardiorespiratory fitness and body composition in the clinical setting, *Comprehensive Therapy*, **6**, 12-27, 1980. Published with permission of The Laux Company, Inc. Harvard, MA.

When studying obese populations, it is often difficult to obtain accurate skinfold measurements for the following reasons: (1) The skinfold may exceed the maximum opening capacity of the caliper; (2) caliper tips may slide on larger skinfolds; and (3) readings tend to decrease with subsequent measurements, which might be associated with edema and repeated compression of the subcutaneous fat (68). To overcome these limitations, Weltman et al. (69, 70) developed and cross-validated body composition prediction equations for obese men and women, using height, weight, and circumference measurements as predictor variables. They found that a combination of the mean of two abdominal girths, height, and weight accurately predicted relative fat in obese males (% fat = 0.31457 [mean Abd] − 0.10969 [Wt] + 10.8336, R = .54, *SEE* = 2.9%) and females (% fat = 0.11077 [mean Abd] − 0.17666 [Ht] + 0.14354 [Wt] + 51.03301; R = .76, *SEE* = 2.9%). (Mean Abd = the average of two circumferences shown as *waist* and *abdomen (b)* in Figure 10.16, Wt = weight, Ht = height.)

BIOELECTRIC IMPEDANCE ANALYSIS

Bioelectric impedance analysis (BIA) is a relatively new technique for estimating body composition in humans

(71). It is based on the principle that the resistance to an applied electric current is inversely related to the amount of the fat-free mass (FFM) contained within the body. This relationship exists because FFM has a greater water and electrolyte content, and therefore a greater conductivity, than adipose tissue and bone. The greater the FFM, the greater the conductivity, and the lower the resistance. Relative body fat can be easily calculated from FFM by this formula: % fat = [(weight − FFM)/weight] · 100.

The specific physical principles of BIA are somewhat complicated and beyond the scope of this chapter. Baumgartner, Chumlea, and Roche (72) have written a detailed but readable review of the theory and engineering behind BIA. Most studies using BIA to estimate body composition have been based on the equation $V = \rho\, L^2/R$; where V represents the volume of the conductor, ρ is the specific resistivity of the tissue being analyzed, L is the length of the conductor, and R is the observed resistance (73). The volume calculated by the previous equation is assumed to represent total body water (TBW), which is highly correlated with FFM (74).

The application of the equation $V = \rho\, L^2/R$ to the estimation of body composition in humans has limitations. It is assumed that the conductor is homogeneous with respect to composition, shape (cross-sectional area), and current density distribution. This is not the case in the human body (75). Stature (S) and not the

Table 10.4   Percent Body Fat Estimation for Men From Age and the Sum of Chest, Abdominal, and Thigh Skinfolds

Sum of skinfolds (mm)	Age to the last year								
	Under 22	23-27	28-32	33-37	38-42	43-47	48-52	53-57	Over 57
8-10	1.3	1.8	2.3	2.9	3.4	3.9	4.5	5.0	5.5
11-13	2.2	2.8	3.3	3.9	4.4	4.9	5.5	6.0	6.5
14-16	3.2	3.8	4.3	4.8	5.4	5.9	6.4	7.0	7.5
17-19	4.2	4.7	5.3	5.8	6.3	6.9	7.4	8.0	8.5
20-22	5.1	5.7	6.2	6.8	7.3	7.9	8.4	8.9	9.5
23-25	6.1	6.6	7.2	7.7	8.3	8.8	9.4	9.9	10.5
26-28	7.0	7.6	8.1	8.7	9.2	9.8	10.3	10.9	11.4
29-31	8.0	8.5	9.1	9.6	10.2	10.7	11.3	11.8	12.4
32-34	8.9	9.4	10.0	10.5	11.1	11.6	12.2	12.8	13.3
35-37	9.8	10.4	10.9	11.5	12.0	12.6	13.1	13.7	14.3
38-40	10.7	11.3	11.8	12.4	12.9	13.5	14.1	14.6	15.2
41-43	11.6	12.2	12.7	13.3	13.8	14.4	15.0	15.5	16.1
44-46	12.5	13.1	13.6	14.2	14.7	15.3	15.9	16.4	17.0
47-49	13.4	13.9	14.5	15.1	15.6	16.2	16.8	17.3	17.9
50-52	14.3	14.8	15.4	15.9	16.5	17.1	17.6	18.2	18.8
53-55	15.1	15.7	16.2	16.8	17.4	17.9	18.5	19.1	19.7
56-58	16.0	16.5	17.1	17.7	18.2	18.8	19.4	20.0	20.5
59-61	16.9	17.4	17.9	18.5	19.1	19.7	20.2	20.8	21.4
62-64	17.6	18.2	18.8	19.4	19.9	20.5	21.1	21.7	22.2
65-67	18.5	19.0	19.6	20.2	20.8	21.3	21.9	22.5	23.1
68-70	19.3	19.9	20.4	21.0	21.6	22.2	22.7	23.3	23.9
71-73	20.1	20.7	21.2	21.8	22.4	23.0	23.6	24.1	24.7
74-76	20.9	21.5	22.0	22.6	23.2	23.8	24.4	25.0	25.5
77-79	21.7	22.2	22.8	23.4	24.0	24.6	25.2	25.8	26.3
80-82	22.4	23.0	23.6	24.2	24.8	25.4	25.9	26.5	27.1
83-85	23.2	23.8	24.4	25.0	25.5	26.1	26.7	27.3	27.9
86-88	24.0	24.5	25.1	25.7	26.3	26.9	27.5	28.1	28.7
89-91	24.7	25.3	25.9	26.5	27.1	27.6	28.2	28.8	29.4
92-94	25.4	26.0	26.6	27.2	27.8	28.4	29.0	29.6	30.2
95-97	26.1	26.7	27.3	27.9	28.5	29.1	29.7	30.3	30.9
98-100	26.9	27.4	28.0	28.6	29.2	29.8	30.4	31.0	31.6
101-103	27.5	28.1	28.7	29.3	29.9	30.5	31.1	31.7	32.3
104-106	28.2	28.8	29.4	30.0	30.6	31.2	31.8	32.4	33.0
107-109	28.9	29.5	30.1	30.7	31.3	31.9	32.5	33.1	33.7
110-112	29.6	30.2	30.8	31.4	32.0	32.6	33.2	33.8	34.4
113-115	30.2	30.8	31.4	32.0	32.6	33.2	33.8	34.5	35.1
116-118	30.9	31.5	32.1	32.7	33.3	33.9	34.5	35.1	35.7
119-121	31.5	32.1	32.7	33.3	33.9	34.5	35.1	35.7	36.4
122-124	32.1	32.7	33.3	33.9	34.5	35.1	35.8	36.4	37.0
125-127	32.7	33.3	33.9	34.5	35.1	35.8	36.4	37.0	37.6

Note. Percent fat calculated by the formula of Siri: percent fat = $[(4.95/D_b) - 4.5] \times 100$, where D_b = body density.
From Pollock, M.L., Schmidt, D.H., and Jackson, A.S.: Measurement of cardiorespiratory fitness and body composition in the clinical setting, *Comprehensive Therapy*, **6**, 12-27, 1980. Published with permission of The Laux Company, Inc., Harvard. MA.

Table 10.5   Percent Body Fat Estimation for Women From Age and the Sum of Triceps, Suprailium, and Thigh Skinfolds

Sum of skinfolds (mm)	Age to the last year								
	Under 22	23-27	28-32	33-37	38-42	43-47	48-52	53-57	Over 57
23-25	9.7	9.9	10.2	10.4	10.7	10.9	11.2	11.4	11.7
26-28	11.0	11.2	11.5	11.7	12.0	12.3	12.5	12.7	13.0
29-31	12.3	12.5	12.8	13.0	13.3	13.5	13.8	14.0	14.3
32-34	13.6	13.8	14.0	14.3	14.5	14.8	15.0	15.3	15.5
35-37	14.8	15.0	15.3	15.5	15.8	16.0	16.3	16.5	16.8
38-40	16.0	16.3	16.5	16.7	17.0	17.2	17.5	17.7	18.0
41-43	17.2	17.4	17.7	17.9	18.2	18.4	18.7	18.9	19.2
44-46	18.3	18.6	18.8	19.1	19.3	19.6	19.8	20.1	20.3
47-49	19.5	19.7	20.0	20.2	20.5	20.7	21.0	21.2	21.5
50-52	20.6	20.8	21.1	21.3	21.6	21.8	22.1	22.3	22.6
53-55	21.7	21.9	22.1	22.4	22.6	22.9	23.1	23.4	23.6
56-58	22.7	23.0	23.2	23.4	23.7	23.9	24.2	24.4	24.7
59-61	23.7	24.0	24.2	24.5	24.7	25.0	25.2	25.5	25.7
62-64	24.7	25.0	25.2	25.5	25.7	26.0	26.7	26.4	26.7
65-67	25.7	25.9	26.2	26.4	26.7	26.9	27.2	27.4	27.7
68-70	26.6	26.9	27.1	27.4	27.6	27.9	28.1	28.4	28.6
71-73	27.5	37.8	28.0	28.3	28.5	28.8	28.0	29.3	29.5
74-76	28.4	28.7	28.9	29.2	29.4	29.7	29.9	30.2	30.4
77-79	29.3	29.5	29.8	30.0	30.3	30.5	30.8	31.0	31.3
80-82	30.1	30.4	30.6	30.9	31.1	31.4	31.6	31.9	32.1
83-85	30.9	31.2	31.4	31.7	31.9	32.2	32.4	32.7	32.9
86-88	31.7	32.0	32.2	32.5	32.7	32.9	33.2	33.4	33.7
89-91	32.5	32.7	33.0	33.2	33.5	33.7	33.9	34.2	34.4
92-94	33.2	33.4	33.7	33.9	34.2	34.4	34.7	34.9	35.2
95-97	33.9	34.1	34.4	34.6	34.9	35.1	35.4	35.6	35.9
98-100	34.6	34.8	35.1	35.3	35.5	35.8	36.0	36.3	36.5
101-103	35.3	35.4	35.7	35.9	36.2	36.4	36.7	36.9	37.2
104-106	35.8	36.1	36.3	36.6	36.8	37.1	37.3	37.5	37.8
107-109	36.4	36.7	36.9	37.1	37.4	37.6	37.9	38.1	38.4
110-112	37.0	37.2	37.5	37.7	38.0	38.2	38.5	38.7	38.9
113-115	37.5	37.8	38.0	38.2	38.5	38.7	39.0	39.2	39.5
116-118	38.0	38.3	38.5	38.8	39.0	39.3	39.5	39.7	40.0
119-121	38.5	38.7	39.0	39.2	39.5	39.7	40.0	40.2	40.5
122-124	39.0	39.2	39.4	39.7	39.9	40.2	40.4	40.7	40.9
125-127	39.4	39.6	39.9	40.1	40.4	40.6	40.9	41.1	41.4
128-130	39.8	40.0	40.3	40.5	40.8	41.0	41.3	41.5	41.8

Note. Percent fat calculated by the formula of Siri: percent fat = $[(4.95/D_b) = 4.5] \times 100$, where D_b = body density.
From Pollock, M.L., Schmidt, D.H., and Jackson, A.S.: Measurement of cardiorespiratory fitness and body composition in the clinical setting, *Comprehensive Therapy*, **6**, 12-27, 1980. Published with permission of The Laux Company, Inc., Harvard, MA.

actual length of the conductor (although stature and conductor length are highly correlated) is used as a measure of conductor length; and the specific resistivity (ρ) varies among individuals, based upon the amount and distribution of tissues and fluids within the body (76). These limitations indicate that S^2/R (the resistive index) does not have the same relationship to TBW or FFM in all individuals. In spite of these limitations, high correlations between S^2/R, TBW, and FFM indicate that S^2/R can be used as a reasonable predictor of TBW and FFM (71, 77-79).

To minimize variability associated with whole-body impedance, several investigators have predicted FFM using impedance measurements from various body segments (79, 80). In some instances the sum of specific segment indices can predict FFM more accurately than S^2/R (81). This approach is more complicated (less efficient) than making a single whole-body measurement.

gmental approach may be beneficial when accu-

Physiological Assessment of Human Fitness

Table 10.6 Selected Validation Statistics for the Prediction of Body Composition From Stature^2/Resistance (S^2/R)

Authors	N	Age (years)	Regression equation	R^2	RMSE
TBW					
Lukaski et al. (71)	37 M	19-42	2.03 + 0.63 (S^2/R)	.90	2.1 L
Kushner & Schoeller (78)	40 M+W	32-54	0.83 + 0.714 (S^2/R)	.94	2.5 L
FFM					
Lukaski et al. (71)	37 M	19-42	3.04 + 0.85 (S^2/R)	.96	2.6 kg
Lukaski et al. (77)	84 M	18-50	5.21 + 0.83 (S^2/R)	.96	2.5 kg
	67 W		4.92 + 0.82 (S^2/R)	.91	2.0 kg
Chumlea et al. (79)	24 boys	9-17	−1.23 + 0.92 (S^2/R)	.88	4.0 kg
	26 girls	9-17	−1.38 + 0.96 (S^2/R)	.84	4.2 kg
	28 M	18-62	3.50 + 0.87 (S^2/R)	.81	2.9 kg
	44 W	18-62	11.55 + 0.69 (S^2/R)	.80	2.7 kg
Cordain, Whicker, & Johnson (101)	30 boys & girls	9-14	6.86 + 0.81 (S^2/R)	.69	4.1 kg

Note. M = men, W = women; RMSE = root mean squared error.
Adapted from Baumgartner et al. (72) with permission.

The segmental approach may be beneficial when accurate measures of stature are difficult to obtain or for estimating body composition in amputees (82).

Validation statistics for selected regression equations developed to predict TBW and FFM from S^2/R are illustrated in Table 10.6. Standard errors of prediction are around 2.5 L for TBW and range from 2.0 kg to 4.2 kg for FFM. The addition of certain anthropometric variables (skinfolds, circumferences), age, and gender can improve the statistical association between S^2/R and body composition (83).Some typical multivariate prediction equations and their associated validation statistics are presented in Table 10.7.

Equipment

A variety of BIA analyzers are commercially available. They range in price from several hundred to several thousand dollars. The differences among BIA analyzers are primarily in the amount of computer hardware and software included. A basic low-cost BIA unit will generally display the measured impedance in ohms. More expensive units may calculate and display parameters such as relative body fat and include a printer to generate reports.

The technology required for BIA instrumentation is not complicated, and the more expensive BIA units do not necessarily provide a more accurate measure of impedance. When a BIA analyzer is used that calculates body composition parameters, validation of the algorithms (prediction equations) employed is critical. Reputable manufacturers should be willing to provide the user with the specific equation(s) used and docu-mentation of independently conducted validation studies. A BIA analyzer should have the capability of displaying impedance in ohms. This enables the user to choose from a variety of published prediction equations. The best prediction equation for a given situation might not be one supplied by the manufacturer. In addition, BIA practitioners may want to take advantage of new and improved equations generated by continued research.

One concern when selecting an equation to predict body composition from BIA is the type of instrument on which the equation was developed. Prediction equations are most accurate when used with data collected on the same instrument as used to develop the equation (84). Therefore, a prediction equation developed on one type of BIA analyzer should not be used with a different analyzer unless the impedance measure can be corrected to account for the difference.

Measurement Procedure

The methodology employed for whole-body BIA is relatively simple. The subject to be measured lies supine on a nonconductive surface. The legs should be abducted so that the thighs do not touch. The arms should also be abducted slightly so that they do not contact the torso. A pair of electrodes (aluminum foil "spot" electrodes are often used) is placed on the ankle and foot and a second pair is placed on the wrist and hand (see Figure 10.22). Each pair of electrodes contains a source and a reference (or detecting) electrode. A low-level electrical current (typically 800 µA at a frequency of 50 kHz) is introduced at the source electrodes, and the voltage drop

Table 10.7   Selected Equations, Cross-Validated, for the Prediction of Body Composition Variables From Impedance, Anthropometric Variables, Age, and Gender

Authors	Age (years)	N	Regression equations	R^2	RMSE
TBW					
Kushner & Schoeller (78)	31.8-53.7	20 M	$0.396 (x_1) + 0.143 (x_2) + 8.399$	.98	1.7 L
	(means for groups differing by obesity and sex)	20 W	$0.382 (x_1) + 0.105 (x_2) + 8.315$	.95	0.8 L
Lukaski & Bolonchuk (77a)	20-73	110 M+W	$0.377 (x_1) + 0.14 (x_2) - 0.08 (x_3) + 2.9 (x_4) + 4.65$	.97	1.5 L
FFM					
Guo, Roche, & Houtkooper (83)	7-25	140 M	$-2.93 + 0.646 (x_2) - 0.116 (x_5)$ $0.375 (x_6) + 0.475 (x_7)$ $+ 0.156 (x_1)$	.98	2.3 kg
		110 W	$4.34 + 0.682 (x_2) - 0.185 (x_5)$ $- 0.244 (x_8) - 0.202 (x_9)$ $+ 0.182 (x_1)$	.95	2.2 kg
Graves et al. (84)[a]	23.4 ± 2.8	46 M	$0.485 (x_1) + 0.338 (x_2) + 5.32$	.75	3.8%
	22.8 ± 3.2	46 W	$0.475 (x_1) + 0.295 (x_2) + 5.49$	.71	3.6%
%Fat					
Guo et al. (83a)	18-30	77 M	$1.50 - 0.279 (x_1) +$ $0.632 (x_8) + 0.346 (x_2)$	.74	3.3%
		71 W	$-8.48 + 0.434 (x_{10})$ $+ 1.341 (x_{11}) - 0.845 (x_1)$ $+ 0.384 (x_2)$	.81	3.2%

Note. M = men; W = women; x_1 = Stature^2/resistance (cm^2/ohms); x_2 = weight (kg); x_3 = age (yrs); x_4 = gender (males = 1, females = 0); x_5 = lateral calf skinfold (cm); x_6 = midaxillary skinfold (cm); x_7 = arm circumference (cm); x_8 = triceps skinfold (cm); x_9 = subscapular skinfold (cm); x_{10} = biceps skinfold (cm); x_{11} = calf circumference (cm); RMSE = root mean squared error.
[a] Cross-validation statistics are for percent fat.
Adapted from Baumgartner et al. (72) with permission.

between the reference electrodes is measured as the bioelectric resistance or impedance (R).

Because bioelectric impedance is related to the length of the conductor, proper placement of the reference electrodes is critical. The most frequently cited landmarks for the placement of the reference electrodes are the distal condyles of radius and ulna (for the wrist) and the most prominent portions of the malleoli of the tibia and fibula (for the ankle) (85). The leading edge (superior linear border) of the reference electrodes should be centered on an imaginary line connecting the centers of (bisecting) these bony protrusions. Displacement of the electrodes even slightly from the specified landmarks can result in relatively large changes in observed resistance and error in the estimation of body composition (86, 87). As previously mentioned, stature is generally used to represent conductor length. This is possible because stature and actual conductor length (the distance between the source and reference electrodes) is highly correlated. The accurate prediction of body composition from BIA therefore requires an accurate measure of stature.

Methodological Considerations

Bioelectric impedance is systematically greater on the left side of the body by 8 to 10 ohms (84, 88). Thus, impedance must be measured on the side for which the prediction equation was developed. For the purpose of standardization, BIA measurements are usually made on the right side of the body.

BIA is not extremely sensitive to age or gender. Although prediction errors of age- and gender-specific regression equations are lower than prediction errors for equations developed on the entire population (89), the improvement in accuracy following the addition of age and gender to prediction equations is usually small (< 2.0 kg of FFM) (72). Of more critical importance than age and gender is the hydration status of the subject

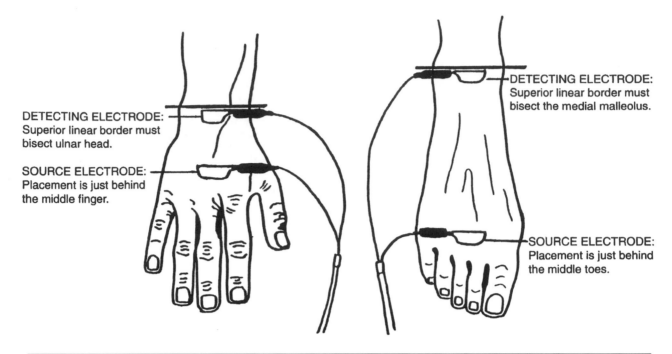

DETECTING ELECTRODE:
Superior linear border must
bisect ulnar head.

SOURCE ELECTRODE:
Placement is just behind
the middle finger.

DETECTING ELECTRODE:
Superior linear border must
bisect the medial malleolus.

SOURCE ELECTRODE:
Placement is just behind
the middle toes.

Figure 10.22   Placement of source and detecting (reference) electrodes (tetrapolar configuration).

(72). Controlling for factors that can affect total body water is important. Because body tissues tend to dehydrate with age, current prediction equations may not be valid when applied to the elderly.

It is prudent to standardize the use of diuretics (90) and other drugs that influence hydration status. BIA measurements should not be taken after strenuous exercise or other conditions that may induce fluid loss (91). Although there is no evidence of cyclical changes in bioelectric impedance associated with menstruation (80), it is recommended that one not take BIA measurements during the week prior to menses, to avoid variability that may be associated with water retention.

Although diurnal variations in BIA have been negligible in some studies (92, 93), Robert et al. (88) found a 10-ohm reduction in impedance over the course of a 9-hour day, and Pollock et al. (unpublished abstract, 1990) found an 18-ohm reduction in bioelectric impedance over the course of a 14-hour day. The change observed by Pollock et al. was twice the magnitude of change seen following exercise-induced dehydration (–9 ohms) in the same study. Diurnal changes in bioelectric impedance may be related to daily shifts in fluid volumes (80). For serial measurements on the same individual, time of day should be consistent, to get the most accurate results.

Bioelectric impedance measures are temperature dependent (94). Temperature-related effects on BIA may be due to changes in fluid volume or distribution associated with changes in temperature. It is recommended that BIA measurements be made at a comfortable and

unchanging ambient temperature. There is currently a lack of information related to the prediction of body composition from BIA in individuals of different ethnic origins, and it is not known whether BIA prediction equations can be applied to different races.

Reliability and Cross-Validation

Bioelectric impedance measurements are highly reliable for both interobserver and intraobserver comparisons (71, 78, 84, 86, 87, 95, 96). Reliability coefficients are typically $r \geq .990$. Lukaski et al. (97) reported $r = .999$ for a single measurement, $r = .995$ for measurements taken 2 hours apart, and $r = .99$ for measurements over 5 days (71).

When BIA prediction equations are validated on independently selected populations (cross-validations), results have been variable. For example, cross-validation of the equation developed by Lukaski et al. (71) for predicting relative fat in men has yielded statistics of $r_{yy}' = .93$, $SEE = 2.7\%$ (77); $r_{yy}' = .87$, $SEE = 4.8\%$ (84); and $r_{yy}' = .71$, $SEE = 6.3\%$ (95). Segal et al. (98) have also reported a relatively high SEE (6.1%) for predicting relative fat with BIA using a cross-validation experimental design. The relatively high prediction errors reported for the BIA technique have been a primary concern related to its use as an acceptable field method of predicting body composition. However, the most recent studies have been more favorable and indicate that BIA can predict body composition with the same degree of accuracy as anthropometric techniques (99, 100). BIA has been shown to be valid for a variety of populations, including children (89, 101), athletes (102), and certain patient populations (103, 104).

ULTRASOUND

During the 1950s, ultrasound was being used in the meat industry to determine body composition of livestock (105-107). In the 1960s researchers began applying the ultrasound method to the assessment of human body composition (108, 109). The first human studies used the A-scan mode, which records depth readings of changes in tissue density. Advances in technology led to the development of the B-scan mode, which provides two-dimensional, cross-sectional images of tissue configuration.

Principles of Ultrasonic Measurements

The following explanation of the principles of ultrasound comes from Cromwell, Weibell, and Pfeiffer (110). Ultrasound is sonic energy at frequencies above the audible range (greater than 20 kHz). Ultrasound exists as a sequence of alternate compressions and rarefactions of a suitable medium (e.g., tissue, bone) and is propagated through that medium at some velocity. Its behavior depends on the frequency (wavelength) of the sonic energy and the density and compliance of the medium through which it travels. Ultrasound can be focused into a beam and therefore obeys the laws of reflection and refraction. Whenever the ultrasound beam passes from one medium to another, a portion of the sonic energy is reflected and the remainder is refracted. The amount of energy reflected depends on the difference in density between the two media and the angle at which the transmitted beam strikes the medium. The greater the difference in media, the greater the amount reflected. Also, the nearer the angle of incidence between the beam and the interface is to 90°, the greater will be the reflected portion.

At interfaces of extreme differences in medium, such as between muscle (density = 1.07 g/cc) and bone (density = 1.77 g/cc), almost all of the energy will be reflected and practically none will continue through the second medium.

The velocity of sound propagation through a given medium varies with its density and elastic properties as well as the temperature. As a general rule, the greater the density, the greater the velocity. For example, fat has a density of 0.90 g/cc and a velocity of 1,440 m/s, whereas muscle, which has a density of 1.07 g/cc, has a velocity of 1,570 m/s. As ultrasound travels through a material, some of the energy is absorbed and the wave is attenuated a certain amount for each centimeter through which it travels. The amount of attenuation is a function of both

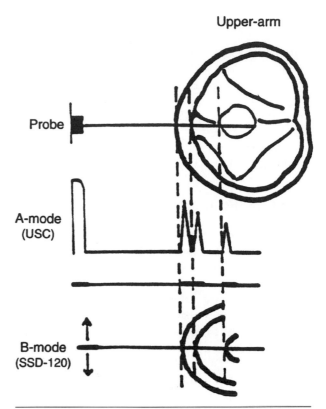

Figure 10.23 Illustration of results obtained from A-mode and B-mode ultrasound. A-mode records depth readings of changes in tissue density; B-mode produces a two-dimensional, cross-sectional image of underlying tissue configuration.

the frequency of the ultrasound and the characteristics of the material. Attenuation increases with higher frequencies. Therefore, the higher the frequency, the less distance it can penetrate into the body. For this reason, lower frequencies are used for deeper penetration.

A-Mode Versus B-Mode Ultrasound

With A-mode ultrasound, a pulse of mechanical vibration is sent out from the sound source (probe) into the subject and is partially reflected by an interface where the specific acoustic impedance of the medium changes (e.g., skin–fat, fat–muscle, and muscle–bone interfaces). The reflected pulse returns along its original path back to the source. The time the echo takes to return gives a measure of the depth of the interface from the surface of the sound source. This information is presented visually on an oscilloscope screen. Because the trace travels across the screen uniformly with time, the distance along the horizontal trace from the zero point to the vertical deflection is proportional to the time interval for ultrasonic waves to pass from the probe to the reflection interface and back again (108). To convert this distance into actual length, the sound velocity of human fat and muscle must be known (1,440 m/s for fat and 1,570 m/s for muscle). It is often difficult to correlate the individual echoes seen along the line with the surfaces that produced them (111). B-mode ultrasound overcomes this difficulty because it allows one to visualize an interface in two dimensions and to see its relation to other interfaces more easily (see Figure 10.23). This is done by coupling the transducer (probe) to an echo camera that converts the reflected impulses into a picture of the internal tissue structures.

Equipment and Methodology

Necessary equipment includes a transducer (5 MHz), echo camera, videographic printer, Vernier caliper, and ultrasound transmission gel (Figure 10.24). The transducer is coupled with the echo camera, which is interfaced to the videographic printer. With B-mode ultrasound, a cross-sectional image of the underlying tissues is produced and printed from the graphic printer. The Vernier caliper is then used to measure the fat layer (distance between skin–fat interface and fat–muscle interface) and the muscle layer (distance between the fat–muscle interface and muscle–bone interface) to the nearest 0.1 mm (Figure 10.25). Figure 10.26 shows a diagrammatic view of the various interfaces of the arm (biceps) and an actual B-mode ultrasonic view. A small amount of ultrasound transmission gel is applied to the head of the transducer prior to taking measurement to assure airless contact with the skin.

Subjects should stand with feet comfortably apart while the measurements are taken. The transducer with gel is then placed gently (to avoid compression of tissue) over the desired sites, perpendicular to the underlying bone (Figure 10.27). The gain knob and distance controls are used to focus the image on the echo camera. When the image is clear, it is frozen on the screen of the echo camera by pressing the freeze button of the videographic printer.

The transducer is placed on the same sites used for skinfolds. The transducer is held horizontally for all of the sites except the subscapular and medial calf, for which the transducer is held vertically. The main advantages of the ultrasound technique as compared to the traditional caliper method are: (1) there is no tissue compression; (2) there is no need to polpate the fat–muscle interface; (3) larger fat layers can be easily measured; and (4) it also provides information on muscle thickness.

Validity and Reliability of Ultrasound

Early studies established the validity of the ultrasound method to estimate subcutaneous fat thickness in humans.

Bullen et al. (108) compared A-mode ultrasonic determinations of subcutaneous fat (abdominal site) to fat thickness measurements obtained by direct needle puncture ($N = 13$). The correlation between the two methods was $r = .97$ over a range of 3 to 40 mm of fat, indicating good agreement. Reliability coefficients of correlation between duplicate ultrasonic measurements ($N = 100$) were also high (triceps, $r = .98$; subscapular, $r = .99$; abdominal, $r = .99$). Booth, Goddard, and Paton (112) also used the abdominal site to compare the A-mode ultrasound technique to electrical conductivity methods ($N = 20$). The correlation between these two methods was $r = .98$ (standard error $= \pm 0.24$ mm).

The results of Ishida et al. (113) also confirmed the high reliability of the ultrasound method. Thirty volunteers (17 men, 13 women) were measured at 14 sites (forearm, biceps, triceps, axilla, subscapular, lumbar, chest [men only], abdomen, suprailiac, quadriceps, hamstrings, suprapatellar, and medial and posterior calf) on 2 separate days. Four identical ultrasound images were printed for each site, and two investigators each measured two of the images. Intratester reliability coefficients ranged from $r = .96$ to $r = .99$, and intertester reliability was greater than .90 at 11 of the 14 sites for fat and at 8 of the 11 sites for muscle. The abdomen, lumbar, and hamstrings sites yielded inconsistent between-day correlations for both fat and muscle. Generalizability theory was used to determine the contribution from testers, days, trials, and subjects to the total variance. For the fat and muscle measurements at each site, less than 2% of the variability was due to the effect of testers, days, and trials. Generalizability coefficients of at least $r = .92$ were obtained for all muscle measurement sites, while coefficients for fat measurements exceeded $r = .90$ for all but the axilla site.

Haymes et al. (114) investigated the validity of B-mode ultrasound by comparing ultrasonic fat thicknesses (at the suprailiac and triceps sites) to fat thicknesses obtained by soft-tissue roentgenograms ($N = 37$). Correlations between fat measurements for these two techniques were considered moderate to high (suprailiac, $r = .78$; triceps, $r = .88$), but were not as high as the correlations obtained by Bullen et al. (108) and Booth, Goddard, and Paton (112).

Fukunaga et al. (115) also studied the validity of B-mode ultrasound by comparing ultrasonically determined fat and muscle thicknesses of the upper arm, thigh, and abdomen to thicknesses obtained by direct cadaver analysis. These three sites were ultrasonically scanned and surgically cut open, and fat and muscle thicknesses were measured directly with slide calipers. The mean fat thickness was 5.0 ± 0.3 mm, according to direct cadaver analysis (D-method), compared to 4.8 ± 0.3 mm as determined by the ultrasound method (U-method). This corresponds to a D $-$ U/D ratio of 2.7%. The mean muscle thickness was 17.5 ± 1.3 mm (D-method), compared to a mean value of 17.0 ± 1.3 mm (U-method) (D $-$ U/D ratio = 1.8%). These investigators concluded that there were no significant dif-

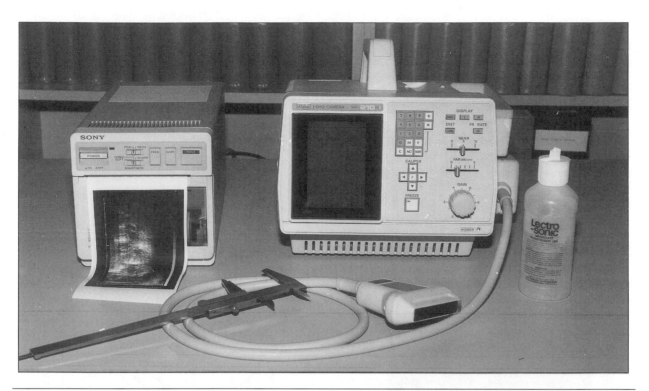

Figure 10.24 Photo of B-mode ultrasound equipment echo camera (right), videographic printer (left), transducer or probe (foreground right), and a Vernier caliper (foreground left).

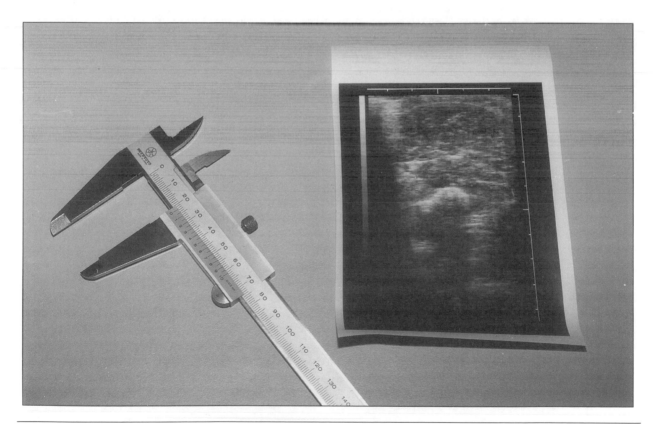

Figure 10.25 Photo of the printout obtained from the videographic printer and a Vernier caliper, which is used to measure the fat thickness (distance A) and the muscle thickness (distance B) to the nearest 0.1 mm.

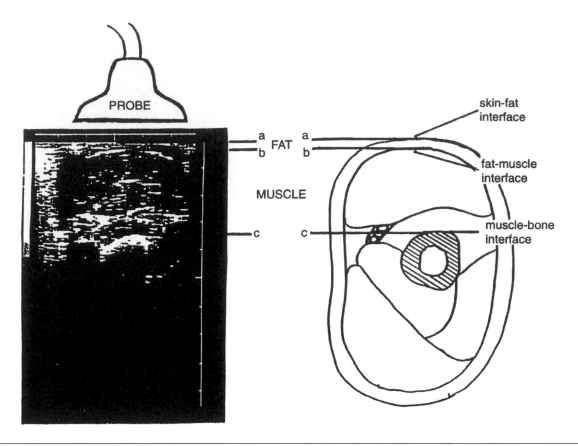

Figure 10.26   Thicknesses of the fat (distance between A and B) and muscle (distance between B and C) layers of the biceps as viewed by B-mode ultrasound.

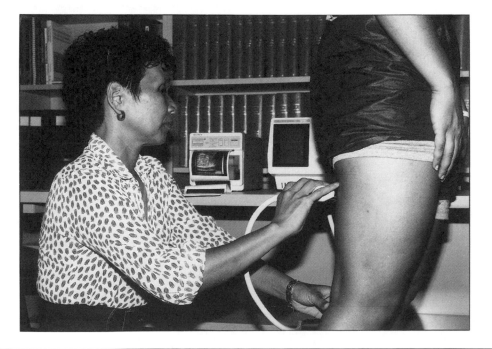

Figure 10.27   Measurement of the posterior thigh site with B-mode ultrasound. A small amount of ultrasonic gel is applied to the head of the transducer, which is then placed gently over the desired site, perpendicular to the underlying bone.

ferences in muscle and fat thicknesses between D and U methods. Therefore, B-mode ultrasound is a valid technique for measuring subcutaneous fat and muscle thickness.

Prediction Equations

Few researchers have attempted to predict body composition from ultrasound measurements. The earliest studies used A-mode ultrasound (109, 116). These studies showed moderate to good prediction estimates of D_b from ultrasonically determined skinfold fat ($R = .81$ and $R = .75$, respectively). More recently, Fanelli and Kuczmarski (117) developed three prediction equations ($N = 124$) for D_b using two B-mode ultrasonic fat measurements: waist and thigh ($R = .81$, *SEE* = 0.0078 g/cc), triceps and waist ($R = .76$, *SEE* = 0.0085 g/cc), and triceps and thigh ($R = .76$, *SEE* = 0.0086 g/cc). Volz and Ostrove (118) studied college-aged women ($N = 66$) and derived two regression equations for predicting D_b from the log transformation of B-mode ultrasound fat measurements: suprailiac ($R = .74$, *SEE* = 0.0074 g/cc) and thigh and suprailiac ($R = .78$, *SEE* = 0.0069 g/cc). Kuczmarski, Fanelli, and Koch (68) studied obese males ($n = 13$) and females ($n = 31$) between the ages of 26 and 69 years. A subject was considered obese if weight-for-height exceeded by at least 20% the upper values listed for a large frame in the 1983 Metropolitan height–weight tables. They developed a regression equation for D_b based on three fat variables: thigh, biceps, and the thigh × biceps cross-product ($R = .82$, *SEE* = 0.0095 g/cc).

Recently, Garzarella et al. (119) developed and cross-validated generalized prediction equations for D_b and FFM using the B-mode ultrasound technique. They studied a sample of 254 women who varied greatly in age (range = 18 to 74 years) and percent fat (range = 9.2% to 52.8%). The "best" D_b equation was the quadratic form of the sum of four ($\Sigma 4$) fat thicknesses (anterior thigh, abdomen, biceps, and triceps) and age [$D_b = 1.08812 - 0.00085 (\Sigma 4) + 0.000002 (\Sigma 4)^2 - 0.00031$ (age)]; $R = .93$, *SEE* = 0.0070 g/cc. The sum of five ($\Sigma 5$) muscle thicknesses (anterior forearm, biceps, triceps, abdomen, and anterior thigh) with age, height, and weight yielded the "best" FFM equation [FFM = $- 44.417 + 0.14276 (\Sigma 5) - 0.06426$ (age) $+ 0.37284$ (Ht) $+ 0.18147$ (Wt)]; $R = .92$, *SEE* = 2.4 kg. These later correlations and standard errors are comparable to results obtained from anthropometric prediction equations.

Sources of Error

Although these data show a reasonably high reliability and validity of the ultrasound technique, certain limitations still exist (120). The appropriate signal frequency has not been well defined. A range of 2.5 to 7.5 MHz has been reported in the literature, with the best predictive accuracy associated with the highest frequency. Another difficulty is the need for uniform and constant pressure when applying the probe to the scan site (114). Changes in pressure by probe application can affect the distribution of adipose tissue and prejudice the ultrasonic determination of adipose thickness. Finally, the landmarks used for measurement sites need to be well defined and standardized so that published prediction equations can be used with better accuracy.

DUAL-ENERGY PROJECTION METHODS

Dual-energy projection methods have been used for over a decade to measure bone and soft-tissue composition *in vivo* (121). There are two types of dual-energy projection methods. Dual-photon absorptiometry (DPA) is based on the differential attenuation by tissues of transmitted photons at two energy levels (122). DPA uses a gadolinium radionuclide (^{153}Gd) and has been widely used for the measurement of regional bone mineral density (BMD) and bone mineral content (BMC), particularly of the spine and proximal femur (121).

Dual-energy X-ray absorptiometry (DEXA) is a recently introduced noninvasive radiologic projection technique. The energy source for DEXA is X-ray rather than the gadolinium used in DPA. This technological change has improved the ability to quantify various parameters of body composition; radiation exposure is minimal, evaluation time is reduced, and precision is improved by enhanced resolution. A Lunar (Madison, WI) DEXA (DPX-L) is shown in Figure 10.28. DPA and DEXA instruments differentiate body weight into three chemical compartments—lean soft tissue, fat soft tissue, and bone (123)—and have the ability to distinguish regional as well as whole-body parameters of body composition. Figure 10.29 illustrates BMD results of an anterior–posterior (AP) spine scan.

Unlike hydrostatic densitometry, DEXA is not limited by the assumptions associated with the two-compartment constant-density model. Tissue densities are measured directly and are differentiated. This is a significant advantage over underwater weighing for the determination of body composition in humans.

Reliability and validity of DPA (124, 125) and DEXA (126, 127) are well established. Precision errors are less than 3% for fat and 1.1 kg and 30 g for muscle and bone, respectively (126). Correlations between body composition parameters as measured by DPA and other methods such as hydrodensitometry and neutron activation analysis are typically greater than $r = .90$ (125, 128, 129). In a

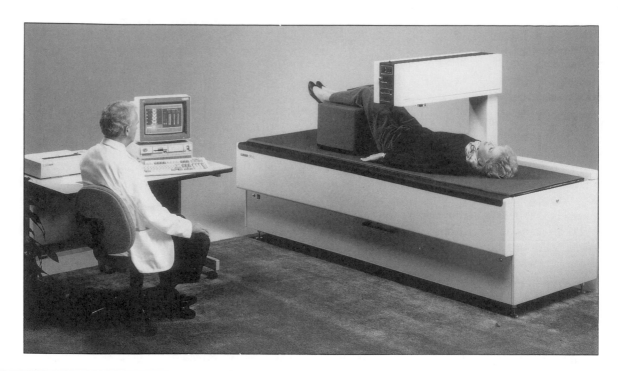

Figure 10.28   Lunar (Madison, WI) DEXA (DPX-L) machine.

recent study that evaluated the interday reliability of 13 bone density parameters measured by DEXA, correlation coefficients were $r = .90$ to $r = .99$, and *SEE* ranged from 0.01 to 0.08 g/cm², which represented less than 4% of the mean density values (130).

Unfortunately dual-energy projection methods are expensive (cost can exceed $60,000) and often require trained radiology personnel. This limits the applicability of DEXA and DPA to clinical and research laboratory settings. As the cost of DEXA becomes less prohibitive, it will likely replace hydrostatic weighing as a criterion measure of body composition in many studies.

COMPARISON AMONG METHODS

The only direct method of evaluating body composition is chemical digestion and subsequent analysis of the tissues. This is obviously not a practical approach in humans. Computer imaging, dual-energy projection, and radioisotope techniques are highly accurate but expensive and require specially trained personnel. For these reasons, hydrostatic densitometry is the most common criterion method of body composition analysis.

Relative fat values derived from hydrostatic weighing have been compared with relative fat from DPA and DEXA in several studies (126, 131, 132). Wang et al. (132) found the reliability of DPA ($r = .97$) to be similar to that of hydrostatic weighing ($r = .95$). Relative fat determined by hydrostatic weighing was related to DPA fat by $r = .87$ and *SEE* = 3.4%. Haarbo et al. (126) found a correlation of $r = .97$ between hydrostatically determined percent fat and percent fat derived from DEXA, but the *SEE* (5.6%) was somewhat higher than that observed by Wang et al. (132). Verlooy et al. (131) reported an $r = .96$ and *SEE* = 1.68% for a comparison of relative fat values obtained by hydrostatic weighing and DEXA.

Hydrostatic densitometry requires relatively expensive, specialized equipment and is time-consuming. Thus, it is not a suitable field method of measuring body composition. Anthropometry and BIA are the most common field techniques used for predicting body composition. Both are relatively simple to perform and can be completed in less than 10 min.

Because skinfolds are more highly correlated with body fat than are other anthropometric measures (circumferences, skeletal diameters), prediction equations for body composition from anthropometry generally include skinfolds (51). As with BIA, the addition of one or more circumference measures to skinfold prediction equations can slightly improve accuracy (39). Anthropometric and BIA techniques for predicting body composition have typically employed hydrostatic densitometry as the criterion method during the development of prediction equations. Thus, the 2.5% error associated with hydrostatic densitometry is inherent in the prediction of relative fat from anthropometry and BIA. An error of ±2.5% is the best possible degree of accuracy one could

AP SPINE RESULTS
LUNAR CORPORATION
313 W. BELTLINE HWY., MADISON, WI 53713

PATIENT ID:	SCAN:	1.2	12/11/91
NAME:	ANALYSIS:	1.2	12/11/91

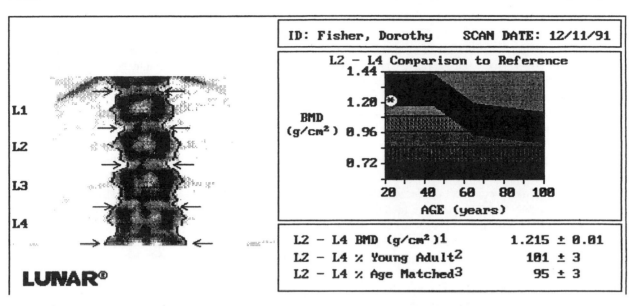

ID: Fisher, Dorothy   SCAN DATE: 12/11/91

L2 - L4 Comparison to Reference

L2 - L4 BMD (g/cm²)[1]	1.215 ± 0.01
L2 - L4 % Young Adult[2]	101 ± 3
L2 - L4 % Age Matched[3]	95 ± 3

Age (years).........	23	Large Standard......	279.25	Scan Mode..............	Fast
Sex.................	Female	Medium Standard.....	209.90	Scan Type..............	DPX-L
Weight (Kg).........	86.0	Small Standard......	148.20	Collimation (mm).......	1.68
Height (cm).........	173	Low keV Air (cps)...	747395	Sample Size (mm).......	1.2x1.2
Ethnic..............	White	High keV Air (cps)..	460239	Current (uA)...........	3000
System..............	7019	Rvalue (%Fat)....... 1.351(20.5)			

REGION	BMD g/cm²	Young Adult[2] %	Young Adult[2] Z	Age Matched[3] %	Age Matched[3] Z
L1	1.128	94	-0.60	88	-1.30
L2	1.251	104	0.43	97	-0.27
L3	1.229	102	0.24	96	-0.46
L4	1.173	98	-0.22	91	-0.92
L1-L2	1.191	104	0.34	97	-0.36
L1-L3	1.205	103	0.29	96	-0.41
L1-L4	1.196	101	0.13	95	-0.57
L2-L3	1.239	103	0.33	97	-0.37
L2-L4	1.215	101	0.12	95	-0.58
L3-L4	1.200	100	-0.00	93	-0.70

1 - See appendix E on precision and accuracy. Statistically 68% of repeat scans will fall within 1 SD.

2 - USA AP Spine Reference Population, Ages 20-45. See Appendix C.

3 - Matched for Age, Weight, Ethnic. See Appendix C.

Figure 10.29   Results of the anterior–posterior (AP) lumbar spine scan.

expect from a prediction technique based on underwater weighing. The accuracy reported for anthropometry and BIA generally ranges from ± 3% to 6% fat overall and from 3% to 4% fat for the most accurate equations. Both BIA and anthropometry tend to overpredict in very lean individuals and underpredict in the obese with equations developed from normal populations. For comparative purposes, the accuracy of predicting relative fat from anthropometric and BIA techniques is listed with age, height, weight, and BMI in Table 10.8 (133).

Population-specific equations are often invalid when applied to persons who do not fit the characteristics of the population from which they were developed. Therefore, selection of the prediction equation is critical for both BIA and anthropometric prediction techniques. Generalized equations that predict body composition with an acceptable degree of accuracy over a wide range of individuals have been developed for skinfold (38, 39) and BIA techniques (89, 134).

Comparisons of body composition derived from anthropometric and bioelectric impedance methods have been made (99, 100, 104). Campos et al. (99) found that D_b, total body water, relative fat, and FFM could be predicted by both anthropometry (weight, height, and two skinfold measures) and BIA with similar accuracy. Kushner and Haas (100) also concluded that there is excellent agreement between the estimation of FFM by BIA and skinfold anthropometry. Schols et al. (104), however, found BIA to be more accurate than skinfold thicknesses for predicting FFM in 32 pulmonary patients. Fuller and Elia (135) studied 24 normal men ($n = 14$) and women ($n = 10$) and found a small advantage for predicting D_b from BIA when compared to the skinfold method described by Durnin and Womersley (61).

Anthropometry is probably the least expensive method of predicting body composition. Additional advantages of anthropometric measurements over BIA include the fact that the measurements provide regional information on body composition and are often of value by themselves for comparative purposes and tracking changes over time. Whole-body resistance in ohms from BIA means little to most individuals by itself.

Predicting body composition from ultrasound measurements is similar in theory to the fat skinfold technique. When compared to anthropometric and bioelectrical impedance (BIA) equations, the ultrasound technique is equally reliable and valid. However, an important advantage that the ultrasound technique has over the other methods is that it provides useful information on muscle thickness. This would be valuable in studying the effects of a resistance-training program on body composition. Circumference measurements alone cannot determine whether a change in circumference was due to an alteration in the amount of fat, muscle, or both. The ultrasound technique, however, can make this distinction. Furthermore, unlike the BIA method, which gives information only on total changes in body composition, the ultrasound technique can tell the specific sites at which the changes occurred in both fat and muscle. A major disadvantage that ultrasound has over anthropometry and BIA is cost (approximately $30,000).

The advantage of BIA over anthropometry and ultrasound is that only a single measurement is required to predict body composition and it is not greatly affected by interinvestigator variability. However, because hydration status can greatly influence BIA measures, careful standardization of factors influencing hydration is important. Neither anthropometry nor BIA are suitable techniques for obtaining criterion measures of body composition for research purposes.

Table 10.8   Correlation and Standard Error of Predicting Relative Fat From Selected Variables

Variable	Women		Men	
	r	SEE(%)	r	SEE(%)
Age	−0.35	6.7	−0.38	7.4
Height	−0.08	7.2	0.01	8.0
Weight	−0.63	5.6	−0.62	6.3
BMI	−0.70	5.1	−0.69	5.8
Σ 7 Skinfolds	−0.85	3.8	−0.88	3.8
BIA	0.71	3.6	0.75	3.8

Note. BMI = body mass index: $Wt(kg)/Ht^2(cm^2)$.
Data for age, height, weight, BMI, and Σ 7 skinfolds from Pollock, Schmidt, and Jackson (133). Published with permission. Data for BIA from Graves et al. (84).

NORMATIVE DATA

Body composition has been evaluated extensively in humans, and normative data are available by age and for a variety of athletic populations (136). For younger women, normative values for percent fat range from 22% to 29%, for younger men from 12% to 15%, for older women from 25% to 34%, and for older men from 18% to 27% (52). Recommended levels of relative fat are 15% for men and 23% for women and are based upon the Behnke and Wilmore (18) models of the reference man and woman. Although relative fat increases as a function of age, there are no known advantages to gaining fat beyond the recommended levels. In fact, increased levels of body fat are associated with an increased risk of cardiovascular and metabolic disease (17). Thus, it is advantageous to maintain a healthy level of relative fat with a combination of sensible diet and physical activity throughout life.

REFERENCES

1. Cureton, K.J., Sparling, P.B., Evans, B.W., Johnson, S.M., Kong, U.D., & Purvis, J.W. (1978). Effect of experimental alterations in excess weight on aerobic capacity and distance running performance. *Medicine and Science in Sports*, **10**, 194-199.

2. Montgomery, D.L. (1982). The effect of added weight on ice hockey performance. *Physician and Sportsmedicine*, **10**(11), 91-99.

3. Farquhar, J.W. (1978). *The American way of life need not be hazardous to your health*. New York: Norton.

4. Hubert, H.A., Feinlab, M., McNamara, P.M., & Castelli, W.P. (1983). Obesity as an independent risk factor for cardiovascular disease: A 26-year follow-up of the participants in the Framingham heart study. *Circulation*, **67**, 968-977.

5. Mayer, J. (1968). *Overweight: Causes, costs, and control*. Englewood Cliffs, NJ: Prentice Hall.

6. Bray, G.A. (1985). Complications of obesity. *Annals of Internal Medicine*, **103**, 1052-1062.

7. Harrison, G.G. (1985). Height-weight tables. *Annals of Internal Medicine*, **103**, 989-994.

8. Millar, W.J., & Stephens, T. (1987). The prevalence of overweight and obesity in Britain, Canada, and United States. *American Journal of Public Health*, **77**, 38-41.

9. Keys, A., Fidanza, F., Karvonen, M.J., Kimura, N., & Taylor, H.L. (1972). Indices of relative weight and obesity. *Journal of Chronic Diseases*, **25**, 329-343.

10. Wilmore, J.H., & Haskell, W.L. (1972). Body composition and endurance capacity of professional football players. *Journal of Applied Physiology*, **33**, 564-567.

11. Brozek, J., Grande, J., Anderson, T., & Keys, A. (1963). Densitometric analysis of body composition: A review of some quantitative assumptions. *Annals of the New York Academy of Sciences*, **110**, 113-140.

12. Siri, W.E. (1961). Body composition from fluid spaces and density. In J. Brozek & A. Henschel (Eds.), *Techniques for measuring body composition* (pp. 223-244). Washington, DC: National Academy of Science.

13. Clarys, J.P., Martin, A.D., & Drinkwater, D.T. (1984). Gross tissue weights in human cadaver dissection. *Human Biology*, **56**, 459-473.

14. Lohman, T.G. (1981). Skinfolds and body density and their relation to body fatness: A review. *Human Biology*, **53**, 181-225.

15. Lohman, T.G. (1986). Applicability of body composition techniques and constants for children and youths. *Exercise and Sports Sciences Reviews*, **14**, 325-357.

16. Garn, S.M. (1973). Adult bone loss, fracture epidemiology and nutritional implications. *Nutrition*, **27**, 107-115.

17. Pollock, M.L., & Wilmore, J.H. (1990). *Exercise in health and disease: Evaluation and prescription for prevention and rehabilitation* (2nd ed.). Philadelphia: W.B. Saunders.

18. Behnke, A.R., & Wilmore, J.H. (1974). *Evaluation and regulation of body build and composition*. Englewood Cliffs, NJ: Prentice Hall.

19. Ward, A., Pollock, M.L., Jackson, A.S., Ayres, J.J., & Pape, G. (1978). A comparison of body fat determined by underwater weighing and volume displacement. *American Journal of Physiology*, **234**, E94-E96.

20. Fahey, T.D., & Schroeder, R. (1978). A load-cell system for hydrostatic weighing. *Research Quarterly*, **49**, 85-87.

21. Girandola, R.N., Wiswell, R.A., & Romero, G. (1977). Body composition changes resulting from fluid ingestion and dehydration. *Research Quarterly*, **48**, 299-303.

22. Katch, F.I. (1968). Apparent body density and variability during underwater weighing. *Research Quarterly*, **39**, 993-999.

23. Goldman, R.F., & Buskirk, E.R. (1961). Body volume measurement by underwater weighing: Description of a technique. In J. Brozek & A. Henshel (Eds.), *Techniques for measuring body composition* (pp. 78-89). Washington, DC: National Academy of Science.

24. Goldman, H.I., & Becklace, M.R. (1959). Respiratory function tests: Normal values of medium altitudes and the prediction of normal results. *American Review of Tuberculosis and Respiratory Diseases*, **79**, 457-467.

25. Buskirk, E.R. (1961). Underwater weighing and body density: A review of procedures. In J. Brozek & A. Henschel (Eds.), *Techniques for measuring body composition* (pp. 90-105). Washington, DC: National Academy of Science.

26. Wilmore, J.H. (1969). The use of actual, predicted, and constant residual volumes in the assessment of body composiiton by underwater weighing. *Medicine and Science in Sports*, **1**, 87-90.

27. Katch, F.I., & Katch, V.L. (1980). Measurement and prediction errors in body composition assessment and the search for the perfect equation. *Research Quarterly for Exercise and Sport*, **51**(1), 249-260.

28. *Clinical spirometry*. (1967). Braintree, MA: W.C. Collins.

29. Craig, A.B., & Ware, D.E. (1967). Effect of immersion in water on vital capacity and residual volume of lungs. *Journal of Applied Physiology*, **23**, 423-425.

30. Werdein, E.J., & Kyle, L.H. (1960). Estimation of the constancy of density of the fat-free body. *Journal of Clinical Investigations*, **39**, 626-629.

31. Keys, A., & Brozek, J. (1953). Body fat in adult men. *Physiological Reviews*, **33**, 245-325.

32. Pascale, L.R., Grossman, M.I., Sloan, H.S., & Frankel, T. (1956). Correlations between thickness of skinfolds and body density in 88 soldiers. *Human Biology*, **28**, 165-176.

33. Pollock, M.L., Laughridge, E., Coleman, B., Linnerud, A.C., & Jackson, A. (1975). Prediction of BD in young and middle-aged women. *Journal of Applied Physiology*, **38**, 745-749.

34. Mendez, J., & Lukaski, H.C. (1981). Variability of body density in ambulatory subjects measured at different days. *American Journal of Clinical Nutrition*, **34**, 78-81.

35. Jackson, A.S., Pollock, M.L., Graves, J.E., & Mahar, M.T. (1988). Reliability and validity of bioelectrical impedance in determining body composition. *Journal of Applied Physiology*, **64**, 529-534.

36. Oppliger, R.A., Looney, M.A., & Tipton, C.M. (1987). Reliability of hydrostatic weighing & skinfold measurements of body composition using generalizability study. *Human Biology*, **59**, 77-96.

37. Lohman, T.G., Roche, A.F., & Martorell, R. (Eds.). (1988). *Anthropometric standardization reference manual*. Champaign, IL: Human Kinetics.

38. Jackson, A.S., & Pollock, M.L. (1978). Generalized equations for predicting body density of men. *British Journal of Nutrition*, **40**, 497-504.

39. Jackson, A.S., Pollock, M.L., & Ward, A. (1980). Generalized equations for predicting body density of women. *Medicine and Science in Sports and Exercise*, **12**, 175-182.

40. Pollock, M.L., & Jackson, A.S. (1984). Research progress in validation of clinical methods of assessing body composition. *Medicine and Science in Sports and Exercise*, **16**, 606-613.

41. Pett, L.B., & Olgilvie, G.F. (1957). The report on Canadian average weights, heights, and skinfolds. *Canadian Bulletin of Nutrition*, **5**, 1-81.

42. Edwards, D.A.W., Hammond, W.H., Healy, M.J.R., Tanner, J.M., & Whitehouse, R.M. (1955). Design and accuracy of calipers for measuring subcutaneous fat thickness. *British Journal of Nutrition*, **9**, 133-143.

43. Sloan, A.W., & Shapiro, A. (1972). A comparison of skinfold measurements in three standard calipers. *Human Biology*, **44**, 29-36.

44. Lohman, T.G., Pollock, M.L., Slaughter, M.H., Brandon, L.J., & Boileau, R.A. (1984). Methodological factors and the prediction of body fat in female athletes. *Medicine and Science in Sports and Exercise*, **16**, 92-96.

45. Gruber, J.J., Pollock, M.L., Graves, J.E., Colvin, A.B., & Braith, R.W. (1990). Comparison of Harpenden and Lange calipers in predicting body composition. *Research Quarterly for Exercise and Sport*, **61**, 184-190.

46. Pollock, M.L., Laughridge, E., Coleman, B., Linnerud, A.C., & Jackson, A.E. (1975). Prediction of body density in young and middle-aged women. *Journal of Applied Physiology*, **38**, 745-749.

47. Pollock, M.L., Hickman, T., Kendrick, Z., Jackson, A., Linnerud, A.G.L., & Dawson, G. (1976). Prediction of body density in young and middle-aged men. *Journal of Applied Physiology*, **40**, 300-304.

48. Jackson, A.S., Pollock, M.L., & Gettman, L.R. (1978). Intertester reliability of selected skinfold and circumference measurements and percent fat estimates. *Research Quarterly*, **49**, 546-551.

49. Munro, A., Joffe, A., Ward, J.S., Syndham, C.H., & Fleming, P.W. (1966). An analysis of the errors in certain anthropometric measurements. *Internationale Zeitschrift Fur Angewandte Physiologic Einschliesslish Arbeitsphysiologic*, **23**, 93-106.

50. Pollock, M.L., Jackson, A.S., & Graves, J.E. (1986). Analysis of measurement error related to skinfold site, quantity of skinfold fat, and sex. *Medicine and Science in Sports and Exercise*, **18**, S32.

51. Jackson, A.S., & Pollock, M.L. (1976). Factor analysis and multivariate scaling of anthropometric variables for the assessment of body composition. *Medicine and Science in Sports*, **8**, 196-203.

52. Katch, F.I., & McArdle, W.D. (1973). Prediction of body density from simple anthropometric measurements in college-age men and women. *Human Biology*, **45**(3), 445-454.

52a. McArdle, W.D., Katch, F.I., & Katch, V.L. (1991). *Exercise physiology: Energy, nutrition, and human performance* (3rd ed.). Philadelphia: Lea & Febiger.

53. Brozek, J., & Keys, A. (1951). The evaluation of leanness-fatness in man: Norms and intercorrelations. *British Journal of Nutrition*, **5**, 194-206.

54. Jackson, A.S., & Pollock, M.L. (1982). Steps toward the development of generalized equations for predicting body composition of adults. *Canadian Journal of Applied Sports Science*, **7**, 189-196.

55. Sloan, A.W., Burt, J.J., & Blyth, C.S. (1962). Estimation of body fat in young women. *Journal of Applied Physiology*, **17**, 967-970.

56. Young, C.M., Martin, M., Tensuan, R., & Blondin, J. (1962). Predicting specific gravity and body fatness in young women. *Journal of the American Dietetic Association*, **40**, 102-107.

57. Young, C.M. (1964). Prediction of specific gravity & body fatness in older women. *Journal of the American Dietetic Association*, **45**, 333-338.

58. Katch, F.I., & Michael, E.D. (1968). Prediction of body density from skinfold and girth measurements of college females. *Journal of Applied Physiology*, **25**, 92-94.

59. Wilmore, J.H., & Behnke, A.R. (1970). An anthropometric estimation of body density and lean body weight in young women. *American Journal of Clinical Nutrition*, **23**, 267-274.

60. Sinning, W.E. (1978). Anthropometric estimation of D$_b$, fat, and LBW in women gymnasts. *Medicine and Science in Sports and Exercise*, **10**, 243-249.

61. Durnin, J.V.G.A., & Womersley, J. (1974). Body fat assessed from total body density and its estimation from skinfold thickness: Measurements on 481 men and women aged from 16 to 72 years. *British Journal of Nutrition*, **32**, 77-92.

62. Sinning, W.E., & Wilson, J.R. (1984). Validity of "generalized" equations for body composition analysis in women athletes. *Research Quarterly*, **55**, 153-160.

63. Smith, J.F., & Mansfield, E.R. (1984). Body composition prediction in university football players. *Medicine and Science in Sports and Exercise*, **16**, 398-405.

64. Bulbulian, R. (1984). The influence of somatotype on anthropometric prediction of body composition in young women. *Medicine and Science in Sports and Exercise*, **16**, 389-397.

65. Thorland, W.G., Johnson, G.O., Tharp, G.D., Fagot, T.G., & Hammer, R.W. (1984). Validity of anthropometric equations for the estimation of body density in adolescent athletes. *Medicine and Science in Sports and Exercise*, **16**, 77-81.

66. Scherf, J., Franklin, B.A., Lucas, CP., Stevenson, D., & Ruberfire, M. (1986). Validity of skinfold thickness measures of formerly obese adults. *American Journal of Clinical Nutrition*, **43**, 128-135.

67. Latin, R.W. (1987). Percent body fat determinations by body impedance analysis and skinfold measurements. *Fitness in Business*, **2**, 24-27.

68. Kuczmarski, R.J., Fanelli, M.T., & Koch, G.G. (1987). Ultrasonic assessment of body composition in obese adults: Overcoming the limitation of the skinfold caliper. *American Journal of Clinical Nutrition*, **45**, 717-724.

69. Weltman, A., Seip, R.L., & Tran, Z.V. (1987). Practical assessment of body composition in obese males. *Human Biology*, **59**, 523-536.

70. Weltman, A., Levine, S., Seip, R.L., & Tran, Z.V. (1988). Accurate assessment of body composition in obese females. *American Journal of Clinical Nutrition*, **48**, 1179-1183.

71. Lukaski, H.C., Johnson, P.E., Bolonchuk, W.W., & Lykken, G.I. (1985). Assessment of fat-free mass using bioelectrical impedance measurements of the human body. *American Journal of Clinical Nutrition*, **41**, 810-817.

72. Baumgartner, R.N., Chumlea, W.C., & Roche, A.F. (1990). Bioelectrical impedance for body composition. In K.B. Pandolf & J.O. Holloszy (Eds.), *Exercise and sport sciences reviews* (pp. 193-224). Baltimore: Williams & Wilkins.

73. Baker, L.E. (1989). Principles of the impedance technique. *Institute of Electrical and Electronic Engineers Engineering in Medicine*, **3**, 11-15.

74. Hoffer, B.C., Meador, C.K., & Simpson, D.C. (1969). Correlation of whole-body impedance with total body water volume. *Journal of Applied Physiology*, **27**, 531-534.

75. Smith, D.N. (1987). Body composition by tetrapolar impedance measurements—correlation or con? In *Proceeding of the VIIth International Conference on Electrical Bio-Impedance*. Portschach, Austria.

76. Rush, S., Abildskoo, J.A., & McFee, R. (1963). Resistivity of body tissues at low frequencies. *Circulation Research*, **12**, 40-50.

77. Lukaski, H., Bolonchuk, W.W., Hall, C.B., & Siders, W.A. (1986). Validation of tetrapolar bioelectrical impedance method to assess human body composition. *Journal of Applied Physiology*, **60**, 1327-1332.

78a. Lukaski, H.C., & Bolonchuk, W.W. (1988). Estimation of body fluid volumes using tetrapolar bioelectrical impedance measurements. *Aviation, Space, and Environmental Medicine*, **59**, 1163-1169.

78. Kushner, R.F., & Schoeller, D.A. (1986). Estimation of total body water by bioelectrical impedance analysis. *American Journal of Clinical Nutrition*, **44**, 417-424.

79. Chumlea, W.C., Baumgartner, R.N., & Roche, A.F. (1988). The use of specific resistivity to estimate fat-free mass from segmental body measures of bioelectrical impedance. *American Journal of Clinical Nutrition*, **48**, 7-15.

80. Chumlea, W.C., Roche, A.F., Guo, S., & Woynarowska, B. (1987). The influence of physiological variables and oral contraceptives on bioelectric impedance. *Human Biology*, **59**, 257-270.

81. Chumlea, W.C., & Baumgartner, R.N. (1990). Bioelectrical impedance methods for the estimation of body composition. *Canadian Journal of Sport Sciences*, **15**(3), 172-179.

82. Vettorazzi, C., Barillas, C., Pineda, O., & Solomons, N.W. (1987). A model for assessing body composition in amputees using bioelectrical impedance analysis. *Federation Proceedings*, **46**, 1186.

83. Guo, S., Roche, A.F., & Houtkooper, L. (1989). Fat-free mass in children and young adults predicted from bioelectrical impedance and anthropometric variables. *American Journal of Clinical Nutrition*, **50**, 435-443.

83a. Guo, S., Roche, A.F., Chumlea, W.C., Miles, D.S., & Pohlman, R.L. (1987). Body composition predictions from bioelectrical impedance. *Human Biology*, **59**, 221-233.

84. Graves, J.E., Pollock, M.L., Colvin, A.B., Van Loan, M., & Lohman, T.G. (1989). Comparison of different bioelectrical impedance anlayzers in the prediction of body composition. *American Journal of Human Biology*, **1**, 603-611.

85. Van Loan, M.D. (1990). Bioelectrical impedance analysis to determine fat-free mass, total body water and body fat. *Sports Medicine*, **10**(4), 205-217.

86. Elsen, R., Siu, M.-L., Pineda, O., & Solomons, N.W. (1987). Sources of variability in bioelectrical impedance determinations in adults. In K.J. Ellis, S. Yasumura, & W.D. Morgan (Eds.), *In vivo body composition studies* (pp. 184-188). New York: Plenum Press.

87. Schell, B., & Gross, R. (1987). The reliability of bioelectrical impedance measurements in the assessment of body composition in healthy adults. *Nutrition Report International*, **36**, 449-459.

88. Robert, S., Zarowitz, B., Pilla, A.M., & Peterson, E.L. (1991). Body composition analysis by bioelectrical impedance: The effects of time of day and body size on estimated gentamicin pharmacokinetics. *Pharmacotherapy*, **11**(2), 122-126.

89. Deurenberg, P., Kusters, C.S.L., & Smit, H.E. (1990). Assessment of body composition by bioelectrical impedance in children and young adults is strongly age-dependent. *European Journal of Clinical Nutrition*, **44**, 261-268.

90. Zebatakis, P.M., Gleim, G.W., Vitting, K.E., Gardemswartz, M., Agrawal, M., Michelos, M.F., & Nicholas, J.A. (1987). Volume changes affect electrical impedance measurement of body composiiton. *Medicine and Science in Sports and Exercise*, **19**, S40.

91. Deurenberg, P., Weststrate, J.A., & van der Kooy, K. (1989). Body composition changes assessed by bioelectrical impedance measurements. *American Journal of Clinical Nutrition*, **49**, 401-403.

92. de Cossio, T.G., Diaz, E., Delgado, H.L., Mendoza, R., & Gramajo, L. (1987). Accuracy and precision of bioelectrical impedance and anthropometry for estimating body composition. In K.J. Ellis, S. Yasumura, & W.D. Morgan (Eds.), *In vivo body composition studies* (pp. 195-200). New York: Plenum Press.

93. Roche, A.F., Chumlea, W.C., & Guo, S. (1986). *Identification and validation of new anthropometric techniques for quantifying body composition* (Technical Report No. TR-86-058). Natick, MA: U.S. Army Natick Research, Development and Engineering Center.

94. Caton, J.R., Mole, P.A., Adams, W.C., & Heustis, D.S. (1988). Body composition analysis by bioelectrical impedance: Effect of skin temperature. *Medicine and Science in Sports and Exercise*, **20**, 489-491.

95. Jackson, A.S., Pollock, M.L., Graves, J.E., & Mahar, M.T. (1988). Reliability and validity of bioelectrical

impedance in determining body composition. *Journal of Applied Physiology*, **64**, 529-534.

96. Siu, M.-L., Elsen, R., Mazariegos, M., Solomons, N.W., & Pineda, D. (1987). Evaluation through sequential determination of the stability of bioelectrical impedance measurements for body composition analysis. In K.J. Ellis, S. Yasumura, & W.D. Morgan (Eds.), *In vivo body composition studies* (pp. 189-194). New York: Plenum Press.

97. Lukaski, H.C., Bolonchuk, W.W., Johnson, P.E., Lykken, G.I., & Sandstead, H.H. (1984). Assessment of fat-free mass using bioelectrical impedance measurements of the human body. *American Society for Clinical Nutrition*, 657-658. (Abstract)

98. Segal, K.R., Gutin, B., Presta, E., Wang, J., & Van Itallie, T.B. (1985). Estimation of human body composition by electrical impedance methods: A comparative study. *Journal of Applied Physiology*, **58**, 1565-1571.

99. Campos, A.C., Chen, M., & Meguid, M.M. (1989). Comparisons of body composition derived from anthropometric and bioelectrical impedance methods. *Journal of the American College of Nutrition*, **8**(6), 484-489.

100. Kushner, R.F., & Haas, A. (1988). Estimation of lean body mass by bioelectrical impedance analysis compared to skinfold anthropometry. *European Journal of Clinical Nutrition*, **42**, 101-106.

101. Cordain, L., Whicker, R.E., & Johnson, J.E. (1988). Body composition determination in children using bioelectrical impedance. *Growth, Development and Aging*, **52**, 37-40.

102. Lukaski, H.C., Bolonchuk, W.W., Siders, W.A., & Hall, C.B. (1990). Body composition assessment of athletes using bioelectrical impedance measurements. *Journal of Sports Medicine and Physical Fitness*, **30**, 434-440.

103. Hannan, W.J., Cowen, S., Freeman, C.P., & Shapiro, C.M. (1990). Evaluation of bioelectrical impedance analysis for body composition measurements in anorexia nervosa. *Clinics in Physical and Physiological Measurement*, **11**(3), 209-216.

104. Schols, A.M.W.J., Wouters, E.F.M., Soeters, P.B., & Westerterp, K.R. (1991). Body composition by bioelectrical-impedance analysis compared with deuterium dilution and skinfold anthropometry in patients with chronic obstructive pulmonary disease. *American Journal of Clinical Nutrition*, **53**, 421-424.

105. Dumont, B.L. (1957, July). *New methods of estimation of carcass quality on live pigs.* Paper presented at the joint FAO/EAAP Meeting on Pig Progeny Testing, Copenhagen, Denmark.

106. Dumont, B.L. (1959). Measure of the fatness of hogs by the method of ultrasonic echoes. *C.R. Academy of Agriculture*, **45**, 628.

107. Claus, A. (1957). The measurement of natural interfaces in the pig's body with ultrasound. *Fleischwirtschaft*, **9**, 552-554.

108. Bullen, B.A., Quaade, F., Oleson, E., & Lund, S.A. (1965). Ultrasonic reflections used for measuring subcutaneous fat in humans. *Human Biology*, **37**, 375-384.

109. Sloan, A.W. (1967). Estimation of body fat in young men. *Journal of Applied Physiology*, **23**, 311-315.

110. Cromwell, L., Weibell, F.J., & Pfeiffer, E.A. (1980). *Biomedical instrumentation and measurement* (2nd ed.). Englewood Cliffs, NJ: Prentice Hall.

111. Newell, J.A. (1961). Ultrasonic localisation. *The British Journal of Radiology*, **34**, 539-546.

112. Booth, R., Goddard, B., & Paton, A. (1966). Measurement of fat thickness in man: A comparison of ultrasound, calipers, and electrical conductivity. *British Journal of Nutrition*, **20**, 719-727.

113. Ishida, Y., Carroll, J.F., Pollock, M.L., Graves, J.E., & Leggett, S.H. (1990). Reliability of B-mode ultrasound in the measurement of body fat and muscle thickness. *Medicine and Science in Sports and Exercise*, **22**, S111.

114. Haymes, E.M., Lundegren, H.M., Loomis, J.L., & Buskirk, E.R. (1976). Validity of the ultrasonic technique as a method of measuring subcutaneous adipose tissue. *Annals of Human Biology*, **3**, 245-251.

115. Fukunaga, T., Matsuo, A., Ishida, Y., Tsunoda, N., Uchino, S., & Ohkubo, M. (1989). Study for measurement of muscle and subcutaneous fat thickness by means of ultrasonic B-mode method. *Japanese Journal of Medical Ultrasonics*, **16**, 50-57.

116. Borkan, C., Halts, D., Cardarelli, J., & Burrows, B. (1982). Comparison of ultrasound and skinfold measurements in assessment of subcutaneous and total fatness. *American Journal of Physical Anthropology*, **58**, 307-313.

117. Fanelli, M.T., & Kuczmarski, R.J. (1984). Ultrasound as an approach to assessing body composition. *American Journal of Clinical Nutrition*, **39**, 703-709.

118. Volz, P.A., & Ostrove, S.M. (1984). Evaluation of a portable ultrasonoscope in assessing the body composition of college-age women. *Medicine and Science in Sports and Exercise*, **16**, 97-102.

119. Garzarella, L., Ishida, I., Graves, J.E., Leggett, S.H., Pollock, M.L., Carroll, J.F., & Feurtado, D. (1991). The development of prediction equations for estimating body composition in females by B-mode ultrasound. *Medicine and Science in Sports and Exercise*, **23**, S90.

120. Lukaski, H.C. (1987). Methods for the assessment of human body composition: Traditional and new. *American Journal of Clinical Nutrition*, **46**, 537-556.

121. Mazess, R.B., Barden, H.S., Bisek, J.P., & Hanson, J. (1990). Dual-energy x-ray absorptiometry for total-body and regional bone-mineral and soft-tissue composition. *American Journal of Clinical Nutrition*, **51**, 1106-1112.

122. Witt, R.M., & Mazess, R.B. (1978). Photon absorptiometry of soft-tissue and fluid content: The method and its precision and accuracy. *Physics in Medicine and Biology*, **23**, 620-629.

123. Heymsfield, S.B., & Waki, M. (1991). Body composition in humans: Advances in the development of multicompartment chemical models. *Nutrition Reviews*, **49**(4), 97-108.

124. Peppler, W.W., & Mazess, R.B. (1981). Total body bone mineral and lean body mass by dual photon absorptiometry. I Theory and measurement procedure. *Calcified Tissue International*, **33**, 353-359.

125. Heymsfield, S.B., Wang, J., Aulet, M. (1990). Dual photo absorptiometry: Validation of mineral and fat measurements. In S. Yasumura & J.E. Harrison (Eds.), *In vivo body composition studies* (pp. 327-337). New York: Plenum Press.

126. Haarbo, J., Gotfredsen, C., Hassager, C., & Christiansen, C. (1991). Validation of body composition by dual energy x-ray absorptiometry (DEXA). *Clinical Physiology*, **11**, 331-341.

127. Mazess, R., Collick, B., Trempe, J., Barden, H., & Hanson, J. (1989). Performance evaluation of dual-energy x-ray bone densitometer. *Calcified Tissue International*, **44**, 228-232.

128. Heymsfield, S.B., Wang, J., Heshka, S., Kehayias, J.J., & Pierson, R.N. (1989). Dual-photon absorptiometry: Comparison of bone mineral and soft tissue mass measurements in vivo with established methods. *American Journal of Clinical Nutrition*, **49**, 1283-1289.

129. Lichtman, S., Heymsfield, S.B., & Kehayias, J.J. (1990). Elemental reconstruction of human composition in vivo. *Federation of American Societies for Experimental Biology*, **4**, A2261.

130. Tucci, J., Carpenter, D., Graves, J., Pollock, M.L., Felheim, R., & Mananquil, R. (1991). Interday reliability of bone mineral density measurements using dual energy x-ray absorptiometry. *Medicine and Science in Sports and Exercise*, **23**(4), S115.

131. Verlooy, H., Dequeker, J., Geusens, P., Nijs, J., & Goris, M. (1991). Body composition by intercomparison of underwater weighing, skinfold measurements, and dual-photon absorptiometry. *The British Journal of Radiology*, **64**, 765-767.

132. Wang, J., Heymsfield, S.B., Aulet, M., Thornton, J.C., & Pierson, R.N. (1989). Body fat from body density: Underwater weighing vs. dual-photon absorptiometry. *American Journal of Physiology*, **256**, E829-E834.

133. Pollock, M.L., Schmidt, D.H., and Jackson, A.S. (1980). Measurement of cardiorespiratory fitness

and body composition in the clinical setting. *Comprehensive Therapy, 6*(9), 12-27.

134. Segal, K.R., Van Loan, M., Fitzgerald, P.I., Hogdon, J.A., & Van Itallie, T.B. (1988). Lean body mass estimation by bioelectrical impedance analysis: A four-site cross-validation study. *American Journal of Clinical Nutrition, 47*, 7-14.

135. Fuller, N.J., & Elia, M. (1989). Potential use of bioelectrical impedance of the 'whole body' and of body segments for the assessment of body composition: Comparison with densitometry and anthropometry. *European Journal of Clinical Nutrition, 43*, 779-791.

136. Wilmore, J.H., & Costill, D.L. (1988). *Training for sport and activity: The physiological basis of the conditioning process* (3rd ed.). Boston: Allyn and Bacon.

CHAPTER *11*

Anthropometry

Robert M. Malina, PhD

University of Texas at Austin

Anthropometry is a series of systematized measuring techniques that express quantitatively the dimensions of the human body. Anthropometry is often viewed as the traditional and perhaps basic tool of biological anthropology, but it has a long tradition of use in physical education and the physical activity and sport sciences, and it is finding increased use in the biomedical sciences. The purposes of this chapter are to

- provide an overview of anthropometry as a method,
- describe a series of dimensions and several ratios that have relevance to the physical activity and sport sciences,
- discuss issues related to measurement variability and quality control in anthropometry, and
- discuss several applications of anthropometry and the concept of reference data.

ANTHROPOMETRY IN THE SPORT SCIENCES

Body size and proportions, physique, and body composition are important factors in physical performance and fitness. Historically, stature and weight, both indicators of overall body size, have been used extensively with age and sex to identify some optimal combination of these variables for grouping children, youth, and young adults in various kinds of physical activities. Body size, particularly weight, is the standard frame of reference for expressing physiological parameters (e.g., $\dot{V}O_2$max as $ml \cdot kg^{-1} \cdot min^{-1}$), whereas skinfold thicknesses are often used to estimate body composition. Anthropometry has long been used in defining overweight and obesity and in establishing the relationship between being overweight and health-related fitness and life expectancy. Anthropometry, thus, is central to many of the concerns of the physical activity and sport sciences.

SUGGESTED MEASUREMENTS AND TECHNIQUES

Anthropometry involves the use of carefully defined body landmarks for measurements, specific subject positioning for these measurements, and the use of appropriate instruments. The measurements that can be taken on an individual are almost limitless in number. Measurements are generally divided into mass (weight), lengths and heights, breadths or widths, depths, circumferences or girths, curvatures or arcs, and soft-tissue measurements (skinfolds). In addition, numerous special measurements for specific body parts can be defined, especially for the head and face, the hand, and the foot. There is no minimum accepted list of measurements that must be taken to define a population.

A key issue in anthropometry is the selection of measurements. This depends on the purpose of the study and the specific questions under consideration. Thus, a necessary preliminary to the application of anthropometry is a thorough logical analysis, beginning with a clear concept of the knowledge to be sought and leading to a selection of the measurements needed to obtain an acceptable answer. *Anthropometry is a method and should be treated as such, a means to an end and not an end in itself.* Each measurement should be selected to provide a specific piece of information within the context of the study design. Thus, *no single battery of measurements will meet the needs of every study.* A corollary is that measurement for the sake of measurement is not acceptable; it makes no sense to take an extensive battery of measurements simply because one has the opportunity to measure.

Anthropometry is noninvasive in a physiological sense. All measurements are external dimensions of the body or its parts. However, anthropometry is invasive in a personal sense: An individual person is being measured. And, in some groups, cultural sanctions may limit which dimensions can be measured.

Although anthropometry is highly objective and highly reliable in the hands of trained anthropometrists, the biological or functional significance of many dimensions has not been adequately established. A key to effective anthropometry lies in understanding the meaning or significance of specific dimensions so that a set can be chosen that effectively answers the question(s) addressed. Measurements differ in their utility, and some have become firmly entrenched in manuals due to blind repetition rather than because they are known to be useful.

Much of the variation in human morphology relates to the development of skeletal, muscle, and adipose tissues, as well as the viscera. The suggested measurements thus focus on bone, muscle, and fat, and provide information on skeletal, muscular, and subcutaneous fat tissues. Regional variation in morphology is also a consideration; thus, both trunk (upper and lower) and extremity (upper and lower) dimensions are suggested. Combinations of dimensions also provide information on body proportions and physique. The suggested dimensions are also selected on the basis of site location and accessibility, although local cultural preferences may, at times, limit the accessibility of some sites for measurement (e.g., chest circumference or some trunk skinfolds in adolescent girls).

Procedures for taking the suggested measurements are from the *Anthropometric Standardization Reference Manual* edited by Lohman, Roche, and Martorell (26). The necessary equipment and methods of measurement are illustrated in the manual. Some of the measurements are also illustrated in Malina and Bouchard (31).

Overall Body Size

Weight and stature (height) are the two most often used anthropometric dimensions. *Body weight* is a measure of body mass. It is a heterogeneous measure, a composite of many tissues that often vary independently. Although weight should be measured with the individual nude, this is often impractical. Hence, weight is frequently taken with the individual attired in ordinary indoor clothing (e.g., gym shorts and T-shirt), without shoes.

Stature, or standing height, is a linear measurement of the distance from the floor or standing surface to the top (vertex) of the skull. It is a composite of linear dimensions contributed by the lower extremities, the trunk, the neck, and the head. Stature should be measured with a fixed stadiometer. If a movable anthropometer is used, one individual should hold the anthropometer so that it is properly aligned while the other positions the subject and takes the measurement. It is measured with the subject in the standard erect posture, without shoes. Weight is evenly distributed between both feet, heels are together, arms are hanging relaxed at the sides, and the head is in the Frankfort horizontal plane.

Stature and weight show *diurnal variation*, or variation in the dimension during the course of a day. This can be a problem in short-term longitudinal studies, in which apparent changes might simply reflect variation in the time of the day at which the measurement was taken. For example, stature is greatest in the morning upon arising from bed, and decreases as the individual assumes upright posture and walks about. The "shrinking" of stature occurs as a result of the compression of fibrous discs of cartilage that separate the vertebrae. With the forces of gravity imposed by standing and walking, the discs are gradually compressed. As a result, stature may diminish by a centimeter or more. The loss of stature is limited to the vertebral column. It is regained by having the individual lie still on a flat surface for about 30 min.

Body weight also shows diurnal variation. The individual is lightest in the morning, specifically after voiding the bladder upon arising. Body weight then increases gradually during the course of the day. It is affected by diet and physical activity. In menstruating girls and women, variation in the phase of the menstrual cycle also affects diurnal variation in body weight.

Specific Segment Lengths

Sitting height is, as the name implies, the height of the individual while sitting. It is measured with an anthropometer as the distance from the sitting surface to the top of the head, with the individual seated in the standard position. The subject sits on a table with the knees hanging freely and directed straight ahead. Hands are on the thighs, and the head is in the Frankfort horizontal plane. The individual is instructed to sit as erect as possible.

This measurement is especially of value when used with stature. Stature minus sitting height provides an estimate of length of the lower extremities (*subischial length*, or *leg length*). Most of the diurnal variation in stature previously discussed occurs in the trunk and thus influences sitting height.

Skeletal Breadths

Breadth or width measurements are ordinarily taken across specific bone landmarks and therefore provide an indication of the robustness or sturdiness of the skeleton. Four of the commonly taken skeletal breadths are the following. *Biacromial breadth* measures the distance across the right and left acromial processes of the scapulae and thus provides an indication of shoulder breadth. *Bicristal breadth* measures the distance across the most lateral parts of the iliac crests and thus provides an indication of the hip breadth. Both measurements are taken from the rear with the upper segment of the anthropometer used as a sliding caliper. The position of the subject is as in the measurement of stature.

Breadth across the bony condyles of the femur (*bicondylar breadth*) and the humerus (*biepicondylar breadth*) provides information on the robustness of the extremity skeleton. The former is measured across the most medial and most lateral aspects of the femoral condyles with the individual seated and the knee flexed 90°; a broad-blade sliding caliper is used. The latter is measured across the epicondyles of the humerus with the elbow flexed 90°; either a broad-blade or a small sliding caliper is used.

Circumferences

Limb circumferences are occasionally used as indicators of relative muscularity. Note, however, that a circumference includes bone, surrounded by a mass of muscle tissue, which is ringed by a layer of subcutaneous fat. Thus, it does not provide a measure of muscle tissue per se. However, because muscle is the major tissue comprising the circumference (except perhaps in the obese), limb circumferences are used to indicate relative muscular development. Circumferences are measured with a flexible, nonstretchable tape. The tape is applied at the appropriate site, making contact with the skin but without compressing the underlying tissue. The two more commonly used limb measurements are the arm and calf circumferences.

Arm circumference is measured with the arm hanging relaxed at the side. The measurement is taken at the point midway between the acromial and olecranon processes. The preceding is occasionally referred to as relaxed arm circumference, because arm circumference is occasionally measured in the flexed state, with the elbow flexed and the biceps muscle maximally contracted. *Flexed arm circumference* is used in the derivation of mesomorphy in the Heath-Carter somatotype protocol, which is discussed later in the chapter.

Calf circumference is measured as the maximum circumference of the calf with the subject in a standing position and the weight evenly distributed between both legs.

Relaxed arm and calf circumferences can be used in combination with arm (triceps and biceps) and calf (medial and lateral calf) skinfolds to provide estimates of muscle circumference and cross-sectional muscle and fat areas (Table 11.1). It should be noted that in surveys of nutritional status, arm circumference is generally corrected only for the thickness of the triceps skinfold (see Table 11.1). Corrected circumferences, though widely

Table 11.1 Calculation of Estimated Limb Muscle Circumferences and Cross-Sectional Muscle and Fat Areas

Using both triceps and biceps, and medial and latral calf skinfolds:

A. Arm muscle circumference (cm) $= C_a - \frac{\pi}{2}(S_t + S_b)$

Arm muscle area (cm^2) $= \frac{1}{4\pi}\left[C_a - \frac{\pi}{2}(S_t + S_b)\right]^2$

where C_a is arm circumference (cm), and S_t and S_b are the triceps and biceps skinfolds, respectively (cm)

B. Calf muscle circumference (cm) $= C_c - \frac{\pi}{2}(S_m + S_l)$

Calf muscle area (cm^2) $= \frac{1}{4\pi}\left[C_c - \frac{\pi}{2}(S_m + S_l)\right]^2$

where C_c is calf circumference (cm), and S_m and S_l are the medial calf and lateral calf skinfolds, respectively (cm)

C. Arm or calf area (cm^2) $= \frac{C^2}{4\pi}$

where C is arm or calf circumference (cm)
D. Arm fat area (cm^2) = arm area − arm muscle area
E. Calf fat area (cm^2) = calf area − calf muscle area

Using only the triceps skinfold:

A. Arm muscle circumference (cm) $= C_a - (\pi S_t)$

Arm muscle area (cm^2) $= \frac{[C_a - (\pi S_t)]^2}{4\pi}$

where C_a is arm circumference (cm) and S_t is the triceps skinfold (cm)
B. Arm area (as above)
C. Arm fat area (as above)

After Forbes (17) and Frisancho (18).

used, have limitations. The procedures assume that the limb is a cylinder and that subcutaneous fat is evenly distributed. The use of the triceps plus biceps skinfolds or the medial plus lateral calf skinfolds adjusts to some extent for the uneven distribution of subcutaneous fat. The size of the bone(s) is not considered, and variation in compressibility of skinfolds is an additional concern.

Thigh circumferences are occasionally utilized in the physical activity and sport sciences, primarily from the perspective of estimating thigh muscle volume. The procedures of Jones and Pearson (24) are often used. They include three thigh circumferences at the gluteal furrow (this is called proximal thigh circumference in Lohman et al. [26]), at a distance one-third of subischial height up from the tibial–femoral joint space, and at the minimum circumference above the knee, and anterior and posterior thigh skinfolds in the midline at the one-third subischial height level.

Given concern for the usefulness of trunk circumferences as indicators of relative fat distribution, *waist* and *hip* circumferences may also be considered. The literature indicates several procedures for the measurement of these girths. Lohman et al. (26) suggest that waist circumference be measured at the level of the natural waist (which is the narrowest part of the torso). A similar measurement, abdominal circumference, is measured at the level of greatest anterior extension of the abdomen (which is usually, but not always, at the umbilicus level). Hip circumference is measured at the level of the maximum protrusion of the buttocks. These circumferences, especially hip circumference, are occasionally taken over light clothing or a measuring gown. More pressure may need to be applied to compress the clothing.

Skinfold Thicknesses

Skinfold thicknesses are indicators of subcutaneous fat, the portion of body fat located immediately beneath the skin. Skinfolds are a double fold of skin and underlying subcutaneous tissue at specific sites. The measurement of a skinfold proceeds as follows. After the site is located and in some cases marked, the double fold of skin and underlying soft tissue are raised with the thumb and index finger of the left hand about 1 cm above (proximal) to the site. The caliper is then applied at the site. The space between the raised fold and the measurement site removes the effect of finger pressure on the caliper reading.

The following skinfold thicknesses are relevant in the physical activity and sport sciences:

- The *triceps skinfold* is measured on the back of the arm over the triceps muscle at the same level as relaxed arm circumference, that is, midway between the olecranon and acromial processes.

- The *biceps skinfold* is measured on the anterior aspect of the arm over the biceps muscle at the same level as relaxed arm circumference.
- The *subscapular skinfold* is measured on the back just beneath the inferior angle of the scapula.
- The *suprailiac skinfold* is measured immediately above the iliac crest in the midaxillary line. A suprailiac skinfold measured over the anterior superior iliac spine is used in the derivation of endomorphy in the Heath-Carter somatotype protocol (see below).
- The *abdominal skinfold* is measured as a horizontal fold 3 cm lateral and 1 cm inferior to the umbilicus.
- The *thigh skinfold* is measured over the anterior aspect of the thigh in the midline midway between the inguinal crease and proximal border of the patella.
- The *medial calf skinfold* is measured on the inside of the calf at the same level as calf circumference, that is, at maximum circumference.
- The *lateral calf skinfold* is measured on the lateral aspect of the calf at the same level as calf circumference.

Skinfolds on the extremities are measured as vertical folds; the subscapular and suprailiac skinfolds are measured following the natural cleavage lines of the skin.

Skinfolds measured on the extremities and on the trunk also provide information on the relative distribution of subcutaneous fat. There is, however, no consensus as to which methods best define and describe subcutaneous fat distribution (46). The sums of several extremity and of several trunk skinfolds expressed as a ratio (the ratio of trunk to extremity skinfolds) are often used to describe relative fat distribution (30, 31). Although ratios have limitations (e.g., they assume that the variables change in a linear manner), they are relatively simple and are useful in surveys.

Principal-components analysis is also used to identify components of fatness and the anatomical distribution of fat (see, for example, refs. 3, 16). The first component relates to overall fatness. Trunk-extremity and upper-lower-extremity components are affected by overall subcutaneous fatness, so it is necessary to control for overall fatness by analyzing residuals of the regression of specific skinfolds (log transformed) on the mean skinfold thickness (log) (see refs. 3, 16).

Skinfolds are often used in the physical activity and sport sciences to predict body density and in turn estimate relative fatness (percent body fat). Many prediction equations are available, but they are sample- or population-specific. Equations should be validated across several samples—their general applicability cannot be assumed without testing on other subjects. Prediction equations generally assume a linear relationship among variables, although a curvilinear relationship between skinfolds and body density is often apparent. Individual differences in relative fat distribution may also influence estimates.

Nevertheless, when use of a prediction equation is necessary, careful attention should be given to the sample that it is based upon, the correlation between predicted and measured body composition values, the standard error of estimate, and the number of measurements. Errors inherent in the measurement of skinfolds and the original body composition procedures must also be considered. Measurement variability associated with anthropometry is discussed later in the chapter.

Overview of Measurements

This brief set of measurements provides information on the size of the individual as a whole (weight and stature) and of specific segments, parts, and tissues. Skeletal breadths describe the overall robustness of the skeleton, limb circumferences provide information on relative muscularity, and skinfold thicknesses are indicators of subcutaneous fat. The specific dimensions include both the trunk and the extremities, because individuals can be similar in overall body size but vary in shape, proportions, and tissue distribution.

RATIOS AND PROPORTIONS

In addition to providing specific information in their own right, measurements can be related to each other in the form of indices or ratios. These are ordinarily calculated by dividing the larger measurement into the smaller measurement. The ratios thus provide information on shape and proportions. The four following ratios are commonly used, although in theory any two measurements can be related to each other.

Body Mass Index

The relationship between weight and stature is commonly expressed in the form of the body mass index (BMI):

$$weight/stature^2$$

where weight is in kilograms and stature is in meters. The BMI grades reasonably well on total body fatness and finds wide use in studies of overweight and obesity, especially in adults. A question that needs consideration is the influence of relative fat distribution on the BMI: Is the BMI a better index of fatness in those with a truncal pattern of fat distribution compared to those with a more peripheral pattern? In a health-related context, one can also inquire whether the BMI has the same implications for individuals of different ethnic groups.

The utility of the body mass index during the transition into puberty and in adolescent males may have limitations. At these times, the relationship between stature and weight is temporarily altered because the growth spurt occurs, on the average, first in stature and then in weight. Further, the adolescent spurt also includes a significant gain in muscle mass.

Sitting Height/Stature

The ratio of sitting height to stature provides an estimate of relative trunk length and, conversely, relative leg length. The ratio is calculated this way:

$$\frac{sitting\ height}{stature} \times 100$$

It basically asks the question: What percentage of height while standing is accounted for by height while sitting? By subtraction, the remaining percentage is accounted for by the lower extremities.

The sitting height/stature ratio is commonly used in nutritional surveys as an indirect indicator of the effects of adverse nutritional circumstances on the lower extremities. Higher ratios tend to be characteristic of chronically undernourished populations. The ratio is also useful in studies of population variation in the proportional contribution of lower extremity length to stature. Mean sitting height/stature ratios are, for example, lower in American Blacks (indicating relatively longer lower extremities) than in American Whites (28). The ratio may also differ among athletes in different sports or events within a given sport.

Bicristal Breadth/Biacromial Breadth

The ratio of bicristal breadth to biacromial breadth relates the breadth of the hips (lower trunk) to that of the shoulders (upper trunk):

$$\frac{bicristal\ breadth}{biacromial\ breadth} \times 100$$

The ratio is a useful indicator of sex differences in the proportional relationship of the shoulders and hips. The ratio is higher, on the average, in girls than in boys at virtually all ages during childhood and adolescence, and this difference persists into adulthood (31). Thus, females have broader hips *relative* to their shoulders, while males have broader shoulders *relative* to their hips.

Biacromial and bicristal breadths are also related in an *index of androgyny*, the degree of masculinity in physique. The index of Tanner (53) is commonly used:

$$(3 \times biacromial\ breadth) - bicristal\ breadth$$

Among female college students and track-and-field athletes, for example, the androgyny index for distance runners (80.0) is quite close to that for nonathletes (79.9), but it is higher (more masculine) in sprinters (82.0), jumpers and hurdlers (84.9), discus and javelin throwers (86.5), and shot-putters (88.9) (38). The value for shot-putters is quite close to that for nonathlete college males.

Waist/Hip

Waist and hip circumferences are expressed as the waist/hip ratio. Waist circumference is an indicator of adipose tissue in the waist and abdominal area; hip circumference is an indicator of adipose tissue over the buttocks and hips. The ratio thus provides an index of relative fat distribution in adults, the higher the ratio the greater the proportion of abdominal fat. Computed tomography has generally confirmed the validity of anthropometric estimates of fat distribution in adults (1). The validity of these circumferences as measures of fat distribution in youth is not known (42).

Limitations of Ratios

Ratios are influenced by the relationship between the two variables and assume that the two dimensions change in a linear manner. Ratios are also affected by the measurement variability associated with each dimension. They may yield spurious results when they are based on different types of dimensions, such as weight and stature or arm circumference and stature, or when the standard deviations of the dimensions differ considerably (52). Note that most ratios are commonly based upon similar measurements (e.g., two lengths or two skeletal breadths). The BMI is an exception, and to overcome some of these problems, stature is squared (see ref. 11).

PHYSIQUE

Physique is the individual's body form, the configuration of the entire body rather than of specific features. Physique is commonly referred to as body build. The physical activity and sport sciences have a long history of studying physique, including relationships between physique and performance (27, 29) and physiques characteristic of athletes in a variety of sports (8, 9, 54). Physique has also been related to various disease states, occupations, and behaviors (14).

The assessment of physique is most often expressed in the context of the *somatotype* as conceptualized by Sheldon (50). An individual's somatotype is a composite of the contributions of three components: *endomorphy* (predominance of digestive organs, softness and roundness of contours throughout the body), *mesomorphy* (predominance of muscle, bone, and connective tissues), and *ectomorphy* (predominance of surface area over body mass, linearity).

The measurements indicated previously include those necessary to estimate the Heath-Carter anthropometric somatotype (9), which has reasonably wide use in the sport sciences. The complete Heath-Carter method actually combines photoscopic and anthropometric procedures; in practice, however, the Heath-Carter method is used primarily in its anthropometric form for the simple reasons that anthropometry is more objective and obtaining standardized somatotype photographs is quite difficult and costly. The measurements and algorithms for estimating the Heath-Carter anthropometric somatotype are summarized in Table 11.2.

Definition of somatotype and procedures for estimating somatotype with the Heath-Carter method are *not identical*

Table 11.2   Estimating Somatotype With the Heath-Carter Anthropometric Method

Somatotype component	Estimation procedure
Endomorphy	$-0.7182 + 0.1451\,(X) - 0.00068\,(X^2) + 0.0000014\,(X^3)$ where X is the sum of the triceps, subscapular, and suprailiac (over the anterior superior iliac spine) skinfolds. X is multiplied by 170.18/stature in cm to yield stature-corrected endomorphy.
Mesomorphy	$(0.858 \times$ biepicondylar breadth $+ 0.601 \times$ bicondylar breadth $+ 0.188 \times$ corrected arm circumference $+ 0.161 \times$ corrected calf circumference $- ($stature $\times 0.131) + 4.50$ Corrected arm circumference is simply flexed-arm circumference (cm) minus the triceps skinfold (cm), while corrected calf circumference is calf circumference (cm) minus the medial calf skinfold (cm).
Ectomorphy	$HWR \times 0.732 - 28.58$ where HWR is height (cm)/cube root of weight (kg). If HWR < 40.75, but > 38.25, Ectomorphy $= HWR \times 0.463 - 17.63$. If $HWR \leq 38.25$, a rating of 0.1 is assigned.

From *Somatotyping—Development and Applications* (p. 374) by J.E.L. Carter and B.H. Heath, 1990, Cambridge: Cambridge University Press. Adapted with the permission of Cambridge University Press.

to the Sheldonian somatotype and procedures (49, 50). Sheldon's method is basically photoscopic or anthroposcopic, based on visual observation and evaluation of three standardized photographs. Configuration of the body as a whole, its contours, reliefs, relative proportions, robustness, delicateness, and so on, serve as criteria (see ref. 31).

By definition, the somatotype is a *gestalt* defined by the contributions of endomorphy, mesomorphy, and ectomorphy. The somatotype should thus be treated as a unit. For example, in estimating the relationship between mesomorphy and strength, the other two somatotype components, endomorphy and ectomorphy, must be statistically controlled. In practice, however, each component is commonly treated as an independent unit in analyses of relationships of somatotype to performance or risk factors for disease, or in multivariate analyses incorporating somatotype components. Carter and Heath (9) provide a summary of traditional methods of analyzing somatotype data, while Cressie, Withers, and Craig (12) describe multivariate methods for analyzing somatotype data.

MEASUREMENT VARIABILITY AND QUALITY CONTROL

Implicit in studies utilizing anthropometric methods is the assumption that every effort is made to ensure reliability and accuracy of measurement and standardization of technique. It is assumed that measurements are made by trained observers. This is essential to obtain reliable and accurate data, and to enhance the usefulness of the data from the comparative perspective. Further, reliable and accurate data are particularly critical in serial studies, short term or long term, in which the definition of rather small changes is necessary and technical errors of measurement can mask the true changes. Therefore, quality control and careful monitoring of the measurement process are essential.

It is perhaps of importance at this point to indicate how one becomes trained in anthropometry. Several suggestions follow.

1. Study the anatomy and anatomic location of the landmarks.
2. Study each measurement. What is specifically being measured, and what information does it provide?
3. Obtain instruction from, and practice under the supervision of, an individual experienced in anthropometry. One can receive much subtle instruction and many measurement tips during practice sessions.
4. Check measurement consistency on a regular basis. This should include both intra- and interobserver consistency.
5. Practice on a regular basis.

Anthropometry is quite easy; however, do not take your skill for granted.

In addition to trained anthropometrists, it is imperative that individuals who record the data are well versed in the measurement procedures and techniques. In addition to transcribing specific measurements as they are called out by the anthropometrist, the recorder is important in monitoring subject positioning, in recognizing spuriously high or low values, and in seeing that all measurements in a specific protocol are taken.

Although anthropometric procedures are reasonably standardized, and in the hands of trained anthropometrists relatively easy to use, variation associated with the process of measurement is a concern. Within-subject variability is of specific interest. It is due to measurement variation (imprecision) and physiological variation (undependability) (19). Undependability is of minor concern for most anthropometric dimensions; imprecision or measurement error is a major concern (39).

Error is the discrepancy between the measured value and its true quantity. Measurement error can be random or systematic. Random error is a normal aspect of anthropometry and results from variation within and between individuals in measurement technique, problems with measuring instruments (e.g., calibration or random variation in manufacture), and error in recording (e.g., transposition of numbers). Random error is nondirectional; that is, it is above or below the true dimension. In large-scale surveys random errors tend to cancel each other and ordinarily are not a major concern. Systematic error, on the other hand, results from the tendency of a technician or a measuring instrument (e.g., an improperly calibrated skinfold caliper or weighing machine) to consistently under- or overmeasure a particular dimension. Such error is directional and introduces bias into the measurement process.

Within-subject variability or imprecision is estimated by taking duplicate measurements on the same individual. The replicate measurements are taken independently, either by the same technician after a relatively short period of time has lapsed (within-technician measurement error) or by two different technicians (between-technician measurement error).

The *technical error of measurement* is a widely used measure of replicability. It is defined as the square root of the sum of the squared differences of replicates divided by twice the number of pairs (i.e., the within-subject variance) (34):

$$\sigma_e = \sqrt{\Sigma d^2 / 2N}$$

The statistic assumes that the distribution of replicate differences is normal and that errors of all pairs can be pooled. It indicates that about two thirds of the time, the measurement in question should fall within the technical error of measurement. (See refs. 39 and 43 for a more comprehensive discussion of measurement variability and quality.)

Technical errors of measurement are reported in the units of the specific measurement. Examples of within-technician (intraobserver) and between-technician (interobserver) technical errors of measurement for Cycle III of the U.S. Health Examination Survey, the U.S. Hispanic Health and Nutrition Examination Survey, and several studies at the University of Texas are summarized in Table 11.3. Estimates of measurement reliability, dependability, and precision in the Second National Health and Nutrition Examination Survey are reported in Marks et al. (39). The various U.S. surveys are discussed in more detail later in the chapter.

Accuracy, another component of the measurement process, is how closely measurements taken by one or several technicians approximate the "true" measurement. This is ordinarily assessed by comparing values obtained by the technician(s) with those obtained by a well-trained anthropometrist (i.e., the standard of reference).

APPLICATIONS OF ANTHROPOMETRY

Anthropometric data have a variety of applications, including description and comparison, evaluation of interventions, and identification of individuals or groups at risk. Anthropometry serves to describe the morphological status of an individual or a sample, or as a basis for comparison of the sample to the population or to other samples—for instance, the growth status of schoolchildren or the growth status of children participating in specific sports.

Anthropometry is often used as an outcome variable in evaluating interventions, such as the effects of exercise and weight reduction on body weight and subcutaneous fatness, or the effects of resistance training on muscle girths. It can also be used as a mediator variable in evaluating interventions; for instance, the effects of exercise and dietary intervention on serum cholesterol may be mediated by their effects on body weight and fatness.

Finally, anthropometry is often used to identify individuals at risk who may require special attention. It is thus used, for example, to screen individuals for obesity and to screen for children who are not growing appropriately for their chronological age. A corollary of this application is the use of anthropometry to identify individuals with specific characteristics deemed appropriate for success in a particular sport.

REFERENCE DATA

Appropriate reference data are necessary for the application of anthropometry. Reference data (i.e., the reference for comparison or for screening individuals or groups) are derived from a representative sample of clinically normal individuals free from overt disease. They are not necessarily ideal, normal, desirable, optimal, or the standard. In a sense, reference data refer to the situation as it is rather than what it should be, that is, the standard. Levels of weight for stature, or of the BMI, or of subcutaneous fatness deemed ideal for good health or for optimal performance and fitness, are standards. The vast majority of anthropometric data are reference values and not standards. As anthropometric features of a population change over time, reference data also change. A key element in selecting reference data is the representativeness of the sample.

For children and youth, reference data are commonly presented in the form of several growth curves or charts showing different percentiles in order to accommodate the range of normal variability. For adults, reference data are often in the form of tables of percentiles. Commonly reported percentiles are the 5th, 10th, 25th, 50th (median), 75th, 90th, and 95th.

The most commonly used reference data in the United States are those based on anthropometric dimensions taken in several national surveys conducted by the National Center for Health Statistics. The surveys are based upon complex, multistage, stratified sampling procedures that result in the selection of a sample that is representative of the noninstitutionalized civilian population of the United States. Cycle I of the Health Examination Survey (HES), 1959-1962, focused on adults 18 through 79 years of age, while Cycles II (1963-1965) and III (1966-1970) focused on children 6 through 11 years and youth 12 through 17 years of age, respectively. These surveys were followed by the first and second National Health and Nutrition Examination Surveys (NHANES I, 1971-1974, and NHANES II, 1976-1980). The former included subjects 1 through 74 years of age, and the latter included subjects 6 months through 74 years of age. The Hispanic Health and Nutrition Examination Survey (HHANES, 1982-1984) used the same sampling strategy but focused on Americans of Hispanic ancestry, 6 months through 74 years of age, in several regions of the United States. The third National Health and Nutrition Examination Survey (NHANES III) began in 1988 and continued through 1994 (25). NHANES III includes individuals 2 months of age and older. HES Cycles I, II, and III and NHANES I and II include adequate numbers of subjects of American Black and White ancestry, while HHANES is limited to Americans of Mexican (five southwestern states—Texas, New Mexico, Colorado, Arizona, and California), Cuban

Table 11.3 Technical Errors of Measurement in the U.S. Health Examination Survey, the U.S. Hispanic Health and Nutrition Examination Survey, and Several Studies at the University of Texas.

Measurement	Intraobserver measurement variation														Interobserver measurement variation				
	1	2	3	4	5	6	7	8	9	10	11	12	13	1	2	6	7	12
Stature	.49	1.28	.48	.54	.55	.43	.33	.35	.34	.26	.25	.19	.30	.68	.82	.46	.20	.21
Sitting height	.53	.57	.55	.69		.42	.48	.38	.31			.20	.23	.70	.57	1.02	.39	.24
Breadths																		
Biacromial	.54	.40	.46	.72	.46	.19	.32	.34	.40	.25	.26	.17	.19	.91	1.05	.30	.26	.30
Bicristal	.71	1.10	.31	.24	.20	.30	.38	.38	.58	.19	.16	.15	.18	1.54	1.70	.35	.22	.27
Bitrochanteric	.52	.98	.33		.29		.35			.19	.06			.84	.79		.26	
Chest			.26							.20	.84							
Bicondylar	.11		.12	.06	.07	.05	.13	.10	.24	.11	.08	.04	.13	.24		.09	.11	.12
Biepicondylar	.12	.28	.09	.07	.07	.05	.12	.10	.06	.06	.05	.04	.12	.15	.20	.07	.08	.07
Bimalleolar	.09									.05	.11			.17				
Bistyloid	.11									.07	.09			.14				
Circumferences																		
Arm, relaxed	.35	.65	.37	.37	.33	.21	.21	.29	.44	.12	.18	.13	.19	.42	1.33	.25	.26	.20
Arm, flexed								.38	.35			.17	.17					.24
Forearm	.30		.24											.58				
Thigh			.89		.36													
Calf	.87	.85	.23	.30	.22	.17	.19	.45	.52	.11	.15	.13	.26	.34	.52	.41	.15	.19
Waist	1.31													1.56				
Hip	1.23													1.37				

(continued)

Table 11.3 *(continued)*

Measurement	Intraobserver measurement variation													Interobserver measurement variation				
	1	2	3	4	5	6	7	8	9	10	11	12	13	1	2	6	7	12
Skinfolds																		
Triceps	.80	1.60	.82	.51	.69	.43	.33	.55	1.59	.36	45	.15	.19	1.89	2.59	1.13	.45	.27
Biceps				.58	.24			.19					.18					
Subscapular	1.83	2.22	.68	.55	.36	.53	.33	.26	3.44			.17	.17	1.53	3.30	1.36	.40	.31
Midaxillary	2.08		.61	.43			.27							1.47			.40	
Juxtanipple				.71														
Suprailiac	1.87	3.25		.95	.51	.49	.33	.13	1.09			.24	.27	2.45	3.90	2.10	.35	.30
Abdominal				.89				.55										
Midthigh				.74	.55													
Medial calf	1.44	2.72	.66	.66	.98	.49		.47	1.40	.29	.33	.21	.28	2.44	3.92	1.85	.27	.27

Units are *cm* for stature, sitting height, skeletal breadths, and circumferences, and *mm* for skinfolds. Several measurements not described in the text are listed in the table. See Lohman, Roche, and Martorell (26) for a description of methods of measurement.

Specific studies indicated in the table:

1. U.S. Health Examination Survey, Cycle III, youth 12-17 years, replicates taken within 2-1/2 weeks after initial measurements, n = 77 intraobserver, n = 224 interobserver. (Johnston, Hamill, & Lemeshow, [23], Malina, Hamill, & Lemeshow [34]. The latter reference also includes eight specific landmark heights [acromial height, tibial height, etc.], chest circumference, and two foot, two breadth, and two facial measurements.)

2. U.S. Hispanic Health and Nutrition Examination Survey, 12-73 years, replicates taken 2-3 weeks after initial measurements, n = 32 intraobserver, n = 50 interobserver. (Chumlea et al. [10])

3. Philadelphia, White boys, 6-12 years, replicates taken after a mean interval of 9 days, n = 43. (Malina & Moriyama [36])

4. Austin, low-socioeconomic-status Mexican American boys, 9-14 years, replicates taken 1 day after initial measurements, n = 25. (Zavaleta & Malina [58])

5. Austin, White age-group swimmers, both sexes, 8-18 years, replicates taken 1-4 weeks after initial measurements, n = 13. (Meleski [40])

6. Tenza, Colombia, rural schoolchildren—replicates for intraobserver estimates taken within day or 1 day after initial measurements, n = 29-34 boys; replicates for interobserver estimates taken within day, n = 52-79 boys and girls (Mueller [41]). Calculated from standard deviations of the differences between replicate measurements.

7. Oaxaca, Mexico, mild to moderately undernourished rural schoolchildren, both sexes, 6-14 years, within-day replicates, n = 40 (24 for skinfolds, males only) intraobserver, n = 11 interobserver (Malina & Buschang, unpublished; see also Buschang [5]). Also includes four craniofacial measurements.

8. Sao Paulo, Brazil, low-socioeconomic-status schoolchildren, 8 years, replicates taken after an interval of about 1 week, n = 23-29. (Rocha Ferreira [45])

9. San Diego, Mexican-American school girls 12-17 years, replicates taken 1 day after initial measurements, n = 30. (Brown [4])

10. Dallas, White males 5-10 years; Austin, White young adults 18-35 years; within-day replicates, n = 18 (Malina & Buschang [32, 33]). Also includes four craniofacial measurements.

11. Dallas, mentally retarded males, 9-52 years, within-day repliates, n = 17. (Malina & Buschang [32, 33]). Also includes four craniofacial measurements.

12. Austin, White university students, 17-21 years, within-day replicates, n = 22 intraobserver, n = 9 interobserver. (Wellens [57])

13. Pere Village, Papua New Guinea, Manus, both sexes, within-day replicates, n = 16-27. (Shoup [51])

(Dade County, FL), and Puerto Rican (New York metropolitan area, including parts of Connecticut and New Jersey) ancestry. NHANES III oversamples Black and Mexican Americans relative to the U.S. population in 1990. Kuczmarski and Johnson (25) provide an overview of the national surveys, the design, quality control, analytic considerations, and specific anthropometric dimensions included in each (see also ref. 22).

Data from these national surveys are available in varied forms and provide good reference data for the U.S. population as a whole, and at times specifically for Americans of Black, White, and Hispanic ancestry. A summary of the available data for the American population is given in the Appendix to this chapter (see ref. 35 for a historic summary of data for Mexican American children and youth, and refs. 37 and 48 for a compilation of anthropometric data on American children and youth since 1940). Less-extensive anthropometric data have been reported for the Canadian population. Data for several dimensions measured in the Nutrition Canada national survey of nutritional status (stature, weight, weight for stature, sitting height) are reported in Demirjian (15) and in the national survey of physical fitness (stature, weight, weight for stature, triceps skinfold, individuals 7-60+ years; stature, weight, sum of five skinfolds [biceps, triceps, subscapular, suprailiac, medial calf], body mass index, youth 7-19 years) are reported by the Canada Fitness Survey (6, 7).

The most commonly used reference data are the "growth charts" for stature and weight based on children 2 through 18 years from HES Cycles II and III and NHANES I (20, 21). Reference data for children birth through 3 years of age, based on a longitudinal study of predominantly White middle-class children from Ohio, are also included. The need for updating the current charts is currently under discussion and might not proceed until NHANES III is concluded.[1] These growth charts for stature and weight are also recommended for international studies of nutritional status of children under 10 years of age (56), noting, of course, that the growth status of children is often used as an indicator of nutritional status.

Percentiles for the BMI are, at present, the most commonly used reference data for adults. The smoothed race/ethnic-specific percentiles for American Blacks and Whites, based on NHANES I (13), and Mexican Americans, based on HHANES (47), are perhaps the best prepared. Frisancho (18) reports percentiles for American Blacks and Whites based on combined data

from NHANES I and II; the percentiles, however, are not smoothed.

There is no formal reference data for somatotype. Petersen (44) presents a large collection of somatotype photographs of a cross-sectional sample of Dutch children, while Tanner and Whitehouse (55) present longitudinal series of somatotype photographs for British children in the Harpenden Growth Study. Sheldon et al. (49) provide a comprehensive collection of somatotype photographs of adult males. Carter and Heath (9), on the other hand, provide a comprehensive summary of available somatotype data for a variety of samples of children and adults, and of athletes in a variety of sports. Anthropometric somatotype data for a national sample of Canadian adults participating in the YMCA-LIFE program (Lifestyle Inventory–Fitness Evaluation) are reported in Bailey, Carter, and Mirwald (2).

SUMMARY

Anthropometry is a series of methods for taking measurements and should be treated as such, a means to an end and not an end in itself. It is highly objective and reliable in the hands of trained anthropometrists. A key to effective anthropometry lies in understanding the meaning of specific measurements so that a set can be chosen that effectively answers the question(s) addressed or meets the needs of the desired application(s).

APPENDIX

Reference data for the American population from several surveys conducted by the National Center for Health Statistics

Health Examination Survey, Cycle I, Adults 18 to 79 Years

Stoudt, H.W., Damon, A., McFarland, R., & Roberts, J. (1965). Weight, height, and selected body dimensions of adults. *Vital and Health Statistics* (Series 11, No. 8).

Roberts, J. (1966). Weight by height and age of adults. *Vital and Health Statistics* (Series 11, No. 14).

Stoudt, H.W., Damon, A., McFarland, R., & Roberts, J. (1970). Skinfolds, body girths, biacromial diameter, and selected anthropometric indices of adults. *Vital and Health Statistics* (Series 11, No. 35).

Health Examination Survey, Cycles II and III, Children and Youth 6 to 17 Years

Hamill, P.V.V., Johnston, F.E., & Grams, W. (1970). Height and weight of children. *Vital and Health Statistics* (Series 11, No. 104).

---

[1]NCHS Growth Chart Workshop, College Park, MD, December 14-15, 1992, sponsored by the Division of Health Examination Statistics of the National Center for Health Statistics.

Hamill, P.V.V., Johnston, F.E., & Lemeshow, S. (1972). Height and weight of children: Socioeconomic status. *Vital and Health Statistics* (Series 11, No. 119).

Hamill, P.V.V., Johnston, F.E., & Lemeshow, S. (1973). Height and weight of youths 12-17 years. *Vital and Health Statistics* (Series 11, No. 124).

Hamill, P.V.V., Johnston, F.E., & Lemeshow, S. (1973). Body weight, stature, and sitting height: White and Negro youths 12-17 years. *Vital and Health Statistics* (Series 11, No. 126).

Johnston, F.E., Hamill, P.V.V., & Lemeshow, S. (1972). Skinfold thickness of children 6-11 years, United States. *Vital and Health Statistics* (Series 11, No. 120).

Johnston, F.E., Hamill, P.V.V., & Lemeshow, S. (1974). Skinfold thickness of youths 12-17 years, United States. *Vital and Health Statistics* (Series 11, No. 132).

Malina, R.M., Hamill, P.V.V., & Lemeshow, S. (1973). Selected body measurements of children 6-11 years. *Vital and Health Statistics* (Series 11, No. 123).

Malina, R.M., Hamill, P.V.V., & Lemeshow, S. (1974). Body dimensions and proportions, White and Negro children 6-11 years. *Vital and Health Statistics* (Series 11, No. 143).

Roche, A.F., & Malina, R.M. (1983). *Manual of physical status and performance in childhood: Volume 1. Physical status.* New York: Plenum Press.

Malina, R.M., & Roche, A.F. (1983). *Manual of physical status and performance in childhood: Volume 2. Physical performance.* New York: Plenum Press.

Both volumes include summary tables of data for a variety of anthropometric variables from Cycle III of the Health Examination Survey.

National Health and Nutrition Examination Survey, I and II, Children, Youth, and Adults, 6 Months to 74 Years

Hamill, P.V.V., Drizd, T.A., Johnson, C.L., Reed, R.B., & Roche, A.F. (1977). NCHS growth curves for children birth-18 years. *Vital and Health Statistics* (Series 11, No. 165). (See also Hamill, P.V.V., Drizd, T.A., Johnson, C.L., Reed, R.B., Roche, A.F., & Moore, W.M. (1979). Physical growth: National Center for Health Statistics percentiles. *American Journal of Clinical Nutrition*, **32**, 607-629.)

The growth curves are based on HES Cycles II and III, and NHANES I data, in addition to Fels Research Institute data for children birth to 3 years.

Johnson, C.L., Fulwood, R., Abraham, S., & Bryner, J.D. (1981). Basic data on anthropometric measurements and angular measurements of the hip and knee joints for selected age groups 1-74 years of age. *Vital and Health Statistics* (Series 11, No. 219).

Abraham, S., Johnson, C.L., & Najjar, M.F. (1979). Weight by height and age for adults 18-74 years. *Vital and Health Statistics* (Series 11, No. 208).

Abraham, S., Johnson, C.L., & Najjar, M.F. (1979). Weight and height of adults 18-74 years of age. *Vital and Health Statistics* (Series 11, No. 211).

Fulwood, R., Abraham, S., & Johnson, C.L. (1981). Height and weight of adults ages 18-74 years by socioeconomic and geographic variables. *Vital and Health Statistics* (Series 11, No. 224).

Abraham, S., Carroll, M.D., Najjar, M.F., & Fulwood, R. (1983). Obese and overweight adults in the United States. *Vital and Health Statistics* (Series 11, No. 230).

Najjar, M.F., & Rowland, M. (1987). Anthropometric reference data and prevalence of overweight. *Vital and Health Statistics* (Series 11, No. 238).

Cronk, C.E., & Roche, A.F., (1982). Race- and sex-specific reference data for triceps and subscapular skinfolds and weight/stature^2. *American Journal of Clinical Nutrition*, **35**, 347-354.

Frisancho, A.R. (1990). *Anthropometric standards for the assessment of growth and nutritional status.* Ann Arbor: University of Michigan Press.

This volume includes combined data, weighted for sample size, from NHANES I and NHANES II (about 82% White, 16% Black, 2% other ethnic groups), and data specifically for American Blacks and Whites. The race-specific data are not weighted for sample sizes. The percentiles are not smoothed.

Hispanic Health and Nutrition Examination Survey, Children, Youth, and Adults, 6 Months to 74 Years

Najjar, M.F., & Kuczmarski, R.J. (1989). Anthropometric data and prevalence of overweight for Hispanics: 1982-1984. *Vital and Health Statistics* (Series 11, No. 239).

Roche, A.F., Guo, S., Baumgartner, R.N., Chumlea, W.C., Ryan, A.S., & Kuczmarski, R.J. (1990). Reference data for weight, stature, and weight/stature^2 in Mexican Americans from the Hispanic Health and Nutrition Examination Survey (HHANES 1982-1984). *American Journal of Clinical Nutrition*, **51**, 917S-924S.

Ryan, A.S., Martinez, G.A., Baumgartner, R.N., Roche, A.F., Guo, S., Chumlea, W.C., & Kuczmarski, R.J. (1990). Median skinfold thickness distributions and fat-wave patterns in Mexican American children from the Hispanic Health and Nutrition Examination Survey (HHANES 1982-1984). *American Journal of Clinical Nutrition*, **51**, 925S-935S.

Martorell, R., Malina, R.M., Castillo, R.O., Mendoza, F.S., & Pawson, I.G. (1988). Body proportions in three ethnic groups: Children and youths 2-17 years in NHANES II and HHANES. *Human Biology*, **60**, 205-222.

REFERENCES

1. Ashwell, M., McCall, S.A., Cole, T.J., & Dixon, A.K. (1986). Fat distribution and its metabolic complications: Interpretations. In N.G. Norgan (Ed.), *Human body composition and fat distribution* (pp. 227-242). Wageningen, Netherlands: Stichting Nederlands Instituut voor de Voeding.
2. Bailey, D.A., Carter, J.E.L., & Mirwald, R.L. (1982). Somatotypes of Canadian men and women. *Human Biology*, **54**, 813-828.
3. Baumgartner, R.N., Roche, A.F., Guo, S., Lohman, T., Boileau, R.A., & Slaughter, M.H. (1986). Adipose tissue distribution: The stability of principal components by sex, ethnicity and maturation stage. *Human Biology*, **58**, 719-735.
4. Brown, K.R. (1984). *Growth, physique and age at menarche of Mexican American females age 12 through 17 years residing in San Diego County, California*. Unpublished doctoral dissertation, University of Texas at Austin.
5. Buschang, P.H. (1980). *Growth status and rate in school children 6 to 13 years of age in a rural Zapotec-speaking community in the Valley of Oaxaca, Mexico*. Unpublished doctoral dissertation, University of Texas at Austin.
6. Canada Fitness Survey. (1983). *Fitness and lifestyle in Canada*. Ottawa: Canada Fitness Survey.
7. Canada Fitness Survey. (1985). *Physical fitness of Canadian youth*. Ottawa: Canada Fitness Survey.
8. Carter, J.E.L. (1984). Somatotypes of Olympic athletes from 1948 to 1976. In J.E.L. Carter (Ed.), *Physical structure of Olympic athletes: Part II. Kinanthropometry of Olympic athletes* (pp. 80-109). Basel: Karger.
9. Carter, J.E.L., & Heath, B.H. (1990). *Somatotyping—development and applications*. Cambridge: Cambridge University Press.
10. Chumlea, W.C., Guo, S., Kuczmarski, R.J., Johnson, C.L., & Leahy, C.K. (1990). Reliability for anthropometric measurements in the Hispanic Health and Nutrition Examination Survey (HHANES 1982-1984). *American Journal of Clinical Nutrition*, **51**, 902S-907S.
11. Cole, T.J. (1991). Weight-stature indices to measure underweight, overweight, and obesity. In J. Himes (Ed.), *Anthropometric assessment of nutritional status* (pp. 83-111). New York: Wiley-Liss.
12. Cressie, N.A.C., Withers, R.T., & Craig, N.P. (1986). The statistical analysis of somatotype data. *Yearbook of Physical Anthropology*, **29**, 197-208.
13. Cronk, C.E., & Roche, A.F. (1982). Race- and sex-specific reference data for triceps and subscapular skinfolds and weight/stature^2. *American Journal of Clinical Nutrition*, **35**, 347-354.
14. Damon, A. (1970). Constitutional medicine. In O. Von Mering & L. Kasdan (Eds.), *Anthropology and the behavioral and health sciences* (pp. 179-205). Pittsburgh: University of Pittsburgh Press.
15. Demirjian, A. (1980). *Nutrition Canada. Anthropometry report: Height, weight and body dimensions*. Ottawa: Health and Welfare Canada.
16. Deutsch, M.I., Mueller, W.H., & Malina, R.M. (1985). Androgyny in fat patterning is associated with obesity in adolescents and young adults. *Annals of Human Biology*, **12**, 275-286.
17. Forbes, G.B. (1978). Body composition in adolescence. In F. Falkner & J.M. Tanner (Eds.), *Human growth: Vol. 2. Postnatal growth, neurobiology* (pp. 119-145). New York: Plenum Press.
18. Frisancho, A.R. (1990). *Anthropometric standards for the assessment of growth and nutritional status*. Ann Arbor: University of Michigan Press.
19. Habicht, J.-P., Yarbrough, C., & Martorell, R. (1979). Anthropometric field methods. In D.B. Jelliffe & E.E.P. Jelliffe (Eds.), *Nutrition and growth* (pp. 365-387). New York: Plenum Press.
20. Hamill, P.V.V., Drizd, T.A., Johnson, C.L., Reed, R.B., & Roche, A.F. (1977). NCHS growth curves for children birth-18 years. *Vital and Health Statistics*, Series 11, No. 165.
21. Hamill, P.V.V., Drizd, T.A., Johnson, C.L., Reed, R.B., Roche, A.F., & Moore, W.M. (1979). Physical growth. National Center for Health Statistics percentiles. *American Journal of Clinical Nutrition*, **32**, 607-629.
22. Interagency Board for Nutrition Monitoring and Related Research. (1992). *Nutrition monitoring in the United States. The directory of federal and state nutrition monitoring activities*. Hyattsville, MD: Department of Health and Human Services.
23. Johnston, F.E., Hamill, P.V.V., & Lemeshow, S. (1972). Skinfold thickness of children 6-11 years, United States. *Vital and Health Statistics*, Series 11, No. 120.
24. Jones, P.R.M., & Pearson, J. (1969). Anthropometric determination of leg fat and muscle plus bone volumes in young male and female adults. *Journal of Physiology*, **204**, 63P-66P.

25. Kuczmarski, R.J., & Johnson, C. (1991). National nutritional surveys assessing anthropometric status. In J. Himes (Ed.), *Anthropometric assessment of nutritional status* (pp. 319-335). New York: Wiley-Liss.

26. Lohman, T.G., Roche, A.F., & Martorell, R. (Eds.). (1988). *Anthropometric standardization reference manual*. Champaign, IL: Human Kinetics.

27. Malina, R.M. (1975). Anthropometric correlates of strength and motor performance. *Exercise and Sport Sciences Reviews*, **3**, 249-274.

28. Malina, R.M. (1991). Ratios and derived indicators in the assessment of nutritional status. In J. Himes (Ed.), *Anthropometric assessment of nutritional status* (pp. 151-171). New York: Wiley-Liss.

29. Malina, R.M. (1994). Anthropometry, physical performance and fitness. In S.J. Ulijaszek & C.G.N. Mascie Taylor (Eds.), *Anthropometry: The individual and the population* (pp. 160-177). Cambridge: Cambridge University Press.

30. Malina, R.M., & Bouchard, C. (1988). Subcutaneous fat distribution during growth. In C. Bouchard & F.E. Johnston (Eds.), *Fat distribution during growth and later health outcomes* (pp. 63-84). New York: A.R. Liss.

31. Malina, R.M., & Bouchard, C. (1991). *Growth, maturation, and physical activity*. Champaign, IL: Human Kinetics.

32. Malina, R.M., & Buschang, P.H. (1980). *Anthropometric asymmetry in normal and mentally retarded males* (Contract No. 26-8220, final technical report). Austin, TX: Department of Anthropology.

33. Malina, R.M., & Buschang, P.H. (1984). Anthropometric asymmetry in normal and mentally retarded males. *Annals of Human Biology*, **11**, 515-531.

34. Malina, R.M., Hamill, P.V.V., & Lemeshow, S. (1973). Selected body measurements of children 6-11 years. *Vital and Health Statistics*, Series 11, No. 123.

35. Malina, R.M., Martorell, R., & Mendoza, F. (1986). Growth status of Mexican American children and youths: Historical trends and contemporary issues. *Yearbook of Physical Anthropology*, **29**, 45-79.

36. Malina, R.M., & Moriyama, M. (1991). Growth and motor performance of black and white children 6-10 years of age: A multivariate analysis. *American Journal of Human Biology*, **3**, 599-611.

37. Malina, R.M., & Roche, A.F. (1983). *Manual of physical status and performance in childhood: Vol. 2. Physical performance*. New York: Plenum Press.

38. Malina, R.M., & Zavaleta, A.N. (1976). Androgyny of physique in female track and field athletes. *Annals of Human Biology*, **3**, 441-446.

39. Marks, G.C., Habicht, J.-P., & Mueller, W.H. (1989). Reliability, dependability, and precision of anthropometric measurements: The Second National Health and Nutrition Examination Survey 1976-1980. *American Journal of Epidemiology*, **130**, 578-587.

40. Meleski, B.W. (1980). *Growth, maturity, body composition, and familial characteristics of competitive swimmers 8 to 18 years of age*. Unpublished doctoral dissertation, University of Texas at Austin.

41. Mueller, W.H. (1975). *Parent-child and sibling correlations and heritability of body measurements in a rural Colombian population*. Unpublished doctoral dissertation, University of Texas at Austin.

42. Mueller, W.H., & Malina, R.M. (1987). Relative reliability of circumferences and skinfolds as measures of body fat distribution. *American Journal of Physical Anthropology*, **72**, 437-439.

43. Mueller, W.H., & Martorell, R. (1988). Reliability and accuracy of measurement. In T.G. Lohman, A.F. Roche, & R. Martorell (Eds.), *Anthropometric standardization reference manual* (pp. 83-86). Champaign, IL: Human Kinetics.

44. Petersen, G. (1967). *Atlas for somatotyping children*. Assen, Netherlands: Van Gorcum.

45. Rocha Ferreira, M.B. (1987). *Growth, physical performance and psychological characteristics of eight year old Brazilian school children from low socioeconomic background*. Unpublished doctoral dissertation, University of Texas at Austin.

46. Roche, A.F., Baumgartner, R.N., & Guo, S. (1986). Population methods: Anthropometry or estimations. In N.G. Norgan (Ed.), *Human body composition and fat distribution* (pp. 31-47). Wageningen, Netherlands: Stichting Nederlands Instituut voor de Voeding.

47. Roche, A.F., Guo, S., Baumgartner, R.N., Chumlea, W.C., Ryan, A.S., & Kuczmarski, R.J. (1990). Reference data for weight, stature, and weight/stature^2 in Mexican Americans from the Hispanic Health and Nutrition Examination Survey (HHANES 1982-1984). *American Journal of Clinical Nutrition*, **51**, 917S-924S.

48. Roche, A.F., & Malina, R.M. (1983). *Manual of physical status and performance in childhood: Vol. 1. Physical status*. New York: Plenum Press.

49. Sheldon, W.H., Dupertuis, C.W., & McDermott, E. (1954). *Atlas of men: A guide for somatotyping the adult male at all ages*. New York: Harper & Brothers.

50. Sheldon, W.H., Stevens, S.S., & Tucker, W.B. (1940). *The varieties of human physique*. New York: Harper & Brothers.

51. Shoup, R.F. (1987). *Growth and aging in the Manus of Pere Village, Manus Province, Papua New Guinea: A mixed-longitudinal and secular perspective*. Unpublished doctoral dissertation, University of Texas at Austin.

52. Tanner, J.M. (1949). The fallacy of per-weight and per-surface area standards and their relation to spurious correlation. *Journal of Applied Physiology*, **2**, 1-15.

53. Tanner, J.M. (1951). Photogrammetric anthropometry and an androgyny scale. *Lancet*, **1**, 574-579.

54. Tanner, J.M. (1964). *The physique of the Olympic athlete*. London: Allen & Unwin.

55. Tanner, J.M., & Whitehouse, R.H. (1982). *Atlas of children's growth: Normal variation and growth disorders*. New York: Academic Press.

56. Waterlow, J.C., Buzina, R., Keller, W., Lane, J.M., Nichaman, M.Z., & Tanner, J.M. (1977). The presentation and use of height and weight data for comparing the nutritional status of groups of children under the age of 10 years. *Bulletin of the World Health Organization*, **55**, 489-498.

57. Wellens, R.E. (1989). *Activity as a temperamental trait: Relationship to physique, energy expenditure and physical activity habits in young adults*. Unpublished doctoral dissertation, University of Texas at Austin.

58. Zavaleta, A.N., & Malina, R.M. (1982). Growth and body composition of Mexican American boys 9 through 14 years of age. *American Journal of Physical Anthropology*, **57**, 261-271.

CHAPTER 12

Static Techniques for the Evaluation of Joint Range of Motion

Peter J. Maud, PhD

University of Texas at El Paso

Miriam Y. Cortez-Cooper, MA, PT

University of Texas Medical Branch at Galveston

The term *flexibility* is commonly used to describe the range of motion about a joint or about a series of joints. Flexibility can be assessed by both static and dynamic means. The purpose of this chapter is to present gross range-of-motion tests for the lower extremities and trunk and to outline accepted methods of measuring joint range of motion utilizing static evaluation techniques. Indirect methods of assessment that use linear displacement, rather than angular displacement, are presented as gross range-of-motion tests, and direct measures are described in detail for using the Leighton flexometer, the inclinometer, and the goniometer. Electrogoniometry and motion photography allow examination of flexibility during dynamic skilled movement; they probably should be the preferred methods for analyzing the contribution of range of motion in the assessment of athletic ability. Description of these methods, however, is beyond the scope of this chapter.

RATIONALE FOR FLEXIBILITY MEASUREMENT

Although flexibility is generally considered one of the five components of physical fitness, its exact contribution to general health is even less clearly defined than its importance to athletic performance. Within the realm of sport there are many activities where high degrees of flexibility in specific joints are desirable for enhanced performance in both quantitative and qualitative athletic activities. While it seems apparent that tight muscles may predispose an athlete to muscle strains and tendon injuries and that highly extensible muscles might lead to joint dislocations and ligamentous sprains, few prospective studies verify this phenomenon (9, 11). The existence of an optimal joint range appears at least to be sport specific and variable on an individual basis. Because flexibility, as defined by joint range of motion, is affected by joint congruence, tendons, ligaments, fascia, joint capsules, and adipose tissue in addition to muscle, a direct relationship between flexibility and injury becomes difficult to establish. The arrangement of muscles in an agonist/antagonist relationship would also tend to suggest that an imbalance of strength or flexibility would predispose an athlete to injury. However, research results do not consistently support this contention either (21, 22). The reader is referred to an excellent review article by Knapik et al. (22) on the contribution of flexibility to the prevention and prediction of athletic injury.

Given this difficulty in quantifying the flexibility necessary for optimal performance and injury prevention, what then is the purpose of flexibility testing for general fitness? Does flexibility become more important in injury prevention as one becomes older? Can the general public engaging in sporadic recreational activities afford to be more or less flexible than the competitive athlete who constantly stresses his or her musculoskeletal system? One partial answer to these questions is that flexibility testing is important in that it establishes a base line of range of motion prior to intervention. This base line data can be compared with normative values for exercise prescription, or kept for future reference when retesting the individual after an intervening exercise program or during rehabilitation following injury. Therefore, the method of measurement chosen should fit the purpose. For example, if an employee in a work-related fitness program decides to begin a weight-training program for the purpose of improving ground strokes in tennis, flexibility testing might be directed toward gross assessment of range of motion of the trunk and extremities. Follow-up measurements of specific joints that are found to be restricted or that will be specifically placed in demand would also be indicated. However, if the same employee complained of a lack of power in his or her serve, detailed shoulder range-of-motion tests, in addition to strength testing, would be incorporated into the assessment.

METHODS OF MEASUREMENT

One of the major problems of flexibility measurement is that flexibility is not a general characteristic but is highly specific to individual joints (8, 10, 12). Therefore, comprehensive flexibility assessment would involve measurement of all joints through a variety of planes, a very time-consuming task. As stated earlier, specific joints need to be isolated for assessment based upon their contribution to health fitness or to athletic performance. Indirect methods are appropriate for large-scale screening or for documentation of change resulting from specific flexibility exercise training programs. Indirect methods have the advantage of ease and speed of measurement, and low cost of equipment. However, where accurate scientific data are required, particularly when comparing between individuals or between groups, or when assessing range of motion to determine whether

there is impairment within a joint, then direct methods of assessment are essential.

Pretest Activity

Regardless of the method chosen for flexibility testing, it is important to establish a standardized procedure for warm-up prior to testing. Leighton (30) advocated no warm-up prior to measurement, but, as has been noted by Hubley-Kozey (16), a warm-up probably should be included for the sake of safety. As warm-up and muscle stretching before measurement may affect test results, it is important to formulate protocols that specify both the type and duration of warm-up and muscle-stretching techniques to be used. Three measurements are usually required at each joint, with the *greatest angle* measured recorded as the degrees of motion for that particular joint. However, it has also been suggested by Hubley-Kozey (16) that three measurements be taken but that the *mean* of the three be recorded. If, as is normally advocated, a warm-up precedes the evaluation, then it would be more appropriate to use the mean of the three measures.

Indirect Measurement Techniques

Several indirect tests have been used to assess flexibility in a variety of joints. Typically these tests involve linear measurement of distances between body segments or from one anatomical reference point to another or to an external object. Probably the most common example of the latter is the sit-and-reach test used to evaluate hamstring and low-back flexibility. A lack of flexibility in these areas alone, or when accompanied by relative weakness in the abdominal muscles, has frequently been cited as a possible cause of low-back pain syndrome (1, 5). However, little clinical evidence supports this claim, and Nachemson (34) did not specifically mention lack of flexibility as a contributor to low-back pain in his recent review of the relationship between low-back pain, exercise, and physical fitness. Recent studies by Jackson and Baker (18) and Jackson and Langford (17), however, have found that although the sit-and-reach test appeared to be a valid measure of flexibility in the hamstring area, it was not necessarily a valid measure of low-back flexibility. It was found that for both young and adult females the sit-and-reach test correlated moderately well with passive hamstring flexibility, $r = .64$ (17) and $r = .70$ (17), respectively, but poorly with low-back flexibility, $r = .28$ (18) and $r = .12$ (17). On the other hand, for adult males the sit-and-reach test correlation was $r = .89$ for hamstring and $r = .59$ for low-back flexibility. Kippers and Parker (20) evaluated a similar test, the standing toe-touch test, and found that although this test was positively related to trunk and hip flexion, it correlated very poorly with vertebral flexion in males.

A more valid description of the sit-and-reach test would be that it assesses the flexibility of the posterior muscles—the hamstrings and the lower middle, and upper paraspinals and calf muscles. Tightness in any of these muscles can limit the subject's ability to reach forward. However, the tightness may be compensated for by one or more of the other muscles being tested, thereby resulting in a "normal" sit-and-reach test score. In Figure 12.1 three subjects are depicted. Subject A has normal flexibility of the back and hamstrings, and the back has a nice, rounded curve. Subject B has the same sit-and-reach score as subject A, but only because she has more flexible hamstrings. Note the "flat" appearance of the lumbar region. Subject C has both poor hamstring flexibility and poor low-back flexibility, giving rise to a low sit-and-reach test score.

Given these examples, it is understandable why correlations between low-back and hamstring flexibility may be low. Therefore, when used in general health and fitness screening, the sit-and-reach test should be evaluated both quantitatively and qualitatively. If indicated, the qualitative aspect of the test would lead the tester to perform more specific tests for low-back or hamstring flexibility. For example, for Subject B in Figure 12.1, the tester would specifically test low-back flexibility using an indirect method such as the modified-modified Schober technique or a direct method such as the double inclinometer technique. Both of these techniques are described later in this chapter.

Differing limb and torso lengths also have an effect on the indirect measurement of flexibility. It has been assumed that anthropometric variables have little effect on sit-and-reach test results (1), although Broer and Galles (6) found that, with extreme body types, test results were affected. Individuals with long trunk and arm measurements but short legs were at an advantage, whereas those with short trunk and arm measurements and long legs were at a disadvantage. Wear (40) reported similar findings.

To eliminate problems associated with differing arm and leg lengths, Hoeger (14) developed a modified sit-and-reach test that standardized the finger-to-box distance to allow for proportional differences between arms and legs. Hoeger and Hopkins (15) demonstrated that the modified procedure eliminates the problem of disproportional limb lengths. It is, therefore, recommended that when a sit-and-reach test protocol is deemed appropriate, the modified procedure of Hoeger (14) be utilized. A description of the test is given in the next section.

Variations in head position have also been found to significantly affect sit-and-reach test results (37). Although these effects are small, they emphasize the importance of exact test description and adherence to protocol.

Despite these problems, the sit-and-reach test is extensively utilized in the assessment of flexibility in both adult and child populations, and extensive norms have been developed (7, 12, 34, 38 42). Because there are several different protocols which use different measuring scales, if this test is used it is essential that a specific test protocol be adhered to and that the appropriate norms for that specific test be identified.

Johnson (19) describes, and gives normative data for, his version of the sit-and-reach test plus eight additional indirect measures. These additional tests include a bridge-up test to measure hyperextension of the spine, front and side splits, shoulder and wrist elevation, trunk and neck extension measured from the prone position, ankle plantar and dorsiflexion tests, and shoulder rotation. All of these tests use the fleximeasure, which

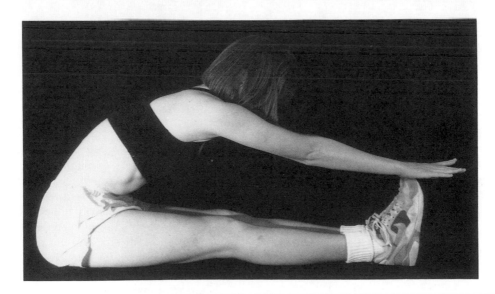

(continued)

Figure 12.1 Flexibility characteristics shown during the sit-and-reach test (subject A, above; *following page*: subject B, top; subject C, bottom).

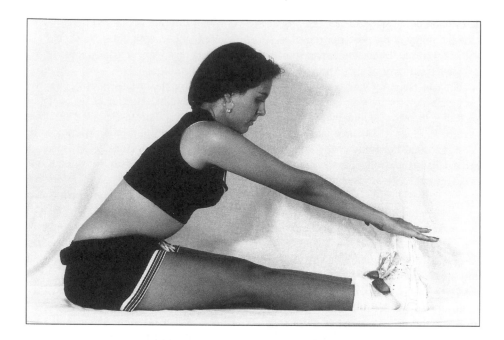

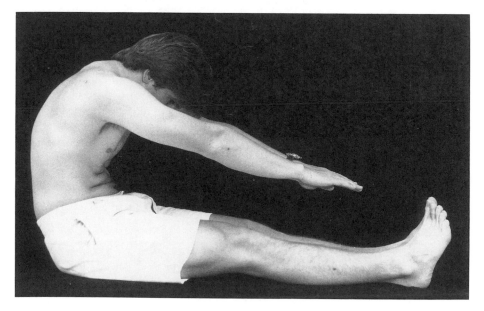

Figure 12.1   *(continued)*

basically consists of a yardstick with an adjustable ruler attached at an angle of 90° by a special sliding aluminum box. This device is designed to facilitate and increase the accuracy and reproducibility of measurement.

The Modified Sit-and-Reach Test

In the modified sit-and-reach test developed by Hoeger (13), the subject sits on the floor with buttocks, shoulders, and head in contact with the wall. The legs are extended, with the knees straight and the soles of the feet placed against a box approximately 12 in. high.

The hands are placed one on top of the other, with neither set of fingers extending beyond the other. A yardstick is placed on top of the box with the zero end toward the subject. The subject reaches forward as far as possible without allowing either head or shoulders to come away from the wall, and the yardstick is positioned and held so that the zero end touches the extended fingers. The yardstick must now be held firmly in place until after completion of the test.

The subject now leans forward slowly, allowing the head and shoulders to move away from the wall and the fingers to slide along the top of the yardstick. Three slow, forward movements are made, and on the third forward motion the subject leans as far forward as possible, holding this position for a minimum of 2 s. A reading is taken of the distance moved by the fingers along the yardstick. Two separate trials are made, and the mean of the two is recorded as the sit-and-reach score. Table 12.1 gives percentile ranks for the test (13).

Modified-Modified Schober

This test, also known as a skin distraction test, was first described by Schober (36) as a means of measuring lumbar flexion. It was later modified by Macrae and Wright (32) and again by Van Adrichem and van der Korst (39) to enhance its reliability and ease of application. Basically, the technique as modified by Macrae and Wright requires that the lumbosacral junction be identified and skin marks made 5 cm below and 10 cm above the lumbosacral junction. A tape measure is placed on the subject's spine between the two skin marks, and the subject flexes forward from a standing position, keeping the knees straight. The new distance between these two skin marks is recorded, to the nearest millimeter, as lumbar flexion. Lumbar extension is measured similarly, with the subject bending backward as far as possible, with the hands on the buttocks. The new distance between the superior and inferior skin marks is recorded, to the nearest millimeter, as lumbar extension. The difficulty in reliability arises from problems with determining the lumbosacral junction. Van Adrichem and van der Korst (39), therefore, modified this technique by using the posterior superior iliac spines (PSIS)

as a reference point for the tape measure. Their modified-modified Schober technique requires that an ink mark be placed on the midline of the lumbar spine between the subject's PSISs. Another mark is made 15 cm above the mark at the PSISs. The tape measure is aligned between the two skin marks with the zero at the inferior skin mark (Figure 12.2, top). The subject flexes forward or extends backward, as previously described, and the difference between the initial length and the new flexed or extended length is recorded (Figure 12.2, bottom).

Direct Measurement Techniques

There are three types of instruments commonly recognized as appropriate for the direct measurement of range of motion: the Leighton flexometer; the typical universal goniometer, which is available in different lengths for measuring both small and large joints; and the clinical goniometer, or inclinometer, as it is termed by the American Medical Association (4) (Figure 12.3).

The Leighton Flexometer

One of the pioneers of flexibility assessment, Jack Leighton, invented and promoted the flexometer, an instrument that has gained universal acceptance for range-of-motion measurement particularly in exercise science research. Leighton has published numerous studies describing his range of motion research (23-30). The flexometer, shown in Figure 12.4, is described by Leighton (31) as follows:

Table 12.1 Percentile Scores for the Modified Sit-and-Reach Test

Percentile rank	Scores (in inches)					
	Men			Women		
	< 35 yrs	36-49 yrs	> 50 yrs	< 35 yrs	36-49 yrs	> 50 yrs
99	24.7	18.9	16.2	19.8	19.8	17.2
95	19.5	18.2	15.8	18.7	19.2	15.7
90	17.9	16.1	15.0	17.9	17.4	15.0
80	17.0	14.6	13.3	16.7	16.2	14.2
70	15.8	13.9	12.3	16.2	15.2	13.6
60	15.0	13.4	11.5	15.8	14.5	12.3
50	14.4	12.6	10.2	14.8	13.5	11.1
40	13.5	11.6	9.7	14.5	12.8	10.1
30	13.0	10.8	9.3	13.7	12.2	9.2
20	11.6	9.9	8.8	12.6	11.0	8.3
10	9.2	8.3	7.8	10.1	9.7	7.5
5	7.9	7.0	7.2	8.1	8.5	3.7
1	7.0	5.1	4.0	2.6	2.0	1.5

From *The Complete Guide for the Development and Implementation of Health Promotion Programs* by W.W.K. Hoeger, 1987, Englewood, CO: Morton Publishing Company. Reprinted by permission.

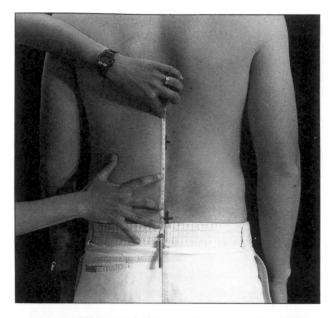

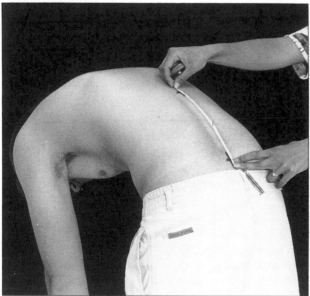

Figure 12.2 The Modified-Modified Schober Test: Van Adrichem and van der Korst variation.

The Leighton Flexometer is basically a gravity-type goniometer. It consists of a weighted 360 degree dial and a weighted pointer in a case. The dial and pointer operate freely and independently, the movement of each being controlled by gravity. The instrument is designed to record movement while in any position that is twenty degrees or more off the horizontal. The zero mark on the dial and the hairline of the pointer move freely to a position of rest and coincide when the instrument is placed in any position off the horizontal as indicated. Independent locking devices are provided for the pointer and the dial which stop all movement of either at any given position. In using the instrument, the Flexometer is strapped to the segment being tested (refer to measurement technique). The dial is locked in one extreme position (i.e., full flexion of the elbow); the movement is made and the pointer locked at the other extreme position (i.e., full extension of the elbow). The direct reading of the pointer on the dial is the arc through which the movement has taken place. A dampening device has been installed to the backs of both dials to reduce oscillation during measurement. (pp. 1-2)

Norms adapted from Leighton (31) are shown in Table 12.2 for males and Table 12.3 for females and are specific to the exact method of measurement described in his manual. A more comprehensive review of normative data available for both athletic groups and the normal population has recently been provided by Hubley-Kozey (16).

The Standard Goniometer

A goniometer is essentially a protractor with two long arms. The stationary arm is structurally a part of the body of the goniometer. The moving arm is attached to the body by a rivet that allows it to move freely. The body of the goniometer, referred to as the fulcrum in this text, can be a semicircle or full-circle protractor that is marked in either 1°, 2°, 5°, or 10° increments. Goniometers can be made of clear plastic or metal, and they come in a variety of sizes to accommodate the different joint sizes (Figure 12.3).

Hubley-Kozey (16) has described some of the limitations of using the standard goniometer. The primary problem is that its reliability is questionable because it is difficult to identify the axis of motion and position of the goniometer arms at certain joints. Use of the goniometer requires certain skills that are essential for maintaining the instrument's reliability and validity. Good palpation skills and knowledge of anatomy are necessary to identify the bony landmarks for alignment of the goniometer's arms and fulcrum. Proper stabilization of the subject's body to prevent excess movement, and thus "extra" range of motion, is also imperative. The goniometer must be read at eye level to prevent errors in reading the scale.

The American Academy of Orthopaedic Surgeons has produced a very useful text (2) that gives average ranges of motion and describes methods of measurement for joints, using the standard goniometer. Detailed descriptions of positioning and stabilization for goniometry, as well as norms, are presented in *Measurement of Joint Motion: A Guide to Goniometry* by Norkin and White (35). The

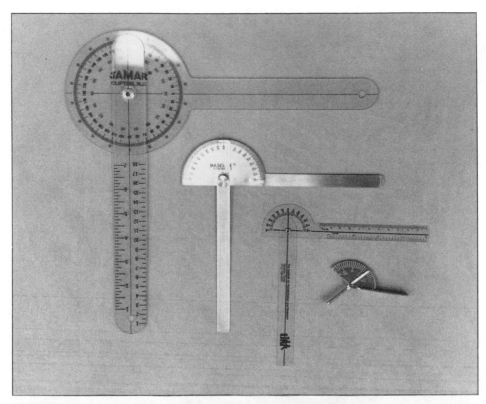

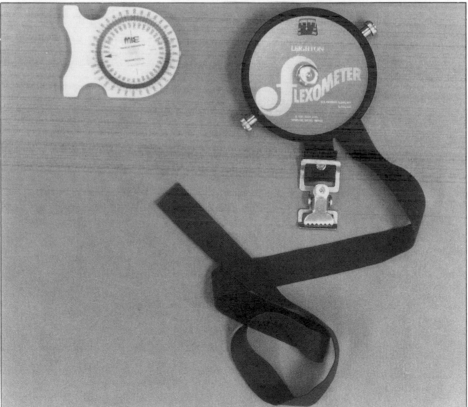

Figure 12.3 Top panel shows typical universal goniometers for measurement of both large and small joints. Bottom panel shows a Leighton flexometer and a clinical goniometer (or inclinometer).

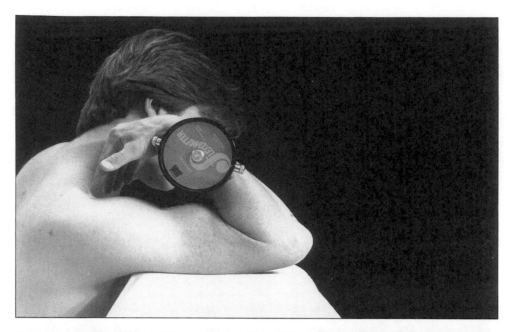

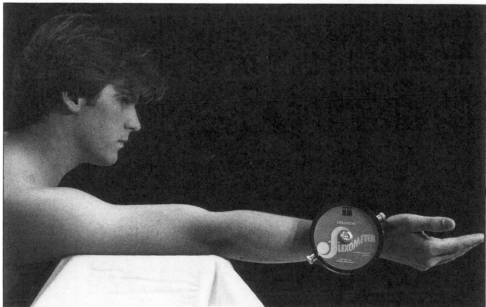

Figure 12.4 The Leighton flexometer being used to measure elbow flexion (top) and extension (bottom).

American Medical Association's text *Guides to the Evaluation of Permanent Impairment* (3rd ed.) (4) gives descriptions of methods of measurement for specific joints as well, but also provides a chart or table of ranges of motion where some degree of impairment is purported to exist. For example if a subject is capable of 60° of motion, the table might indicate that this represents an 11% impairment to total movement of the joint.

Table 12.4 shows average range of motion for selected joints, excluding the spine, according to the American Academy of Orthopaedic Surgeons text (2), and a range of motion below the average indicated by the American

Medical Association (4) as having the minimum percent of impairment. For example, if the average range of motion is listed as 80%, then the text might indicate that a minimal degree of impairment occurs if the subject can only manage 70° of movement. It is suggested that measured ranges of motion at or below the level designated as comprising minimal impairment could be used as a guide to indicate undesirably low levels of range of motion. Both sides should be evaluated to determine whether the restricted joint movement is general or specific to one side only.

Table 12.2 Norms for Joint Range of Motion Using the Leighton Flexometer—Males

Joint measurement	Low	Mod. low	Average	Mod. high	High
Neck					
Flexion/extension	< 107	107-128	129-142	143-160	> 160
Lateral flexion	< 74	74-89	90-106	107-122	> 122
Rotation	< 141	141-160	161-181	182-201	> 201
Shoulder					
Flexion/extension	< 207	207-223	224-242	243-259	> 259
Adduction/abduction	< 158	158-171	172-186	187-200	> 200
Rotation	< 154	154-171	172-192	193-210	> 210
Elbow					
Flexion/extension	< 133	133-143	144-156	157-167	> 167
Forearm					
Supination/pronation	< 151	151-170	171-191	192-211	> 211
Wrist					
Flexion/extension	< 112	151-131	132-152	153-172	> 172
Ulnar/radial deviation	< 64	64-77	78-92	92-105	> 105
Hip					
Flexion/extension	< 50	50-67	68-88	89-106	> 106
Adduction/abduction	< 41	41-50	51-61	61-71	> 71
Rotation	< 59	59-78	79-99	100-119	> 119
Knee					
Flexion/extension	< 122	122-133	134-146	147-157	> 157
Ankle					
Plantar/dorsiflexion	< 48	48-58	59-71	72-82	> 82
Inversion/eversion	< 30	30-41	42-56	57-68	> 68
Trunk					
Flexion/extention	< 45	45-62	63-83	84-101	> 101
Lateral flexion	< 74	74-89	90-106	107-122	> 122
Rotation	< 108	108-126	127-147	148-166	> 166

Note. All data are reported in degrees.
From *Manual of Instruction for Leighton Flexometer* by J.R. Leighton, 1987, Author. Adapted by permission.

The goniometer is not generally advocated for measurement of range of motion of the spine (4), although earlier editions of the AMA text (3) had described goniometric methods. Rather, use of the clinical goniometer or inclinometer is preferred. Mayer (33) suggests that the use of an inclinometer for the measurement of range of motion in the spine provides the only valid technique to differentiate between true lumbar motion as compared to hip motion. However, Williams et al. (41) claim that the modified-modified Schober technique is more reliable than the double inclinometer method. No goniometric description of spinal range-of-motion testing will be included in this chapter.

The Inclinometer

The AMA text (4) uses the term *inclinometer* to describe what has otherwise been called a "clinical" goniometer

or a gravity-and-compass goniometer (Figure 12.6) (16). Basically it works similarly to the Leighton flexometer except that it is handheld rather than strapped into position as with the Leighton model. Because the inclinometer can be used in place of either the clinical goniometer or the Leighton flexometer, no further description of movement at joints to be measured will be given except for selected measurements of the spine. The spinal motion measurements are basically as described in the AMA text (4). Although methods were described for using either a single inclinometer or two instruments, only the preferred, two-instrument method of evaluation will be described (except for the measurement of cervical rotation, where only one inclinometer is required).

Table 12.5 adapted from the AMA (4) text gives the range of motion below which impairment may be

Note. The inclinometer method allows differentiation between the thoracic and the lumbosacral regions of the vertebral column.

Table 12.3 Norms for Joint Range of Motion Using the Leighton Flexometer—Females

Joint measurement	Low	Mod. low	Average	Mod. high	High
Neck					
Flexion/extension	< 125	125-141	142-160	161-177	> 177
Lateral flexion	< 84	84-99	100-116	117-132	> 132
Rotation	< 158	158-177	178-198	199-218	> 219
Shoulder					
Flexion/extension	< 226	226-242	243-261	262-278	> 278
Adduction/abduction	< 167	167-180	181-195	196-209	> 209
Rotation	< 189	189-206	207-227	228-245	> 245
Elbow					
Flexion/extension	< 133	133-143	144-156	157-167	> 167
Forearm					
Supination/pronation	< 160	160-179	180-200	201-220	> 220
Wrist					
Flexion/extension	< 136	136-155	156-176	177-196	> 196
Ulnar/radial deviation	< 75	75-88	89-101	102-117	> 117
Hip					
Flexion/extension	< 82	82-99	100-120	121-138	> 138
Adduction/abduction	< 45	45-54	55-65	66-75	> 75
Rotation	< 90	90-109	110-130	131-150	> 150
Knee					
Flexion/extension	< 134	134-144	145-157	158-168	> 168
Ankle					
Plantar/dorsiflexion	< 56	56-66	67-79	80-90	> 90
Inversion/eversion	< 39	39-50	51-65	66-77	> 77
Trunk					
Flexion/extention	< 30	30-47	48-68	69-86	> 86
Lateral flexion	< 104	104-119	120-136	137-152	> 152
Rotation	< 134	134-152	153-173	174-192	> 192

Note. All data are reported in degrees.
From *Manual of Instruction for Leighton Flexometer* by J.R. Leighton, 1987, Author. Adapted by permission.

considered to exist for selected measurements of motion of the spine.

Other Methods of Range-of-Motion Assessment

Other methods of measuring static-joint range of motion include still photography and radiography, both of which have the advantage of providing a permanent record of the measurement. However, both of these methods, particularly the latter, prove to be relatively expensive, and radiography has the added disadvantage of exposure to radiation.

Neck, Flexion and Extension

Flexometer

Starting Position.   The subject lies on a bench in the supine position with the arms at the side of the body.

The shoulders are touching the edge of the bench, and the head and neck project beyond it. The flexometer is attached to either side of the head, over the ears.

Movement.   The head is raised to a position as near to the chest as possible, and the dial locked in position. The head is then lowered as far back as possible and the pointer locked. A reading is then taken.

Stabilization.   The buttocks and shoulders must remain in contact with the bench during movement, and the lumbar region of the back is not allowed to arch.

Inclinometer

Starting Position.   The subject is seated in a chair with the thoracic and lumbar spine in contact with the back of the chair and the head in the neutral position. Two inclinometers are used and oriented in the sagittal plane. One is placed over the T1 spinous process (the location is previously marked on the skin), and the other is placed

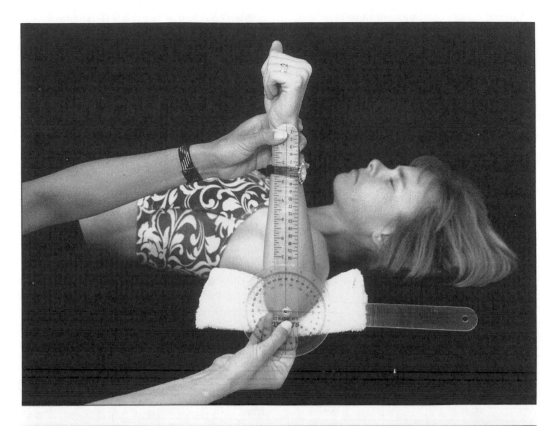

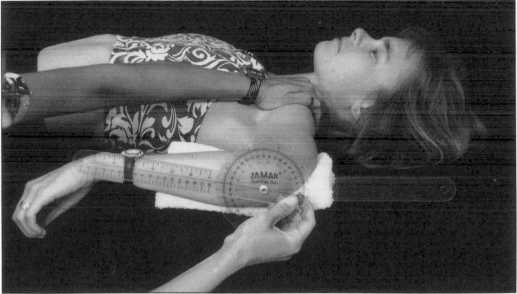

Figure 12.5   Initial (top) and final (bottom) positions for measurement of internal rotation using the goniometer. Notice in panel *a* how correct alignment of the goniometer arms is critical for an accurate baseline measurement of shoulder internal rotation. In panel *b*, stabilization of the shoulder of the subject is necessary to avoid the shoulder rolling up from the table and giving a falsely greater reading of internal rotation.

Table 12.4 Normal Range of Motion and Range at Which Impairment Exists for Selected Joints

Joint	Normal range[b]	Range at which impairment exists
Shoulder		
Flexion	167	160
Extension	62	40
Abduction	184	160
Internal rotation	69	60[a]
External rotation	104	60[a]
Elbow		
Flexion/extension	141	130
Forearm		
Supination	81	60
Pronation	75	70
Wrist		
Flexion	75	50
Extension	74	50
Ulnar deviation	35	25
Radial deviation	21	15
Hip		
Flexion	121	90
Extension	12	20
Adduction	27	10
Abduction	41	30
Internal rotation	44	30[a]
External rotation	44	40[a]
Knee		
Flexion/extension	143	140[a]
Ankle		
Plantarflexion	56	30
Dorsiflexion	13	10
Inversion	37	20
Eversion	21	10

Note. All data are reported in degrees. Data are from references 2 and 4.
[a]Method of measurement description differs between the two texts. Values given are relative to the methods described in the chapter and are similar to those described in the AMA text.
[b]Mean values.

over the occiput of the head. The inclinometers are now set to the zero position.

Movement. The subject flexes the neck maximally, and the reading is taken from both inclinometers. The reading from T1 is subtracted from the reading over the occiput, with the difference recorded as degrees of cervical flexion. The subject then returns the head to the neutral position so that both inclinometers return to the zero reading, and then the neck is extended maximally. Readings are again taken from both inclinometers, and the difference between the two readings is recorded as degrees of cervical extenison.

Table 12.5 Range at Which Impairment May Exist for Selected Measures of Spine Motion

Joint	Range at which impairment may exist
Neck	
Flexion	< 40
Extension	< 50
Right lateral flexion	< 30
Left lateral flexion	< 30
Right rotation	< 60
Left rotation	< 60
Thoracic region	
Flexion/extension	< 30
Right rotation	< 20
Left rotation	< 20
Lumbosacral region	
Right lateral flexion	< 20
Left lateral flexion	< 20

Note. All data are reported in degrees. Data are from reference 4.

Note. If, during extension, the positioning of the inclinometers causes them to contact each other and prevent maximum extension, then the T1 inclinometer should be moved laterally to avoid contact and the location marked. Care should be taken to ensure that when the inclinometer is moved, it is still maintained in the sagittal plane.

Neck, Lateral Flexion

Flexometer

Starting Position. The subject is seated in a low-backed armchair with back straight, upper arm hooked over the back of the chair, and the hands grasping the chair arms. The flexometer is attached to the back of the head.

Movement. The head is moved sideways to the extreme left and the dial is locked. The head is then moved in an arc to the extreme right and the pointer is locked. A reading is then taken.

Stabilization. It is important that body position in the chair not be changed during movement and that the shoulders not be raised or lowered.

Inclinometer

Starting Position. The starting position is as for flexion/extension except that the inclinometers are aligned in the coronal plane.

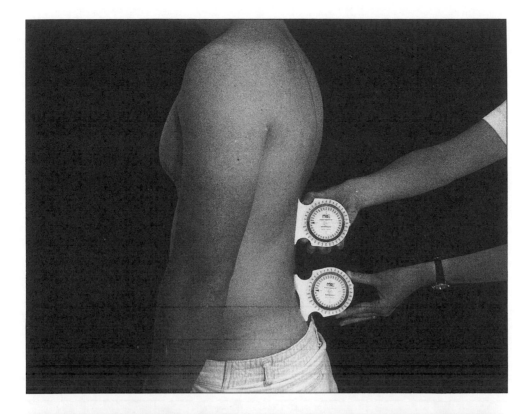

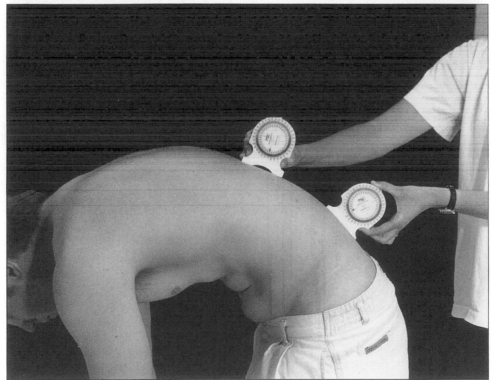

(continued)

Figure 12.6 Panels on this page show how two inclinometers can be used to measure lumbosacral flexion. Panels on following page show measurement of lumbosacral extension.

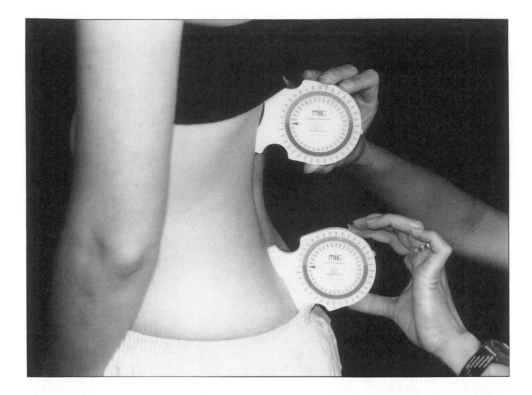

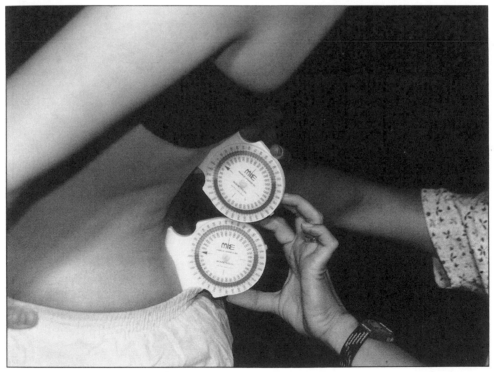

Figure 12.6   *(continued)*

Movement. The subject maximally flexes the neck laterally to the left, and readings are taken from both inclinometers. The difference between the two readings is recorded as maximal cervical left lateral flexion. The subject then returns the head to the neutral position, so that both inclinometers return to the zero setting, and then maximally laterally flexes the neck to the right. The inclinometers are again read, with the difference between the two readings recorded as maximal cervical right lateral flexion.

Neck, Rotation

Flexometer

Starting Position. The subject lies on a bench as for neck flexion and extension, except that the flexometer is attached to the top of the head.

Movement. The head is rotated to the extreme left, and the dial is locked in position. The head is then rotated to the extreme right, and the pointer is locked. A reading is then taken.

Stabilization. Shoulders must remain in contact with the bench.

Inclinometer

Starting Position. The subject lies supine on a flat table. (The shoulders of the subject should be exposed, so that any excessive shoulder rotation may be noted and avoided.) Only one inclinometer is required, and it is placed in the coronal plane on top of the head with the base "near the back of the head approximately in line with the cervico-occipital junction" (5, p. 83). The inclinometer is set to the zero position, with the head of the subject perpendicular to the table.

Movement. The subject rotates the head maximally to the right, and the inclinometer reading is recorded as maximal cervical right rotation. The subject returns the head to the neutral position, so that the inclinometer returns to the zero setting, and then maximally rotates the head to the left. The inclinometer reading is recorded as maximal cervical left rotation.

Shoulder, Flexion and Extension

Flexometer

Starting Position. The subject stands against a wall at a corner in such a way that the head, shoulders, buttocks, and heels are touching the wall, with the arm

on the side to be measured projecting just beyond the corner. The flexometer is attached to the side of the arm.

Movement. The arm is moved forward and upward in the sagittal plane to the extreme flexed position. The palm of the hand should now be positioned against the side of the wall and the dial locked in position. The arm is then moved downward and backward to the extreme extended position, with the palm of the hand sliding against the wall. The pointer is then locked and a reading is taken.

Stabilization. The heels, shoulders, and buttocks must remain in contact with the front of the wall at all times, and the palm of the hand must be in contact with the side of the wall when the dial and pointer are locked. The elbow must be kept straight at all times. If the subject is unable to flex the shoulder far enough so that the palm of the hand can contact the side wall, then the subject should be tested using the alternate technique described by Leighton (30).

Goniometer

Starting Position. The subject may stand or lie supine with the arms by the side of the body, palms against the sides of the thighs. This is the neutral or zero position. The stationary arm of the goniometer is aligned with the mid-axillary line of the thorax. The fulcrum is close to the acromion process. The moving arm is aligned with the lateral midline of the humerus, using the lateral epicondyle of the humerus as a bony landmark or reference point. For measurement of extension, the subject may stand or lie prone.

Movement. Flexion is recorded as the maximal forward and upward movement of the arm from the neutral position. Extension is recorded as the maximal backward and upward movement of the arm from zero.

Stabilization. The subject should not be allowed to arch the back.

Shoulder, Adduction and Abduction

Flexometer

Starting Position. The subject stands upright and sideways to a wall with arms at the side of the body, feet together, and knees and elbows straight. The shoulder of the side not to be measured is in contact with the wall, and the fist on that side is doubled with the knuckles facing forward, the fist in contact with both the hip and the wall. The flexometer is fastened on the back of the arm on the side to be measured.

Movement.   The hand on the side that is to be measured is positioned against the side of the thigh and the dial is locked in position. The arm is then abducted to the extreme position and the pointer locked. A reading is then taken.

Stabilization.   The fist on the side not being measured must be kept in contact with the side of the wall at all times, and the knees, body, and elbows kept straight throughout the whole movement. It is important that the arm movement take place in the frontal plane only and that no forward or backward movement occur. The heels must remain in contact with the floor at all times.

Goniometer

Starting Position.   The neutral position is with the subject either supine or sitting with the arms at the side, hands supinated. The stationary arm of the goniometer is placed just lateral to the anterior chest wall, parallel to the midline of the body. The fulcrum is placed over the anterior aspect of the acromion process. The moving arm is aligned with the midline of the humerus, using the medial epicondyle as a reference.

Movement.   Abduction is recorded as the maximal movement of the arm in the coronal plane from neutral. Adduction is recorded as the return of the shoulder from full abduction.

Stabilization.   The subject should not be allowed to lean laterally.

Shoulder, Rotation

Flexometer

Starting Position.   The subject stands against a wall at a corner in such a way that the shoulder of the side to be measured extends just beyond the projecting corner. The arm on the side to be measured is abducted to 90° and the elbow flexed to 90°. The arm of the side not to be measured is kept by the side of the body, and the shoulders, buttocks, and heels are kept in contact with the wall. The flexometer is attached to the side of the forearm.

Movement.   The arm is internally rotated to the extreme position, and the dial is locked. The arm is then maximally rotated externally and the pointer is locked. A reading is then taken.

Stabilization.   The arm on the side being measured must be kept parallel to the floor and the elbow kept flexed at 90° at all times. The shoulders, buttocks, and heels should remain in contact with the wall throughout the movement.

Goniometer

Starting Position.   The neutral position is with the subject lying supine, the arm abducted to 90° and the elbow flexed to 90° with the forearm upright and perpendicular to the ground. The stationary arm of the goniometer is placed perpendicular to the ground but pointing downward. The fulcrum is placed over the olecranon, between the medial and lateral epicondyles of the humerus. The moving arm is aligned with the lateral surface of the ulna, using the ulnar styloid process as the reference point.

Movement.   External rotation is recorded as the maximal movement of the forearm from the upright, neutral position to a position of backward rotation. Internal rotation is recorded as the maximal movement of the forearm toward a forwardly rotated position.

Stabilization.   During internal rotation, do not allow the subject's scapula to rotate forward up off the table or the back to arch during external rotation.

Elbow, Flexion and Extension

Flexometer

Starting Position.   The subject sits facing a table with the arms on the limb to be measured lying flat with the posterior surface in contact with the table and the elbow extending just beyond the edge of the corner of the table. The flexometer is attached to the posterior surface of the wrist.

Movement.   The forearm is flexed to the extreme position, and the dial is locked in position. The forearm is then extended maximally, and the pointer is locked. A reading is then taken.

Stabilization.   No movement of the arm is permitted during the flexion/extension movement at the elbow.

Goniometer

Starting Position.   In the neutral position, the subject is either lying supine, with the arm at the side of the body and the hand supinated, or sitting with the arm flexed to 90° with the elbow joint fully extended. The stationary arm of the goniometer is aligned with the midline, lateral surface of the humerus, with the acromion process used for a reference point. The fulcrum is placed over the lateral epicondyle of the humerus. The moving arm is aligned with the midline, lateral surface of the radius, using the radial styloid process as a reference point.

Movement. Flexion is recorded as the maximal movement of the forearm from neutral toward the humerus. Extension is the return of the forearm from the fully flexed position to neutral.

Note. Because hyperextension is sometimes present at the elbow, it is important to position the subject so that the surface that is supporting the arm does not limit full extension. A towel roll might be needed just proximal to the elbow. Neutral is zero degrees, so hyperextension would be recorded as a negative number.

Forearm, Pronation and Supination

Flexometer

Starting Position. The subject is seated in a standard chair with back straight against the chair, forearms resting on the chair arms. The fist of the arm to be measured is doubled and extended just beyond the edge of the chair arm, and the wrist is held straight. The strap of the flexometer is grasped in such a manner that the flexometer is fastened to the front of the fist.

Movement. The forearm is supinated maximally and the dial is locked. The forearm is then pronated to the extreme position and the pointer is locked. A reading is then taken.

Stabilization. No body or arm movement is permitted during supination/pronation of the forearm.

Goniometer

Starting Position. The neutral position is with the subject seated, the arm by the side of the body, and the elbow flexed to 90° with the thumb pointing upward (the palm is facing in). The stationary arm of the goniometer is aligned with the lateral midline of the humerus for pronation and with the medial midline for supination. The fulcrum is placed lateral to the ulnar styloid process for pronation and medial to the radial styloid process for supination. The moving arm is placed across the flat part of the wrist just proximal to the ulnar styloid process on the dorsal surface for pronation and on the palmar surface for supination.

Movement. Pronation is recorded as the movement of the forearm from the neutral position to a position in which the palm of the hand is facing the floor. Supination is recorded as the movement of the forearm to a position in which the palm of the hand is facing upward.

Stabilization. The subject should not be allowed to rotate the humerus during measurement. Be particularly aware of this substitution when measuring pronation, as the subject might tend to allow the elbow to come away from the body.

Wrist, Flexion and Extension

Flexometer

Starting Position. The subject is seated as for forearm supination/pronation, with the exception that the forearm is supinated so that the palm of the hand is turned upward. The flexometer is fastened to the lateral side of the fist.

Movement. The wrist is flexed to the extreme position and the dial is locked in position. The wrist is then maximally extended, and the pointer is locked. A reading is then taken.

Stabilization. The forearm must remain in contact with the chair arm at all times.

Goniometer

Starting Position. The neutral position is with the subject seated next to a table, arm abducted to 90° and elbow flexed to 90°, with the forearm in neutral supination/pronation and resting on the table. The wrist and hand extend just beyond the edge of the table, with the palm facing downward. The stationary arm of the goniometer is aligned with the lateral midline of the ulna using the olecranon process as a reference point. The fulcrum is placed on the lateral surface of the wrist, just distal to the ulnar styloid process. The moving arm is aligned with the lateral midline of the fifth metacarpal.

Movement. Wrist flexion is recorded as the movement of the wrist from the neutral position to a position of full flexion, with the palm of the hand directed down and toward the table. Wrist extension is recorded as the movement from the neutral position to full extension, with the palm of the hand facing forward.

Stabilization. Make sure the forearm remains in contact with the surface of the table at all times.

Wrist, Ulnar and Radial Deviation

Flexometer

Starting Position. The subject is seated in the same position as for forearm supination and pronation, except that the posterior surface of the hand to be measured is perpendicular to the floor, the flexometer is fastened to the back of the hand, and the fist is doubled.

Movement. The hand is radially flexed to the extreme position, and the dial is locked in position. The hand is then ulnarly flexed maximally and the pointer locked. A reading is then taken.

Stabilization. The forearm must remain in contact with the chair arm throughout the movement, and no degree of supination or pronation may take place.

Goniometer

Starting Position. The neutral position is the same as for wrist flexion and extension; however, the wrist and hand may be supported on the table. The stationary arm of the goniometer is aligned with the dorsal midline of the forearm, using the lateral epicondyle of the humerus for a reference point. The fulcrum is placed over the dorsal midline of the wrist. The moving arm is aligned with the dorsal midline of the third metacarpal.

Movement. Ulnar deviation is recorded as the movement from neutral to a position in which the hand is maximally directed toward the outside. Radial deviation is recorded as the movement from neutral to a position in which the hand is maximally directed toward the inside.

Stabilization. The subject should not be allowed to pronate or supinate the forearm during measurement.

Hip, Flexion and Extension

Flexometer

Starting Position. The subject stands erect with feet together, knees straight, arms extended over the head, and hands with palms turned upward. The flexometer is attached at the side of the body at the height of the umbilicus.

Movement. The subject bends backward to the extreme extended position and the dial is locked. The subject then flexes maximally at the hips and the pointer is locked. A reading is then taken.

Stabilization. The knees must remain straight and locked throughout the movement. The feet must not be moved, and the toes and heels must remain in contact with the floor.

Goniometer

Starting Position. The neutral position is with the subject prone, with the hip in 0° abduction/adduction and 0° internal/external rotation. The stationary arm of the goniometer is aligned with the lateral midline of the pelvis. The fulcrum is placed over the greater trochanter. The moving arm is aligned with the lateral midline of the femur, using the lateral femoral epicondyle as a

reference point. For hip flexion, the same goniometric alignments are used, except that the subject lies supine.

Movement. Hip extension is recorded as the maximal upward movement of the femur from the neutral position (prone). Hip flexion is recorded as the maximal movement of the femur toward the chest from the neutral position.

Stabilization. It is extremely important that the subject not be allowed to bring the pelvis up off of the table or arch or flex the lumbar spine. For hip flexion, the leg not being tested may be flexed at the hip and knee, with the foot placed flat on the table to help stabilize the pelvis.

Hip, Adduction and Abduction

Flexometer

Starting Position. The subject stands erect with feet together, knees straight, and arms by the side of the body. The flexometer is attached to the posterior surface of either leg.

Movement. The dial is locked with the subject in the starting position. The leg that does not have the flexometer attached is moved in a frontal plane sideways to the extreme abducted position. The pointer is then locked and a reading is taken.

Stabilization. The body must remain upright, the knees straight, and the feet parallel throughout the movement.

Goniometer

Starting Position. The neutral position is with the subject supine and the hip in 0° internal/external rotation and 0° flexion/extension. Both legs are positioned in midline relative to the torso. The stationary arm of the goniometer is aligned across the pelvis, "connecting" the left and right anterior superior iliac spines. The fulcrum is placed over the anterior superior iliac spine of the leg being measured. The moving arm is aligned with the anterior midline of the femur, using the midline of the patella for reference. For hip adduction, the same goniometric placements are used, except that the subject's other leg is abducted so as not to interfere with the movement of the leg being tested. The neutral position is still with the leg to be measured in midline.

Movement. Hip abduction is recorded as the maximal movement of the thigh away from the midline of the body. Hip adduction is recorded as the maximal movement of the thigh across the midline.

Stabilization. The subject should not be allowed to rotate the pelvis or internally or externally rotate the thigh.

Hip, Rotation

Flexometer

Starting Position. The subject is seated on a bench with the leg of the hip to be measured resting on the bench with knee straight and the foot of that leg projecting over the edge of the bench. The flexometer is attached to the plantar surface of the foot. The other leg is extended downward with the foot resting on the floor.

Movement. The leg of the hip to be measured is rotated externally to the extreme position and the dial is locked. The leg is then internally rotated maximally and the pointer is locked. A reading is then taken.

Stabilization. The knee and ankle joints must remain locked throughout the movement, and the position of the hips must remain unchanged.

Goniometer

Starting Position. The neutral position is with the subject seated (hips at 90° flexion and 0° flexion abduction/adduction, and knees at 90° flexion). A small towel roll is placed beneath the distal thigh of the leg to be tested; this ensures that the thigh is parallel to the surface upon which the subject is seated. The stationary arm of the goniometer is held downward, perpendicular to the floor. The fulcrum is placed over the anterior surface of the patella. The moving arm is aligned with the midline of the tibia, using the crest of the tibia and the midpoint of the two malleoli as reference points.

Movement. Hip external rotation is recorded as the maximal movement of the thigh from the neutral position to a position in which the thigh is rolled outward. Hip internal rotation is recorded as the movement of the thigh from neutral to a position of maximal inward rotation.

Stabilization. The subject should not be allowed to let the pelvis rotate up off of the table or chair or to lean to one side, especially during hip internal rotation.

Knee, Flexion and Extension

Flexometer

Starting Position. The subject lies prone on a bench with the patella and the leg extending just over the edge. The arms are placed alongside the body, with the hands gripping the sides of the bench. The flexometer is

attached to the outside of the ankle on the limb to be measured.

Movement. The knee is maximally flexed and the dial is locked in position. The knee is extended to the extreme position and the pointer is locked. A reading is then taken.

Stabilization. The positioning of the thigh must remain unchanged during the movement.

Goniometer

Starting Position. The neutral position is the same as for the flexometer. The stationary arm of the goniometer is aligned with the lateral midline of the thigh, using the greater trochanter as a reference point. The fulcrum is placed over the lateral epicondyle of the femur. The moving arm is aligned with the lateral midline of the fibula, using the lateral malleolus as a reference point.

Movement. Knee flexion is recorded as the movement of the lower leg from the neutral position to a position in which the lower leg and heel are maximally drawn toward the buttocks.

Stabilization. The subject should not be allowed to internally or externally rotate the thigh. Hyperextension is frequently encountered in the knee and is recorded as a negative number (see elbow extension).

Ankle, Plantarflexion and Dorsiflexion

Flexometer

Starting Position. The subject is seated on a bench; the leg of the ankle to be measured is extended with the knee straight. The foot projects over the end of the bench, and the flexometer is attached to the medial edge of the foot. The other leg is extended downward, with the foot resting on the floor.

Movement. The ankle is plantarflexed maximally, and the dial is locked in position. The ankle is then dorsiflexed to the extreme position, and the pointer is locked. A reading is then taken.

Stabilization. The knee of the limb being measured must be kept straight throughout the movement and the foot not allowed to turn sideways.

Goniometer

Starting Position. The neutral position is with the patient seated, knee flexed to 90°, and ankle in 0° inversion/eversion. The plantar surface of the foot is placed parallel to the ground. The knee is flexed to eliminate tightness of the gastrocnemius muscle as a limit to true ankle dorsiflexion. However, dorsiflexion is often measured with the knee at 0° and 90° flexion to determine if in fact the gastrocnemius is tight. The stationary arm is aligned with the lateral midline of the fibula, using the fibular head as a reference point. The fulcrum is placed over the lateral malleolus. The moving arm is aligned parallel with the lateral aspect of the fifth metatarsal.

Movement.   Ankle dorsiflexion is recorded as the maximal movement of the foot upward from the neutral position. Ankle plantarflexion is recorded as the maximal movement of the foot downward from the neutral position.

Stabilization.   The subject must not be allowed to invert or evert the foot.

Ankle, Inversion and Eversion

Flexometer

Starting Position.   The subject is seated on a bench, with knees projecting over the edge and legs perpendicular to the floor. The calves of the legs should be in contact with the end board of the bench. Low-cut shoes should be worn; the flexometer is attached to the front of the foot.

Movement.   The foot is inverted maximally, and the dial is locked in position. The foot is then maximally everted, and the pointer is locked. A reading is then taken.

Stabilization.   The leg must not be changed during the movement. To prevent unwanted movement, the leg may be held by the investigator.

Goniometer

Starting Position.   The neutral position for inversion and eversion is the same as for dorsiflexion and plantarflexion. The stationary arm of the goniometer is aligned with the anterior midline of the tibia, using the crest of the tibia as a reference point. The fulcrum is placed over the anterior ankle joint, using the midpoint of the malleoli as a reference point. The moving arm is aligned with the anterior surface of the second metatarsal.

Movement.   Ankle inversion is recorded as the maximal movement of the foot inward from neutral, and ankle eversion is recorded as the maximal outward movement of the foot.

Stabilization.   The foot should not be allowed to move into extreme plantarflexion during inversion, or extreme dorsiflexion during eversion.

Trunk, Flexion and Extension

Flexometer

Starting Position.   Starting position is as for hip extension and flexion, except that the flexometer is attached to the side of the body at the level of the nipple.

Movement.   The movement is as for hip extension and flexion.

Stabilization.   To obtain measurement of trunk extension and flexion alone, the score obtained for hip extension and flexion must be subtracted.

Lumbosacral Flexion and Extension

Note: The modified-modified Schober test (41) is purported to be a reliable alternative test for measurement of lumbosacral flexion and extension.

Inclinometer

Starting Position.   The subject stands with knees straight, weight evenly distributed, and hands resting on hips. The T12 spinous process is located and a skin mark is made, with a second mark made at the midpoint of the sacrum. Both inclinometers are aligned in the sagittal plane, one over the spinous process of the T12 and the other the midpoint of the sacrum. With the trunk in neutral position, the inclinometers are set to zero.

Movement.   The subject flexes maximally at the hips, the inclinometers are read, and the reading from the midpoint of the sacrum is subtracted from the one obtained at T12. The resultant difference is recorded as maximal lumbar flexion. The subject then returns to the neutral position, where both inclinometers are at the zero setting. The subject then extends backward as far as possible, and the inclinometers are again read. The reading from the midpoint of the sacrum is subtracted from the one obtained at T12, and the difference is recorded as the maximal lumbar extension.

Note.   According to the AMA text (4), "Perceived lumbar flexion is actually a compound movement of both the lumbar and the hips (measured at the sacrum), in which hip flexion normally accounts for at least 50% of total flexion" (p. 89). For this reason the AMA developed criteria to validate the lumbar flexion test, which necessitates the measurement of a straight-leg raise of the tightest leg. The lumbar flexion test is invalid if the joint range of motion for the straight-leg raise exceeds the total of sacral flexion and extension by 10° or more. For measurement of the straight-leg raise, the subject lies supine with the knees of both legs extended. The inclinometer is placed on the tibial spine of one leg and set at zero, and the leg is raised by the investigator. At the position of maximal hip flexion, the inclinometer is read. The leg not being tested remains flat on the floor. The knees of both legs are kept straight throughout the test.

Trunk, Lateral Flexion

Flexometer

Starting Position.   The subject stands erect with feet together, knees straight, and arms at sides. The flexometer is attached to the middle of the back at nipple level.

Movement.   The subject laterally flexes at the trunk to one side to the extreme position, and the dial is locked. The subject then laterally flexes to the other side maximally, and the pointer is locked in position. A reading is then taken.

Stabilization.   Both feet must remain flat on the floor during the movement and the knees kept straight. No forward movement is allowed, but slight backward extension is permissible.

Lumbosacral Lateral Flexion

Inclinometer

Starting Position.   The starting position is as for lumbar flexion/extension except that the inclinometers are aligned in the coronal plane.

Movement.   The subject flexes maximally to the right lateral side and the inclinometer readings are recorded. The sacral reading is subtracted from the T12 reading, and the difference is recorded as maximum right lateral flexion. The subject then returns to the neutral position, with the inclinometers at the zero position, and then flexes maximally to the left. The inclinometer readings are taken, and the sacral reading is subtracted from the T12 reading. The difference is recorded as the maximum left lateral flexion. Hubley-Kozey (16) describes a modified technique using the Leighton flexometer, which allows measurement of separate motions, such as flexion and extension, rather than the total range from extreme flexion to extreme extension as described by Leighton (31). This modified technique uses the zero

or starting positions similar to those described and recommended by the American Academy of Orthopaedic Surgeons (2), which is an advantage when evaluating possible joint restrictions at either end of the total range.

Trunk, Rotation

Flexometer

Starting Position.   The subject lies supine on a bench with legs together. The knees are positioned directly above the hips, and the legs are positioned parallel to the floor. An assistant is required to hold the subject's shoulders. The flexometer is attached to the posterior surface of the legs, midway between ankle and knee, with the strap passing around both legs.

Movement.   The trunk is rotated to one side maximally and the dial locked in position. The trunk is then rotated maximally to the other side and the pointer is locked. A reading is then taken.

Stabilization.   It is essential that the subject's shoulders not be allowed to move away from the bench during movement. The degree of flexion at the hips and knees must be maintained during movement and not allowed to either increase or decrease.

Thoracic Flexion and Extension

Inclinometer

Starting Position.   The subject, seated, is instructed to sit upright with the shoulders pulled back and hands resting on the hips. The T1 and T12 spinous processes are located, and skin marks are made to identify the sites. One inclinometer is placed over the T1 spinous process and the other over the T12 spinous process; both are set to zero and oriented in the sagittal plane.

Flexion.   The subject then is instructed to maximally flex the thoracic spine. (Some flexion at the hips is permitted.) Readings are taken from both inclinometers. The T12 reading is subtracted from the T1 reading, and the difference is recorded as maximal thoracic flexion.

Thoracic Rotation

Inclinometer

Starting Position.   The subject stands and flexes at the hips so that the thoracic spine is horizontal to the floor. Skin marks are made over the T1 and T12 spinous processes. The inclinometers are then aligned vertically in the coronal plane over the T1 and T12 processes. With the trunk in the neutral rotational position, the inclinometers are set to zero.

Rotation. The subject rotates the trunk maximally to the right, and readings are taken from both inclinometers. The T12 reading is subtracted from the T1 reading, and the difference is recorded as maximal right thoracic rotation. The subject then returns to the neutral position so that the inclinometers return to the zero setting. The subject then rotates the trunk maximally to the left, and readings are taken from both inclinometers. The T12 reading is subtracted from the T1 reading, and the difference is recorded as maximal left thoracic rotation.

Alternate Methods of Measurement

Alternate methods using the Leighton flexometer are available for shoulder flexion/extension, shoulder adduction/abduction, shoulder rotation, hip flexion, hip extension, trunk flexion/extension, and knee rotation (31).

Hubley-Kozey (16) describes a modified technique using the Leighton flexometer which allows measurement of separate motions, such as flexion and extension, rather than the total range from extreme flexion to extreme extension as described by Leighton (31). This modified technique uses zero or starting positions similar to those described and recommended by the American Academy of Orthopaedic Surgeons (2), which is an advantage when evaluating possible joint restrictions at either end of the total range.

REFERENCES

1. *AAHPERD technical manual: Health realted physical fitness.* (1984). Reston, VA: American Alliance for Health, Physical Education, Recreation and Dance.
2. American Academy of Orthopaedic Surgeons. (1994). *The clinical measurement of joint motion.* Chicago: Author.
3. American Medical Association. (1984). *Guides to the evaluation of permanent impairment* (2nd ed.). Chicago: Author.
4. American Medical Association. (1988). *Guides to the evaluation of permanent impairment* (3rd ed.). Chicago: Author.
5. Blair, S.N., Falls, H.B., & Pate, R.R. (1983). A new physical fitness test. *The Physician and Sports Medicine,* **11,** 87-95.
6. Broer, M.R., & Galles, N.R.G. (1958). Importance of relationship between various body measurements in performance of the toe-touch test. *Research Quarterly,* **29,** 253-263.
7. *Canadian standardized test of fitness (CSTF) operations manual (for 15 to 69 years-of-age).* (1987). Ottawa, ON: Minister of State, Fitness and Amateur Sports.
8. Corbin, C.B., & Noble, L. (1980). Flexibility: A major component of physical fitness. *The Journal of Physical Education and Recreation,* **51,** 23-24, 57-60.
9. Cowan, D., Jones, B., Tomlinson, P., Robinson, J., & Polly, D. (1988). *The epidemiology of physical training injuries in U.S. Army infantry trainees: Methodology, population, and risk factors* (Tech. Rep. No. T4-89). U.S. Army Research Institute of Environmental Medicine.
10. Dickinson, R.V. (1968). The specificity of flexibility. *Research Quarterly,* **39,** 729-794.
11. Ekstrand, J., & Gillquist, J. (1983). The avoidability of soccer injuries. *International Journal of Sports Medicine,* **4,** 124-128.
12. Golding, L.A., Myers, C.R., & Sinning, W.E. (1989). *The Y's way to physical fitness.* Champaign, IL: Human Kinetics.
13. Hoeger, W.K. (1987). *The complete guide for the development and implementation of health promotion programs.* Englewood, CO: Morton.
14. Hoeger, W.K. (1991). *Principles and labs for physical fitness and wellness.* Englewood, CO: Morton.
15. Hoeger, W.K., & Hopkins, D.R. (1990). Comparisons of the sit and reach and the modified sit and reach flexibility tests. *Medicine and Science in Sports and Exercise,* **22**(Suppl. 2), S10.
16. Hubley-Kozey, C.L. (1990). Testing flexibility. In J.D. MacDougall, H.A. Wenger, & H.J. Green (Eds.), *Physiological testing of the high-performance athlete* (pp. 309-359). Champaign, IL: Human Kinetics.
17. Jackson, A., & Langford, N.J. (1989). The criterion-related validity of the sit and reach test: Replication and extension of previous findings. *Research Quarterly for Exercise and Sport,* **60,** 384-387.
18. Jackson, A.W., & Baker, A.A. (1986). The relationship of the sit and reach test to criterion measures of hamstring and back flexibility in young females. *Research Quarterly for Exercise and Sport,* **57,** 183-186.
19. Johnson, B.L. (1972). *Flexomeasure instructional manual.* Portland, TX: Littleman Books.
20. Kippers, V., & Parker, A. (1987). Toe touch test: A measure of its validity. *Physical Therapy,* **67,** 1680-1684.
21. Knapik, J.J., Bauman, C.L., Jones, B.H., Harris, J.M., & Vaughan, L. (1991). Preseason strength and flexibility imbalances associated with athletic injuries in female collegiate athletes. *American Journal of Sports Medicine,* **19,** 76-81.

22. Knapik, J.J., Jones, B.H., Bauman, C.L., & Harris, J.M. (1992). Strength, flexibility and athletic injuries. *Sports Medicine,* **14**(5), 277-288.

23. Leighton, J.R. (1955). An instrument and technique for the measurement and range of joint movement. *Archives of Physical Medicine and Rehabilitation,* **36**, 24-28.

24. Leighton, J.R. (1956). Flexibility characteristics of males ten to eighteen years of age. *Archives of Physical Medicine and Rehabilitation,* **37**, 494-499.

25. Leighton, J.R. (1957). Flexibility characteristics of four specialized skill groups of college athletes. *Archives of Physical Medicine and Rehabilitation,* **38**, 24-28.

26. Leighton, J.R. (1957). Flexibility characteristics of three specialized skill groups of champion athletes. *Archives of Physical Medicine and Rehabilitation,* **38**, 580-583.

27. Leighton, J.R. (1964). Flexibility characteristics of males six to ten years of age. *Journal of the Association for Physical and Mental Rehabilitation,* **18**, 19-25.

28. Leighton, J.R. (1964). A study of the effect of progressive weight training on flexibility. *Journal of the Association for Physical and Mental Rehabilitation,* **18**, 101-105.

29. Leighton, J.R. (1965). A comparison of the flexibility characteristics of weight training perfectionists with flexibility characteristics of four specialized skill groups of college athletes. *Journal of the Association for Physical and Mental Rehabilitation,* **19**, 47.

30. Leighton, J.R. (1966). The Leighton flexometer and flexibility test. *Journal of the Association for Physical and Mental Rehabilitation,* **20**, 86-93.

31. Leighton, J.R. (1987). *Manual of instruction for Leighton flexometer.* Author.

32. Macrea, I.F., & Wright, V. (1969). Measurement of back movement. *Annals of Rheumatological Disease,* **28**, 584-589.

33. Mayer, T.G. (1990). Discussion: Exercise, fitness and back pain. In C. Bouchard, R.J. Shephard, T. Stephens, J.R. Sutton, & B.D. McPherson (Eds.), *Exercise, fitness, and health: A consensus of current knowledge* (pp. 541-546). Champaign, IL: Human Kinetics.

34. Nachemson, A.L. (1990). Exercise, fitness and back pain. In C. Bouchard, R.J. Shephard, T. Stephens, J.R. Sutton, & B.D. McPherson (Eds.), *Exercise, fitness, and health: A consensus of current knowledge* (pp. 533-540). Champaign, IL: Human Kinetics.

35. Norkin, C.C., & White, D.J. (1985). *Measurement of joint motion: A guide to goniometry.* Philadelphia: Davis.

36. Schober, P. (1937). The lumbar vertebral column in backache. *Munchener Medizinisch Wochenschrift,* **84**, 336-338.

37. Smith, J.F., & Miller, C.V. (1985). The effect of head position in sit and reach performance. *Research Quarterly for Exercise and Sport,* **56**, 84-85.

38. Summary of findings from national children and youth fitness study. (1985). *Journal of Physical Education, Recreation and Dance,* (January), 44-90.

39. Van Adrichem, J.A.M., & van der Korst, J.K. (1973). Assessment of the flexibility of the lumbar spine: A pilot study in children and adolescents. *Scandinavian Journal of Rheumatology,* **2**, 87-91.

40. Wear, C.L. (1963). Relationships of flexibility measurements to length of body segments. *Research Quarterly,* **34**, 234-238.

41. Williams, R., Binkley, J., Bloch, R., Goldsmith, C.H., & Minuk, T. (1993). Reliability of the modified-modified Schober and double inclinometer methods for measuring lumbar flexion and extension. *Physical Therapy,* **73**, 26-37.

42. *Youth fitness in 1985. The President's Council on Physical Fitness and Sports school population fitness survey.* Washington, DC: President's Council on Physical Fitness and Sports.

CHAPTER 13

Practical Considerations for Fitness Field-Testing of Athletes

Jack T. Daniels, PhD

State University of New York, Cortland

Carl Foster, PhD

Milwaukee Heart Institute

Athletic performance relies on an understanding of not only how the body reacts to training and competition intensities of exercise (as measured in a well-controlled laboratory setting), but also how these intensities of exercise might elicit different reactions under more real-life competitive conditions. The quest for understanding what the body is experiencing during athletic competition can often best be accomplished by studying athletes as they perform in their own environment. Field-testing presents its own array of demands upon investigator and athlete alike. It is the purpose of this chapter to generate an awareness of field-specific research demands.

Few things are more useful in bridging the gap between the sport scientist and coaches and athletes than performing thoughtful research in the field under conditions that are representative of what athletes experience in training and competition. Although they are paragons of consistency, laboratories can be intimidating places for the athlete. The laboratory is the domain of the scientist: Protocol rules; both the test circumstances and the methods of producing work are unfamiliar to most athletes (Figure 13.1). In the pool, on the track, on the ice in a lake are where athletes are in their own milieu and feel in charge. In those environments, such unfamiliar technologies as heart rate monitors, blood lactate analyzers, gas collection devices, or even muscle biops-

ies become much more meaningful and acceptable to athletes. Because the session occurs in the athlete's environment, there is less sense of missing some aspect of regular training by participating in a testing program. Predictably, this results in more compliance and interest. Another advantage of field-testing is that it allows more investigators to participate in research. The limitations on bringing state-of-the-art technology into the field mean that research questions have to be asked more simply. It's easy to have a basic exercise laboratory for the field study of athletes for less than $5,000—so research is possible even if you don't have the capital for a mass spectrophotometer. Lastly, field-testing makes investigators more honest. In a fully equipped laboratory

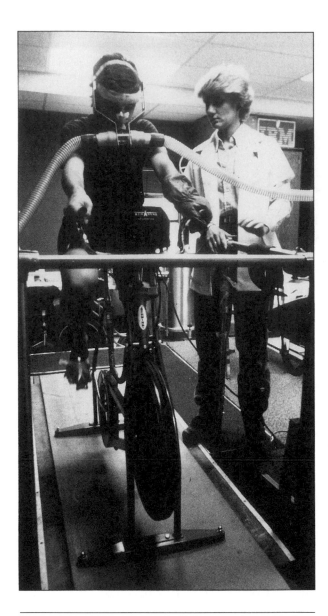

Figure 13.1 The well-equipped laboratory: home for the scientist, alien territory for the athlete.

it's easy to be lulled by the "friendliness" of our computerized hardware and software. Sometimes we forget the calculations necessary to perform studies or, more importantly, the assumptions involved in the study. When errors occur, we often don't recognize them, and many times they can't be solved by a technocrat. A visit to the field makes us appreciate where we are coming from and what we are measuring, and forces us to think about how we are measuring it.

Field-testing brings unique problems for the investigator. The valve that doesn't work, the hose forgotten, the spilled chemical are farther away than the next room in the laboratory. It takes some planning to keep from forgetting the relevant tools. Electrical outlets might not be the sort you need, environmental conditions can be unpredictable (or harder to measure), even the right kind of water might not be available. Most of these problems are easy enough to solve with a little planning before you go into the field.

Particularly relative to athletes, it is important to keep in mind why you are doing your study. If the purpose of the study is to test a hypothesis, then the athletes should know that they are research subjects, that the results might not be available to them immediately, and that they might benefit only in the longer term. They are the same kind of laboratory animal you recruit for any experiment. They should know that you are there to serve the needs of the experiment and that they are agreeing to volunteer. On the other hand, if science is a desired by-product of a service function that you are providing to the athlete and coach, you need to remember that the short-term needs of the athlete and coach are far more important than answering potential experimental questions. Particularly as you work with more and more accomplished athletes, you need to remember that their competitive lifetimes are short, and that lack of understanding and consideration on your part are likely to be poorly tolerated.

GENERAL PRINCIPLES FOR THE FIELD LABORATORY

You are going to be working in an environment that is likely as alien to you as the laboratory is to the athlete. Carefully consider how you plan your studies, so that you can accomplish your goals. We will discuss specific techniques later, but certain general prinicples should always be kept in mind.

Timing

Provide for considerably more time per test than you would in the lab or than you anticipate the test will take. Assume that you will spend half your day fixing things that break because you are moving them about. Allow for the unexpected in your scheduling so you don't make athletes spend half the day waiting around to be studied.

The Nature of Athletes

Understand that most athletes, particularly young athletes, are very social creatures. Assume that they will show up in groups and that you won't have the peace and quiet of the laboratory that you are accustomed to. If controlled conditions, privacy, or confidentiality is of particular importance, you must specifically plan for it. This new "laboratory" is likely to be noisy, often filled with music of a variety that you may be too old to appreciate (Figure 13.2).

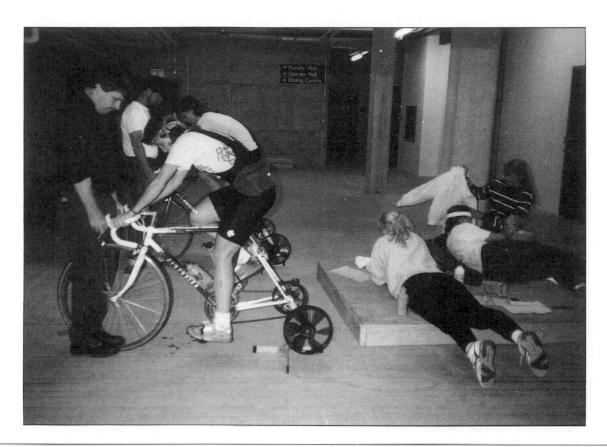

Figure 13.2   Field-testing in the basement of a dorm at the University of Calgary. The wind-load simulators that the athletes use to train on have been converted for use as ergometers. Other athletes are lying around the testing area. One has been recruited to record data while the other two play with the infant child of one of the investigators.

Schedules

Rely as little as possible on external groups for scheduling. If you can't meet with coaches and athletes before the testing session to set up a master schedule, assume that whatever could go wrong with scheduling will. Plan breaks into the schedule so you can catch up after disruptions. And expect to spend some considerable time sitting and waiting.

Insofar as you can control scheduling, pick a time of day when conditions are likely to be favorable for your testing. For outdoor testing, typically early morning and early evening weather is more predictable than midday, when wind and cloud cover are more variable.

Planning and Packing

Prepare a detailed list of facilities, equipment, and conditions that you need for testing and what each subject should provide. Be specific about each subject's needs (shoes, warm-ups, equipment, etc.). Use a checklist when you pack your equipment; if you forget something, you can't go to the next room to retrieve it.

Athlete Requirements

Spell out details of any dietary or training requirements or constraints that will be expected of the athletes or coaches. Your expectations can present a particular problem at training camps, where athletes are typically working particularly hard and might be more tired than usual. Sometimes your most important function is to insist on a rest day for the "integrity" of your testing, but which the athletes need to adapt to the coach's schedule.

Finances

Be clear about expenses for the entire project. Do you expect to pay subjects? If so, you must be sure it is legal for each particular (possibly amateur) athlete to accept money. Who pays the subjects' room and board and transportation? Who pays your expenses? All these answers should be absolutely clear.

Pilot Testing

Run through several complete pilot tests yourself or with dummy subjects to identify and address any problems before involving athletes in any real tests. Also work through how you plan to give feedback to coaches and athletes. You have much less time for analysis than you might prefer, and producing "pretty" results may be very difficult. If you have thought through your feedback information, "quick and dirty" now is often preferable to "elegant" 6 weeks later. Program your computer before you get to the field. Preprinted forms to convey results can be very useful.

Securing Equipment

Consider your security needs for equipment you must leave at the test site when you are not actually conducting tests. It's easy to misplace items in field situations simply because the testing area is different from your home laboratory. In your practice trials and in setting up your field-testing area, aim for consistency, as this will reduce loss of equipment.

Transportation

Know how long it will take to transport equipment, samples, subjects, and so on from the test site to other important facilities such as dorms, showers, or toilets. Try to have more than enough transportation available to make trips back and forth.

Waste Disposal

Determine how you will dispose of any hazardous materials you will use. Bloodstained gauze, needles, and lances are all hazardous. They cannot be disposed of in public trash. Make sure you have containers in which all hazardous materials can be safely stored and transported back to your home laboratory or to other proper disposal areas. If you plan to use a local disposal site such as a hospital, make your arrangements before you show up with a trunkful of containers with hazardous materials.

Permission

Performing research in the field usually means getting permission to use facilities of one kind or another (e.g., a swimming pool, running track, laboratory, or classroom that can be used as a field lab). As collegial as your peers may be at professional meetings, they will rarely be enthusiac about lending you their lab for 10 days. They have their own laboratory agendas. Well ahead of time, work out details of all tests with some local authority. If this isn't feasible, show up at the testing venue a day early and be prepared to be creative. We've used everything from the basement of a college dorm

(Figure 13.2), to local tracks (Figure 13.3, top), to college classrooms, to our dormitory room (Figure 13.3, bottom), to shower rooms as the "lab."

SPECIFIC FIELD-TEST CONDITIONS AND CONSIDERATIONS

Testing on or in Water

Equipment must remain functional in high humidity and when wet. Many investigators rely on tape to prepare and repair equipment, but most tapes do not work well when moist or wet. Duct tape is an exception and will remain secure underwater if it is applied before the surface or tape first become wet (Figure 13.4).

Take precautions to make all pieces of equipment secure or at least retrievable if dropped or mishandled around water. Losing a nose clip during a test is always frustrating, but it can be a real problem if the nose clip goes to the bottom of a lake where it can't be retrieved. Securing the nose clip to the subject's head gear or a larger piece of equipment with dental floss can help save time or even the whole study. Even large items like gas collection valves can profitably be attached to yourself or the boat with dental floss.

Any apparatus used for inspiration or expiration of air during exercise while in or under the water must be airtight and capable of withstanding whatever pressure it is subjected to. Any water leaking into any part of the subject's air-supply tubing can cause considerable concern, especially for the subject who is not comfortable being tested doing intense exercise in the water. In addition to being reliable and watertight, any equipment worn by subjects in the water should be designed to offer limited resistance to moving through the water and also must not obstruct the subject's vision.

Equipment worn in the water should be easily removable by the subject or anyone else in a position to help in an emergency. Equipment worn by subjects should be constructed so that it neither weighs the subject down nor adds to the subject's buoyancy; performance must remain realistic.

Data-recording forms invariably get wet when used around water. Use paper that is a little heavier grade and cover it with a clear plastic cover. Ballpoint pens work better than felt pens or pencils on damp paper. For extreme circumstances, you might use a non-water-soluble grease pen on a plastic slate (but you can't write much down because you have to write big, and cleaning the slate may require bringing some alcohol swabs).

You must take special precautions to prevent liquid samples, such as blood or urine, from being diluted with

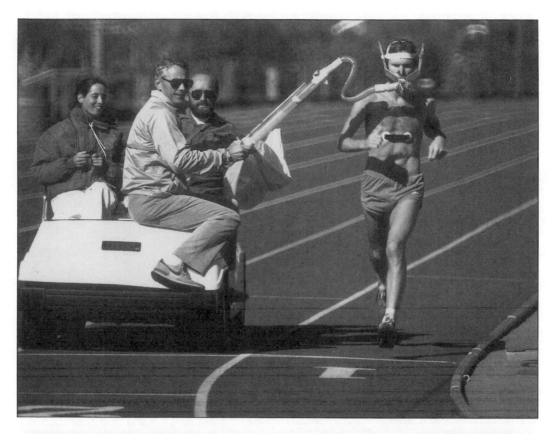

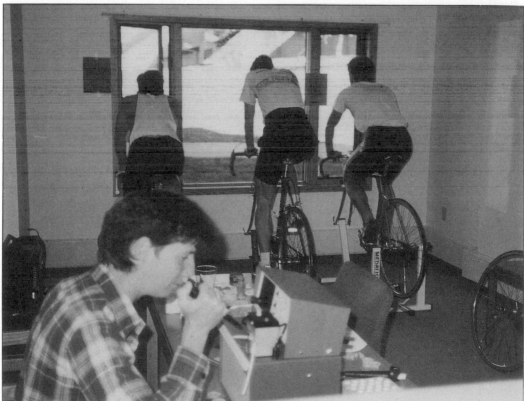

Figure 13.3 Prepare for and be creative when doing field research. Have the proper staff and equipment ready, and calibrate equipment ahead of time.

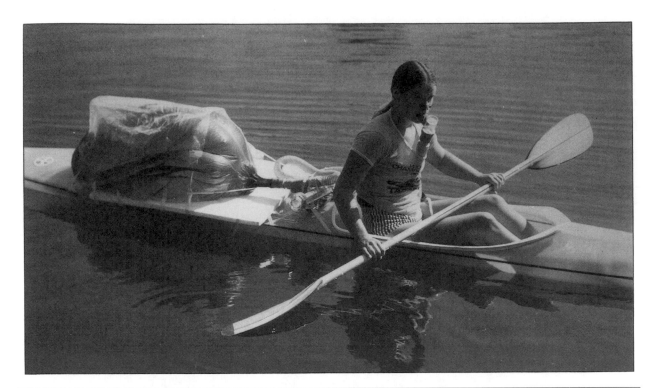

Figure 13.4 This apparatus for collecting expired air in the field is well secured to the boat with duct tape. The hose is secured under the subject's clothing, which can be a safety hazard if the subject capsizes and is unable to right the boat. In cases like this the collection valve is usually spring-loaded and has a stopwatch attached so that the subject can instantly initiate and terminate data collection.

water. This can easily happen with the finger-stick blood samples that are currently popular, unless particular care is taken to dry the skin surface prior to each sampling. It is common, even after the subject's hand has been dried, for water to drip from the hair or other parts of the body and rewet the hand. Several small washcloths may be more practical than a few towels, which will get soaked quickly anyway.

If tests on or in the water are designed to assess the subject's reaction to performing at a variety of speeds, it is imperative that speed of movement can be accurately measured and controlled. Make it clear to the subjects exactly when during the test speed is required, how much speed is required, and how that speed can be controlled. Will there be pace lights, or some sound to follow, or will pace be given in terms of time per measured distance covered? If pace lights are not available, it can be adequate to give time at each pool length, in a pool, but in open water the situation is quite different. Paddlers and rowers must have buoys or a clearly visible line, alongside of which they travel, to help them control speed. If a line is used, it must be taut and firmly anchored at each end, so that movement of the line is not counted as movement through the water. Provide markers of varied designs and colors at relatively short intervals for more accurate control of speed.

Testing in the Cold

Everything can freeze. Blood samples can freeze in capillary tubes while being taken from the finger. The term *hyperemic finger tip* is close to meaningless in a cold environment. Breathing valves can freeze between or even during tests. Batteries, heart rate monitors, and analyzers can suddenly give much less power than when warm. Do everything you can to protect your equipment from the cold and to keep its exposure of short duration. For instance, insulated containers can prevent freezing (Figure 13.5).

Subjects can freeze. Make sure they don't. Provide ways they can keep warm when they are waiting their turns, during recovery intervals, and between tests. Provide warming tents, shelters, and extra clothing. Construct minienvironments for taking blood samples and keeping subjects comfortable between tests. If prolonged testing might produce sweat and wet clothes, all subjects should have several changes of clothing.

Investigators can freeze, too. The subjects are usually exercising, which can help keep them warm. They may show up at the venue, do their thing, and leave, while you are waiting for the next subject and not moving around much. Think of the weather as being much colder than it actually is, because you're going to be standing out in it

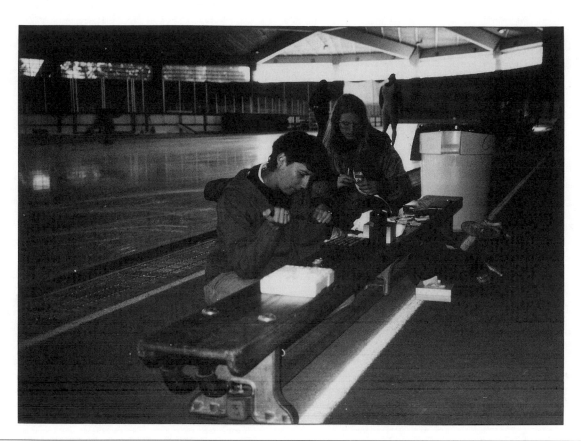

Figure 13.5   Data collection at the Olympic Oval at the Univeristy of Calgary. Even though this is an "ideal" winter sports venue, it is still rather cool (11 °C). The collector's insulated carryall allows the samples to be stored at a higher temperature.

for quite a while. If you're not used to cold weather, its going to be a long day, and your judgment and good humor are going to be mightily tested. Wear multiple layers of clothing, heavy boots, good gloves or mittens, and something warm on your head—a hat *and* a hood.

Testing in the Heat

In a warm environment, heat can accumulate, and the temperature can change significantly over a short period of time. If control over heat exposure is important, allow considerable time for testing, because you may be limited to a narrow temperature "window" each day.

Like water, sweat can contaminate blood samples. Make sure the subject's skin is well dried prior to blood sampling. (This can be important even in cold environments, where mittens or hats can make fingertips or earlobes sweaty.) The lactate concentration in sweat is usually much higher than in blood, and sweat contamination may spuriously elevate lactate concentrations.

Maintain a source of shade near the testing site. This not only allows control of radiant exposure to the subject, it provides a location for cooling and may be critical to the use of some instruments, such as dry gas meters.

When measuring gas volumes in warm (or any other) environments, control for constancy of the environment for a few moments before measurement. Exposure of instrumentation, or even meteorological balloons, to direct sunlight can confound results (Figure 13.6). If you aren't sure there's an adequate source of shade at your testing site, take one with you—an extra-large beach umbrella, for instance (with a method for weighting it down against the wind).

Know and allow for the temperature limits of your instrumentation. In a cold environment, keep instruments in a warming house or your hotel room. In a warm, shady environment the limits of enzymatically driven instruments may be exceeded even when you are relatively comfortable. Portable lactate and glucose analyzers might not remain stable beyond about 85 °F. Likewise it is very important to have a portable cooling device for storing temperature-sensitive samples. For more prolonged storage, you could rent a portable refrigerator or freezer from an appliance store.

Heat stress, and the physiological responses to it, are very dose dependent, so it is important to have a way to assess the magnitude of stress. A thermometer, a sling psychrometer, and a scale for measuring changes in body weight should be used frequently.

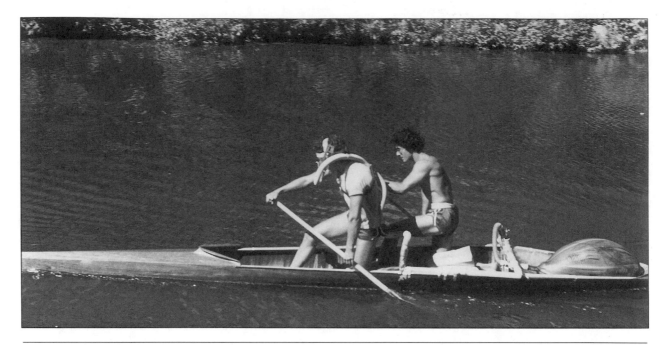

Figure 13.6   Data collection in the field. Note that the collection balloon is exposed to direct sunlight. Before measurements of gas volume can be made, the balloon needs to be transferred to a well-shaded area for several minutes. The dry gas meter used to measure gas volumes in the field must be carefully shielded from direct sunlight, or given up to 30 min to stabilize if exposed accidentally.

Tests at Altitude

The single greatest need for altitude studies is for a reliable source of uncorrected (for sea level) "station" barometric pressure. Portable barometers can be bought from the same scientific supply house that provided your main laboratory barometer. They are usually restricted to relatively low (< 1,500 m) or relatively high (> 1500 m) altitudes. Alternatively, flight service stations are normally good sources of local station pressure, but if you don't specify that you want uncorrected for sea level pressure, you will get a sea level pressure, under the relative altitude conditions. Once you convince the station technician that you want uncorrected station pressure, indicate for what time of day you want that pressure (it is usually recorded every hour). If it is given in inches of mercury, you can convert it to millimeters (mmHg) by multiplying inches by 25.4. It may be useful to remember that standard sea level pressure is 760 mmHg, or 29.92 in.

It is particularly important to unpack all equipment and supplies very carefully, but promptly, upon arrival at altitude. If you are coming from sea level or an altitude different from the one where testing will take place, the pressure in storage vessels, sealed containers, and analyzers will be affected at the new altitude by the change in barometric pressure. Get all supply vessels and equipment "acclimatized" to the new pressure as soon as possible.

Pay particular attention to the hydration status of your subjects. Because of the low relative humidity and strong radiant exposure at altitude, fluid losses may be large and not very obvious. Dehydration may influence your results almost as much as the reduced barometric pressure, particularly during the first few days at altitude.

Beyond an altitude of about 10,000 ft (3,000 m) be alert for changes in mental status, your subjects' and your own. In the unacclamatized individual, rapid ascent to altitudes of this magnitude can impair mental functioning. If your procedures are not rote, consider taking along supplemental O_2.

Because of the dryness of the air during the winter at altitude, you may have a considerable problem with static electricity. Your laboratory equipment, particularly computerized equipment, may function much less well than usual. Portable room humidifiers can help you maintain an environment suitable for contemporary electrical equipment; they will also make you more comfortable during sleep.

MEASURING RESPIRATORY METABOLISM

Equipment Checklist

____ Headgear
____ Rubber connecting hose

___ Breathing valves (with built-in clocks, if possible)
___ Mouthpieces
___ Nose clip
___ Provision for cleaning and disinfecting breathing valves and mouthpieces (usually a portable basin, dish soap, and a disinfectant solution; hydrogen peroxide sometimes works in the absence of Cidex)
___ Flexible hose with connectors to join mouthpiece and collection valve; collection valve with rubber connector hose
___ Collection bags (usually meteorological balloons)

  • Vacuum-cleaner hose connectors to provide rigid neck for bag
  • Numbers on bags
  • Rubber stoppers with glass tubing, rubber tubing, and clamps for sampling aliquots of expired gas

___ Storage syringes for gas samples (30- to 100-ml, glass)

  • Sleeve of syringe should be oiled with mineral oil to prevent gas leaks
  • Three-way Luer stopcock for syringe
  • Numbers on syringes
  • Syringe rack to hold and transport syringes

___ Dry gas meter (calibrated in laboratory to lab gasometer)

  • Thermometer in dry gas meter to measure temperature of gas as it is measured
  • Hose to connect bags to inlet port

___ Charts and recording forms

  • Water vapor pressure chart
  • Data collection and recording sheets
  • Pens, pencils, magic markers, grease pens
  • Clipboards with clear covers and rubber bands

___ Gas analyzer (Lloyd Gallenkamp or micro Scholander)

  • Reference manual
  • Mercury
  • Distilled water
  • Stopcock grease (usually Apezion or another nonsilicone grease)
  • Canula for entering reagents
  • Pipe cleaners
  • Dilute H_2SO_4 in eyedropper bottle
  • Funnel
  • Rubber bands
  • Hemostats
  • Copper wire
  • Cleaning soap
  • 10-ml syringes and tubing
  • 30- to 100-ml glass syringes
  • Glassware for preparing reagents

  • Reagents
  • Mineral oil
  • Balance scale for reagents

If an electronic analyzer is used, bring your own calibration tanks

___ Scales for weighing subjects, including some known weight for calibration checks
___ Barometer (or phone number where local station pressure can be obtained)
___ Sling psychrometer for measuring humidity and temperature
___ Wind gauge
___ Large beach umbrella to protect from sun
___ Vehicle to assist in collections

  • Fuel (electric golf carts have many advantages but must be "charged" frequently)
  • Clearance to drive on track or road for tests
  • Driver and assistants

Marking of Collection Venue

For tracks and pools, standard course marking is usually evident. For roads or supplemental marking, take along a long metric tape measure and brightly colored tape for marking the site (alternatively, take cones or buoys that can be placed and removed easily).

Method for Pacing Subjects

Pacing usually requires auditory or visual feedback to subjects at fairly frequent intervals (every 100 m, running; every 25 m, swimming). Try blowing a whistle when the subject should be at the marker, or give "splits" against a known "split schedule.") If the subjects are moving fairly rapidly, it is helpful to have two investigators with headphones (headphones are available at electronics stores). One investigator takes the split and radios the second, who then provides feedback to the subject. It is also helpful to use hand signals to indicate that a subject is below (hand low), on (hand level), or over (hand high) the desired pace. If money is no object, pacing lights synchronized to the desired pace are state of the art. As a general rule, the more frequent the feedback to the subject, the more even the pace.

MEASUREMENT
OF HEMODYNAMICS
IN THE FIELD

During the last 25 years the development of radiotelemetry pulse monitors has greatly changed the field evaluation of athletes. Older systems depended on relatively powerful, and heavy, transmitters to transmit an ECG waveform to a base station that could be carried with the investigator into the field. This base station could then be used to write an ECG tracing from which heart rate could be recorded. This basic technology is still available, and transmitters are much lighter nowadays.

Beginning about 1960, tape recorders attached to ECG leads were employed to record ambulatory ECGs. Holter monitors today are fairly advanced and of reasonably small size. In most cases two ECG leads can be recorded with enough fidelity to make diagnoses of exercise-induced ischemia as well as of dysrhythmias. These systems can essentially record every heartbeat for periods exceeding 24 hours. With rapid scanning systems, virtually any information regarding the heart rate or ECG can be retrieved. These systems depend on a hard-wire attachment from the subject to the recorder and a recorder large enough to accommodate a cassette tape recorder, which renders them somewhat impractical for many athletic settings.

Approximately 5 years ago, small-scale radio transmitters designed to transmit over a distance of less than 5 ft to a recorder worn by the subject radically changed the capabilities of field evaluation of heart rate (Figure 13.3a). With current microchip technology, several hours of averaged heart rate data can be recorded for essentially instantaneous retrieval to a laptop computer. These systems have virtually taken the work out of measuring heart rate in the field. Simply start the watch, punch the event marker at appropriate times to indicate correlation with events occurring during data collection (beginning and end of intervals, collection of lactate, completion of laps, etc.), and the data can be retrieved later at the investigator's convenience. These systems are generally accurate and easy to use. Most now use a chest strap (or disposable electrodes) to sense ventricular depolarization and to hold the transmitter. The subject wears the receiver on the wrist. In aquatic environments, or wherever the receiver is likely to get wet, a frozen-food baggie can provide protection without compromising function. Given the limited transmission range, there is not usually too much trouble with interference from one subject to another, provided the subjects are reasonably aware of the need to avoid close contact.

Blood pressure can be measured in the field with about the same ease as the recording of ambulatory heart rates for clinical purposes. The monitors are not unreasonably bulky, and the microchip technology for the automated detection of Karotkov sounds is getting better. For highly competitive or strenuous athletic pursuits the system is not yet suitable, but its development is making good progress.

There are even portable gamma scintillation cameras suitable for measuring left-ventricular ejection fraction and relative changes in left-ventricular volume during ambulatory activities and moderate exercise. Although these systems are currently designed primarily for clinical needs, their possibilities for field research at the other end of the exercise spectrum are very clear.

MEASUREMENT OF BLOOD LACTATE

Blood collection in the field is fairly easy today (Figure 13.7). Capillary blood samples may be obtained easily from a fingertip puncture. In cold environments it is particularly important to have the athlete wear warm gloves to optimize blood flow to the hand. Even so, some of the assumptions regarding the degree of hyperemia in the fingertip are probably violated in this setting. With the use of gloves, or in warm weather environments, care must be taken to remove sweat from the sampling site. Given contemporary knowledge of the risk of blood-borne infections, the investigator should certainly wear gloves and follow a detailed protocol for infection control.

The development of the enzyme electrode system for measuring blood lactate (or other blood-borne constituents) has also greatly changed the possibilities for field

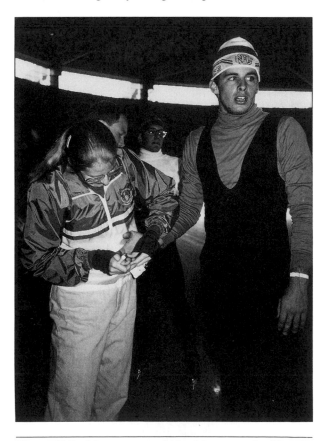

Figure 13.7 Measurement of blood lactate at the Olympic Oval at the University of Calgary.

evaluation of the athlete. Enzymatic laboratory chemistry methods have been available for years, as has the possibility of securing deproteinized blood samples in the field. However, the time required to analyze samples made serious field studies of large numbers of athletes less than feasible. The enzyme electrode system allowed the development of portable analyzers that could be used with the simple injection of a blood sample or a blood sample/buffer mixture. These systems are currently small enough to fit into a small backpack or under an airplane seat. Deproteinized buffered samples are usually stable for at least 24 hours, longer if refrigerated. In many cases, portable analyzers depend on a source of distilled or deionized water for mixing reagents. In the field, an adequate source of distilled water is available at most grocery stores.

OTHER USEFUL ITEMS FOR YOUR TRAVELING LABORATORY

Doing field research is something like being a good scout—your motto has to be Be Prepared. You have to be prepared to pretend you are McGyver and can assemble a mass spectrophotometer from baling wire, duct tape, and three mirrors using only your Swiss Army knife, all the while suspended by one foot below a ski lift rigged to explode. Many of the factors that you tend to take for granted in your home laboratory cannot be assumed in the field. It is worthwhile to have a traveling box with support equipment. This box might include the following items.

- Electrical surge protector with multiple plugs (outside of the U.S. and Canada, you may need a transformer to convert power sources for U.S.-made instruments)
- Electrical adapter to allow grounded plugs to be attached to non-3-prong sockets
- Electrical extension cords, at least two

- Extra batteries for all battery-powered equipment, such as lactate analyzers and heart rate monitors
- Flashlight
- Blank computer disks, computer paper, extra printer cartridge
- Clerical supplies for organizing data (preformated data collection forms, graph paper, three hole punch, stapler, staple remover, paper clips, whiteout, tabbed organizer pages, 3-ring binders, ruler, plastic page protectors, multicolored pens and magic markers, scissors, small knife [Swiss Army knives are perfect], rubber bands, string, etc.)
- Metric tape measure
- Marking tape of several colors
- Various types of other tape (plastic, adhesive, duct)
- Small toolkit including regular and Phillips screwdrivers, Allen and regular wrenches of several sizes, pliers (regular and needlenose)

Portable spectrophotometers can often be rented from local clinical laboratories at a fairly reasonable cost. These should allow analysis of at least some blood samples in the field. Make sure your analysis mode is kit-oriented so that you aren't mixing a lot of chemicals in the field.

Portable refrigerators, freezers, dehumidifiers, humidifiers, and such can often be rented from appliance stores. The availability of dry ice is unpredictable, particularly in small towns. Call ahead to make sure you can get it in the quantity you need. Be careful about storing dry ice in your car or hotel room. Waking up in the middle of the night hyperventilating because your room is full of CO_2 is no fun.

Lastly, bring at least two or three mirrors. Why? Because a good bit of your "magic" will need to be "done with mirrors." Even if the protocol gets broken, or the data don't present themselves in the way you anticipated and planned for, a little creative thought and the careful use of your magical mirrors will help you make the best of a bad situation. For us this is absolutely critical, for we are ever mindful that most good science depends on a creative response to serendipity (or disaster).

CHAPTER 14

Understanding Measurement Concepts and Statistical Procedures

Barry B. Shultz, PhD
William A. Sands, PhD
University of Utah

Exercise speicialists must evaluate and on occasion carry out treatment effectiveness research. This chapter presents the basic steps in designing and analyzing a training program intended to enhance physical fitness. Emphasis is given to designing sensitive studies, being aware of threats to internal and external validity, and considering the special data analysis problems that occur in treatment effectiveness research.

Statistical procedure and experimental design are only two different aspects of the same whole, and that whole is the logical requirements of the complete process of adding to natural knowledge by experimentation.

Fisher (1)

The overriding theme of this text has been the measurement and assessment of fitness parameters. Each of the preceding chapters dealt with the tools and techniques used by exercise specialists to quantify various fitness parameters. Although statistical procedures are used by exercise specialists to study fitness, physiologists did not begin to use statistics for this purpose until the 20th century (2). It has even been suggested that the tools of data analysis can determine what problems scientists

study and how they study these problems (3). Therefore, like any tool, statistical tools must be used appropriately.

Chapter 14 will focus on the use of inferential statistics to assess the effectiveness of various training programs or interventions. This type of research is referred to as treatment effectiveness research (TER) (4) or outcome evaluation research (5). Even though TER can be conducted under the tightly controlled conditions of a laboratory, generally it is conducted in the real world of clinical settings and fitness centers.

The purpose of TER is to discover training programs that work in general for a particular population. It is usually applied research and is conducted to facilitate the decision-making process for questions like these: Should I buy this piece of equipment because it will result in greater strength gains than the equipment I am currently using? Should I use this new aerobic-training program or continue with my present program? Does the time of day I exercise affect the metabolic cost of my exercise?

Initially the exercise specialist might be concerned with determining whether a training program or intervention can bring about change in one or more fitness parameters. If the program is already known to be effective, then comparing this program to an alternative program would be an appropriate second step. For both of these questions, especially when training is conducted in field settings, the preferred research approach is to give each subject a pretest on all fitness parameters of interest, randomly assign them to groups (when possible), implement the treatment (new program vs. traditional program), and then give a posttest to all subjects. Campbell and Stanley (6) referred to this design as a pretest–posttest control group design (see Figure 14.1). This chapter was written with this design in mind, although the simpler posttest-only design will be discussed also for didactic purposes. Other questions and designs are possible, and the material in this chapter will often apply to them.

The purpose of this chapter is to cover a number of design and statistical issues in TER. The intention is not to teach these techniques but merely to develop a conceptual understanding of the issues. References have been included to provide further direction for the interested reader. The chapter has four sections. The first section deals with the role of hypothesis testing in experimental research and the problems that can be created when inductive inferences are made from data to hypothesis or theory. The second section deals with design sensitivity and the importance of planning in experimental research. The third section covers threats to valid inferences and their role in eliminating competing, plausible hypotheses in fitness research. The last section briefly outlines some statistical issues specific to fitness research.

EXPERIMENTATION, HYPOTHESIS TESTING, AND SCIENCE

The process of determining if a treatment was the cause of an effect in a fitness parameter involves experimentation. True experimental research is concerned with cause-and-effect relationships and requires randomization, control, and comparison (7). In field studies these qualities are often not possible and thus the resultant research is called quasi-experimental. The primary reason for quasi-experimental research is the inability to randomly assign subjects to groups. In this case the appropriate experimental design is a nonequivalent control group design (8).

Randomization, perhaps Fisher's greatest contribution to statistical science, is the assignment of subjects to groups by chance. Control is holding constant or varying systematically variables in the physical or experimental environment to remove or compare their effect on the amount of observed variation. The researcher attempts to maximize variance within the substantive (treatment) variable, minimize error variance, and prevent variance from extraneous variables (9). In other words, the experimenter determines what will be manipulated, what will be held constant, and what will be eliminated from the testing environment. However, only a small set of these sources of variance can be controlled in any one study. This lack of closure (10) means that cause-and-effect relationships can be discovered only through repeated testing and accumulated evidence (11) or corroboration (12). Finally, for a true experiment to exist, there must be a comparison. The treatment group must be compared to another group that is treated exactly like the treatment group except they do not receive the treatment.

Hypothesis Testing and Significance Testing

Together, hypothesis testing and tests of significance constitute the primary data-analytical system in the behavioral sciences. Although Fisher made a distinction between these terms (*hypothesis testing* and *tests of significance*), in current practice they are used interchangeably. The name *hypothesis test* merely gives greater emphasis to the deductive aspect of science, and the term *significance test* emphasizes the inductive aspect. Hypothesis testing involves deductively generating scientific hypotheses and then determining the degree of agreement or disagreement between the researcher's expectations and the actual outcome of the study (13). The inductive reasoning behind hypothesis testing is provided by tests of significance (14). Additionally, the test of significance provides the rules that are used to reject, or fail to reject, the statistical null hypothesis.

Although often referred to as tests of significance, the longer phrase *tests of statistical significance* (TOSS) is being used here because the failure to explicitly refer to *statistical* significance has been a source of misinterpretation (15) and criticism (16, 17) in behavioral research. A clear understanding of what TOSS mean, how they have been misinterpreted, and how they fit into the scientific method is needed.

The term *significance* in *test of significance* is derived from the concept of level of significance. However,

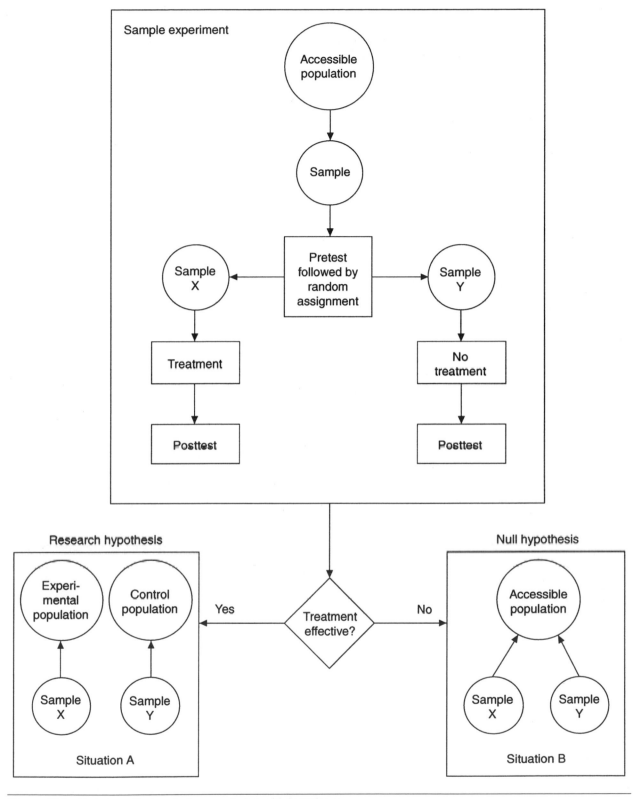

Figure 14.1   Pretest–posttest control group design with hypotheses.

confusion exists as to what this means. Some researchers associate level of significance with alpha, or the probability of a Type I error, whereas other researchers (18, 19) associate level of significance with the p value, or associated probability (17). The p value is one outcome of a statistical test and is generally provided in most computer printouts. Specifically, it is the probability that the results (or a more extreme value) will be produced by chance (sampling fluctuation) under the assumption that the null hypothesis is true (20). A p value is a conditional probability, namely, the probability of data (D) or an outcome of a particular value or more extreme, assuming the null hypothesis (H_0) is true. The p value can be expressed as $P(D/H_0)$.

The outcome of the statistical test is then compared to the worst-case percentile (21) or the maximal risk the researcher is willing to tolerate for falsely rejecting the statistical null hypothesis. The worst-case percentile reflects alpha, or the decision (D^*) to reject the null based on a particular outcome assuming the null hypothesis to be true, and can be expressed as $P(D^*/H_0)$. This decision means the researcher has concluded that some effect exists. The decision will be an error, a Type I error, if and only if the null hypothesis is actually true. Because alpha values are designated prior to data collection under the assumption that the null is true, they are conditional prior probabilities. Using a relative-frequency interpretation of probability, it is clear that alpha is equal to the number of incorrect rejections of the statistical null hypothesis across a series of experiments. Because researchers test both true and false null hypotheses, the actual alpha level, or overall prior probability (20), is less than the nominal level.

The phrase *test of significance* has another implication that has led to misinterpretation. The concept of significance implies that the results are meaningful, important, or large. Examples of this interpretation occur in many articles when results are reported to be *highly* significant (22). This often leads to equating statistical significance with scientific significance (23) and an assumption that there is evidence in support of the research hypothesis (24, 25). In fact, statistical significance is concerned with whether a relationship is big enough that it *needs* explanation, whereas substantive or scientific significance is concerned with whether the relationship is *worth* explaining. It is perhaps for this reason that Kish (23) recommended that TOSS be called tests against the null hypothesis (TANH).

The confusion created by the misinterpretation and misuse of TOSS has lead some researchers to claim that the adoption of TOSS has slowed the rate of knowledge acquisition (24, 25). Others have advocated that behavioral scientists (including biological scientists) abandon TOSS altogether (15, 26). Still others see them as having an important role in theory-corroboration research but

a limited role in descriptive research (27). The reality of the situation is that TOSS are so ingrained in the scientific process that they will continue to be used even if the promises of the method are never fulfilled (28).

So what do TOSS tell the researcher? Statistical significance occurs when the probability is low that a difference in sample means would be this large or larger under the assumption that the null is true. Statistical significance means some effect probably exists and it reflects statistical rareness (15). It can also indicate the direction of the relationship (29). So what do TOSS tell the researcher? They merely gives the researcher permission to proceed and explain a finding.

Misinterpreting Significance Tests

The tendency to equate statistical significance with substantive significance has created misunderstanding and exaggerated claims for TOSS. These claims have resulted in myths and illusions that have been perpetuated by researchers. Carver (15) identified the following three fantasies or myths associated with TOSS: (a) the odds-against-chance fantasy, (b) the reliability fantasy, and (c) the valid-research-hypothesis fantasy.

The level of significance does not tell the researcher the probability of committing a Type I error (20) or that the results are due to chance (15). The null hypothesis represents the probability of all possible hypothetical outcomes of size N. Hence it is associated with sampling errors or chance factors. Researchers are ultimately interested in the truth of hypotheses, and many think that the significance level tells them the probability that the null hypothesis is true given the results of their study; in other words: $P(H_0/D^*)$. This is the conditional posterior probability of having made a Type I error. Although researchers employing classical statistical inference would like to attach a probability statement to this finding, only Bayes' theorem can provide insight into this statement (20, 30), and even then not all researchers support this contention. Alpha, a prior conditional probability ($P[D^*/H_0]$), and the posterior probability of having made a Type I error ($P[H_0/D^*]$) are not algebraically equivalent. Therefore, the truth of the null hypothesis cannot be known through classical statistical techniques.

If two samples were drawn from the same population and the treatment had no effect (Figure 14.1, Situation B), the sample means probably would not be identical but would not differ by more than would be expected due to sampling fluctuations and measurement error. That is, the differences in sample means would be attributed to chance or sampling errors. When statistically significant differences in sample means occur, it is more likely that a treatment effect exists, although a Type I error is possible. Many researchers assume that the decision to "accept" the null means that chance is the only possible explanation. To make this statement would require that we know the probability that the null hypothesis is true given the evidence provided by our study, or $P(H_0/D^*)$. However, as has just been shown, this is a posterior conditional probability and is not appropriate in classical statistics. In reality, the easiest way to fail to reject the null is to underpower the study and then misinterpret the results as being due solely to chance.

The second fantasy is concerned with research reports that summarize the results of TOSS by stating that a significant difference represents a reliable difference (15). The impression is that if the study were repeated, the same results would occur. In fact, replication depends on whether the important variables have been controlled and manipulation occurs in the exact same way when the experiment is repeated. The confusion may come from the fact that the sampling distribution for the summary statistic of interest represents an infinite number of hypothetical replications of the same experiment. Thus, a particular training program may be found to be statistically different from another program, but this result might not be repeated with another population or another instructor. Even though the null hypothesis has been rejected, the study should be replicated before generalizing the results. Although replication has been an important principle in scientific inference, this aspect of behavioral research has been neglected and often discouraged by journal editors and thesis advisors (31, 32).

Finally, the results of TOSS do not automatically validate the researcher's hypothesis (15). This is the result of confusing statistical inference with scientific inference. The researcher is interested in determining if the data supports his or her scientific hypothesis or theory. Statistical significance, however, is associated with the data and not the research hypothesis (33). The rejection of the statistical null hypothesis means that *some* alternative hypothesis is a more likely explanation of the data than the statistical null hypothesis. The statistical and scientific hypotheses are related only in the agricultural model of science (27), that is, when the substantive treatment is used as the experimental manipulation.

In theory-corroboration research, the statistical alternative hypothesis might have little to do with the research or substantive hypothesis of interest (25, p. 824; 34). If the difference between the experimental group and the control group is large enough to reject the null hypothesis, then other plausible rival hypotheses must still be eliminated before support can be given to the specific research hypothesis proposed by the investigator. For the statistician there are only two hypotheses, the statistical null hypothesis and the alternative hypothesis,

but for the scientist there are many potential research hypotheses. The inability to predict specific alternative hypotheses means there exists a wide range of alternative research hypotheses potentially capable of explaining the data. It is illogical to think that all potential values of group differences would support only the researcher's hypothesis. Rejection of the statistical null hypothesis may increase the statistician's belief in the statistical alternative, that some difference exists, but it does little to signal which research alternative is most likely. In fact, some researchers question whether TOSS can be used as evidence for the research hypothesis at all (35). It is only after ruling out other plausible hypotheses and replicating the results in a number of different situations that an increase in confidence may be placed in the research hypothesis (36).

Some researchers compound the valid-research-hypothesis fantasy by extending belief in the hypothesis to belief in the theory. This is accomplished by deducing a hypothesis from a theory. The hypothesis is a proper subset of the theory and can be used to specify an expected outcome. Next, an experiment is set up to provide evidence for the prediction, and if the statistical null is rejected, support for the theory is assumed. TOSS have been used to support both the hypothesis and the theory, and in essence a double hurdle has been jumped (37). The statistical alternative hypothesis has been used not only to invalidly affirm the research hypothesis but to invalidly affirm the theory.

Statistics and Science

The role of TOSS in the method of science is also misunderstood by many researchers. Despite the warnings of philosophers of science, a confirmation bias, confirming theories rather than falsifying them, has become the predominant approach to scientific inquiry in the behavioral sciences (12, 38, 39). The logic behind this approach is to assume that a theory or hypothesis (antecedent) is correct and then generate an expected experimental outcome (consequent). TOSS provide the minor premise in the logical argument (conditional or implicative syllogism) used in theory testing. Therefore, rejection of the statistical null hypothesis provides support for the statistical alternative hypothesis. An assumption is made that this evidence supports the outcome predicted by the theory and thus affirms the consequent. Conceptually the major premise of the conditional argument states that *if* the researcher's theory or hypothesis is true, *then* this expected outcome should result. If the minor premise, results of TOSS, supports the expected outcome, then the conclusion is that the theory is supported. Unfortunately this is an invalid form of logic (5) called affirming the consequent.

The method of science preferred by philosophers of science is modus tollens, denying the consequent (24, 25). In this approach a prediction (consequent) is generated from a theory (antecedent), and if the evidence refutes the prediction, the theory is refuted. This method of doing science is typical of the physical sciences and results in a reasonably rapid acquisition of knowledge and the elimination of inadequate theories (25, 40). This is most easily done by associating the researcher's hypothesis with the null hypothesis and predicting an outcome that cannot occur. If the study produces the value that cannot occur, then the hypothesis is falsified. This is a modified form of modus tollens and results in denying the consequent.

Some researchers have been under the impression that rejecting the statistical null hypothesis constitutes what Popper (12) referred to as falsification. However, Popper advocated falsifying the researcher's hypothesis, not the statistical null. Fisher, who was trained in logic, realized that a valid form of logic could be obtained by falsifying a hypothesis. He created the null hypothesis (the only hypothesis that exists in his approach to statistical inference) for this reason. In the Neyman-Pearson approach to statistical inference, the researcher's hypothesis is associated with the alternative, and the null hypothesis is falsified. Many researchers believe that this weakens our current approach to science, because point null hypotheses can never be true (41, 42) and therefore are thought to be a straw man (21), although not all researchers agree (43).

Many researchers have been confused by the hybrid science of statistics being taught and published in popular textbooks (28). The contributions of Bayes' theorem, Fisher's significance testing, and Neyman-Pearson's decision theory have been combined into an objective, mechanical form of inductive inference that is contrary to symbolic logic and devoid of the contradictions and controversies of these three approaches to statistical inference. Researchers act as if disproving the null (Fisher's term) is evidence of a posterior or inverse probability (Bayes' theorem). Disproving the null is considered a positive result. Failure to disprove the null (accepting the null, Neyman-Pearson's term) is considered a negative result. However, a positive result means that the null hypothesis has been rejected, not that the researcher's hypothesis has been supported. The confusion created by mixing these approaches and ignoring controversies has seriously limited the development of research in the behavioral sciences (28).

Meehl (24) referred to this confusion as a methodological paradox. Research in the behavioral sciences seems to have focused on increasing power and precision to eliminate a weak hypothesis (null hypothesis or straw man) that few believe to be true (see the criticism of the null hypothesis covered earlier) and use the evidence from TOSS to confirm the researcher's hypothesis—whereas, in the physical sciences, increasing the power, control, and precision of experiments increases the risk of refuting theories or hypotheses. It has also been argued that this is an issue of estimation procedures of statistical inference versus significance testing rather than an issue of natural sciences versus behavioral sciences (44).

The practical implication of eliminating weak hypotheses is that behavioral researchers seem to be content to test rather trivial questions, such as, Is exercise better than no exercise? The bias against publishing nonsignificant results (32, 45) has resulted in fewer risks of refutation (25), and some argue that rejection of the null hypothesis merely reflects the size of the sample and the power of the test. Editors of some journals have treated TOSS as a necessary but not sufficient condition for an effect (32, 44, 46). This has supported and perpetuated the confirmation bias approach to research (38) and resulted in the questionable research practices alluded to previously. The rejection of a null hypothesis has a limited role in hypothesis testing and merely answers the question, Is there a big enough relationship here that needs explanation? (23). Whether this *statistically* significant difference is worth explaining is an issue of substantive significance (11) and is not a statistical issue. After all, the purpose of a scientific investigation is to convince the reader that the data support the conclusions of the researcher and could not be supported by other explanations (36).

DESIGN SENSITIVITY

Design sensitivity is the ability of an experimental design to detect true treatment effects, if they exist. In essence, design sensitivity can be equated with the concept of power. Fisher (1) used the term *sensitivity* in much the same way as modern data analysts use the term *power*.

Although researchers are interested in detecting true differences if they exist, they are also concerned with making valid inferences. These two concepts, design sensitivity and validity of inferences, are dealt with in this and the next section. There is a certain reciprocal relation between the two concepts. Lipsey (4) introduced the concept of design sensitivity, which he equated with statistical conclusion validity, as an aspect of internal validity. He treated design sensitivity as the foundation on which valid inferences must be based, and he viewed statistical conclusion validity as an aspect of design sensitivity (p. 12). Cook and Campbell (47) viewed statistical power, another name for design sensitivity, as one of three factors determining covariation (pp.

39-41). First, covariation is equated with establishing statistical conclusion validity, suggesting that in evaluating an experiment the investigator needs to determine if the experiment is sensitive enough to detect covariation. Second, if there is sufficient sensitivity, the investigator determines whether there is evidence to infer that the presumed cause and effect covary. The third factor is the magnitude of the covariation. The first question deals with design sensitivity, the second with statistical conclusion validity, and the third is concerned with practical (rather than statistical) significance. The remainder of this section will focus on design sensitivity as the foundation upon which inferences about TER are built. However, the relationship of design sensitivity to other sources of internal and external validity must not be forgotten.

Designing sensitive TER requires four steps (4). First, the researcher must work from a theory (model) or conceptual framework. Second, the researcher must select one or more optimal outcome measures to reflect any treatment effects. Third, the researcher should specify the effect size the research is designed to detect. Last, the researcher should conduct a power analysis. Because the last three factors are closely tied to the concept of power, they will be covered in a single section.

Conceptual Framework of Fitness

It is the job of the scientist to observe the natural world, develop a model or hypothesis relating the causes and effects of the observation, and then test the model to see if the model is supported by experimental evidence. In short, the scientist seeks to explain natural phenomena by a simplifying model, idea, or construct. Vogel (48) wrote about scientific biological models.

> Explanation requires simplification, and nothing is so un-simple as an organism. And the most immediate sort of simplification is the use of non-living models, whether physical or (even) mathematical.
>
> Science is in fact, utterly addicted to models for simplification and generalization. Even a tiny aspect of the world is just too complex to yield to simultaneous and systematic analysis of all of its diverse characteristics. . . . Simplification and abstraction have marked all progress in science; one begins very simply and then adds elements of complication as necessary and possible. (p.11)

Model or hypothesis development is an early and critical step in the scientific method. A model of natural phenomena is necessary to identify the underlying structure of the natural world, and the research or assessment process. A model is like a jigsaw puzzle, with individual experiments corresponding to the individual elements or pieces of the puzzle. Even the individual elements of the puzzle are smaller-scale models integrated into the whole model. This kind of cascade of models from large to small and back again is inherent in science and in the understanding of the real world. According to the writings of Hutton in 1956, "The model so becomes a link between theory and experiment. We explain and test the theory in terms of the model" (49, p. 116). If research is to be efficient and effective, it must proceed from a model. Each model must be carefully tested, supporting or refuting the overlying structure or larger model. In short, a model is what the investigator tests.

The search for a model of physiological fitness is young and inconclusive. Many research- and assessment-oriented models have been proposed (50-57). A categorization of models was discussed by Lachman (49) and included four types of models: (a) models providing modes of representation, (b) models functioning as rules of inference, (c) models providing interpretation, and (d) models providing pictorial visualization.

An example of a model of representation is the common fitness profile of athletes (58-62). This type of model represents the magnitude of certain fitness characteristics that a group of athletes or students has, and is therefore representational.

An example of an inferential model of fitness is the dose–response relationship of training type and magnitude to fitness qualities attained (63, 64). The inferential model seeks to describe cause-and-effect relationships. This type of model manipulates some variable while observing the effects on another variable. The inferential model provides the rules of what will happen when such a manipulation occurs.

A model of interpretation offers the rules of translation from one form of description or inference to another, such as an analogy. For example, the interpretation of a mathematical formula requires a "key" or "legend" to tell the reader what the symbols mean. An example of an interpretation model in a fitness setting is the classification of fitness in terms of field-test results. Norms and measures of variability can give the investigator a means of interpreting the distribution of scores obtained by translating them to high, medium, or low (or some other scheme of fitness magnitude). The interpretation of test results, qualitative description based on quantitative data, and diagnosis rely on a translation model.

The fourth type of model is one of pictorial visualization, or graphic representation. Graphs and figures of various types are often used to show models of some physiological relationships or relative magnitudes. There are many examples of these models in physiology. For example, a graphic description of a model of energy system contribution to effort has been provided by Fox (65). Fox's model shows how the ATP-PC, anaerobic, and aerobic energy systems blend as a function of performance time and effort adaptation by a simple, but profound, line drawing.

The development or choice of the correct model is much of what underlies science. Inappropriate models have been used in the past, such as lactic acid as a metabolic "poison," muscle fiber types as predictive of athletic potential, and muscle contraction as due to by some pneumatic principle rather than to sliding filaments. Science progresses by the selection and testing of these models. This is followed by acceptance or refutation of various proposed models as theories. Fitness models have been built around the idea of the contribution of different energy systems to performance. Moreover, the prevailing model of fitness implies that fitness is composed of several components. Each of the previous chapters of this book has dealt with individual components of physiological fitness. A possible model for physical fitness, and thus a guide for TER, might consist of the components listed in Table 14.1.

The model in Table 14.1 is proposed as a possible simplified, global model of physiological fitness. Each of the six components is operationally defined. To be a model, the proposed model must be capable of being placed within one of the four categories previously described. This model fits in the representational category and represents fitness as a construct. Each component is also a model, representing a part of the total construct of fitness. The proposed fitness model must also be testable. Can an investigator perform tests on the various

Table 14.1 A Simplified Physical Fitness Model

Fitness parameter	Definition
Strength (alactic isometric)	The peak force or torque developed during a maximal isometric voluntary contraction
Power (alactic isotonic)	The time rate at which mechanical work is performed
Muscular endurance (lactic isotonic)	The ability of a muscle or muscle group to perform repeated contractions against a light load for an extended period of time
Maximal aerobic power	The maximum rate at which energy can be released from the oxidative process exclusively
Flexibility	The range of motion of a joint or a related series of joints
Body composition	The relative content of lean body mass, essential fat mass, and nonessential fat mass

components of the model and determine fitness from nonfitness? One must arbitrarily assign magnitudes of these components as representative of fitness and nonfitness, or one must map the results onto a continuum from low fitness to high fitness.

Current approaches to the assessment of physiological fitness use models such as this. It is not impossible to approach research without the traditional models described earlier (66), but these new models or shifts in paradigms will require model development of their own. It is important to keep the large models of the natural world in mind while reducing problem complexity by approaching smaller, scaled-down models for investigation. The interactions of other knowledge areas and the intrusion of other models on a proposed investigation are profound. The place of the experimental model in the whole of the understanding of a phenomenon must be determined and kept firmly in mind while pursuing experiment size questions. To test these models, sensitive designs must be developed.

Concept of Power

Power is an often-neglected concept in TER. By definition, power is the probability of rejecting the null hypothesis when the null is false (67). In other words, if a treatment effect really exists and you conclude on the basis of your statistical test that a difference this large could not have occurred by chance, assuming the null to be true, then your test has sufficient power. The lack of attention to power is probably the result of an overreliance on the Fisherian approach to significance testing or a lack of understanding of how to specify an exact alternative hypothesis so that the Neyman-Pearson approach can be used (68).

A statistical test that has sufficient power implies that a correct inference has been made. However, not all inferences drawn from statistical tests are without error. The concept of power is most closely associated with beta or Type II error. When a true treatment effect exists but the researcher fails to reject the null hypothesis, a false inference or conclusion has been made. Because TOSS result in binary decisions (reject or fail to reject the null hypothesis) and only two states of nature can exist (null is true or null is false), two errors are possible (see Figure 14.2). However, in any single study only one type of error actually occurs.

Unfortunately, there are no widely accepted values for power as there are with Type I errors (69, 70). Traditionally accepted values of alpha include .05 and .01, although more liberal (e.g., .1) (71, 72) or more conservative (e.g., .001) values are often suggested (73). Acceptable levels of power can be derived from the intuitions of researchers and the fact that power is the

		Status of the null hypothesis in the population	
		Null true	Null false
Researcher's decision based on sample data	Do not reject the null	1 – Alpha Correct decision $P(D-|H_0)$	Beta Type II error $P(D-|H_1)$
	Reject the null	Alpha Type I error $P(D+|H_0)$	1 – Beta Power $P(D+|H_1)$

Figure 14.2   Conditional probabilities of traditional statistical inferences.

complement of Type II errors. Greenwald (45) found that in a survey of 95 authors and reviewers of psychological journals the average satisfactory level for a Type I error was .046 and for a Type II error .274. Several experts (41, 68, 74) have recommended similar values, stating that Type I errors are four times as serious as Type II errors. Therefore, if the researcher typically sets alpha equal to .05, then beta would be .20. Based on this apparent consensus, Cohen (67) has recommended that a minimal standard for power be set at .80.

There are occasions when a different level of power might be acceptable. These levels of power are determined by subtraction after establishing error rates. Some researchers have recommended that error values be selected based on a cost-benefit analysis of the errors. Others have suggested that the purpose of the research might influence error rates and hence the desired level of power.

The consequences of a Type I error would be that an ineffective treatment was falsely concluded to be effective. Clinical technicians and exercise specialists would begin to use a treatment that was actually incapable of enhancing fitness for groups of subjects similar to the original study. This could mean that ineffective equipment might be purchased for training and trainers educated in ineffective methods. Clients exposed to such

a program would suffer from a lack of results and lose their good will toward the specialist. Other researchers might also try to replicate the treatment effects or explore ways to "enhance" the effect by altering treatment dimensions. But what is the cost of this error in terms of financial and human resources? Whatever the costs, they seem sufficient to require that researchers act conservatively.

What are the consequences of a Type II error? In this case, a real treatment effect has been missed. A treatment that can positively affect fitness parameters is abandoned for lack of statistical significance. It is important to remember that the conclusion that the treatment was ineffective is actually an improper conclusion. In fact we cannot conclude that our treatment was effective, just that a difference exists and needs an explanation. If there is an absence of sample differences, we must conclude that we cannot reject the null hypothesis. When Type II errors occur, the potential client suffers the cost if the treatment is effective. Lipsey (4) argued that in TER, Type II errors were just as serious as Type I errors. For this reason he argued that power should be set at .95.

Other researchers (75) have argued that, due to the uncertainty of inductive inferences, data analysts should take a conservative approach to setting error rates. If the purpose of the research is to demonstrate that one program is better than another, based on the research hypothesis, then the researcher must guard against Type I errors. However, when a researcher is trying to confirm a no-difference hypothesis, then Type II errors are more important. Until the cost of Type I and Type II errors can be estimated in behavioral research, it might be best to design experiments for alpha = .05 and power = .80, when testing for differences. The case for testing no-difference hypotheses requires special considerations and will be covered under statistical issues.

Power in Treatment Effectiveness Research

Power is a function of sample size, significance level, and the population effect size (76, 77). Each of these will be discussed in the following paragraphs. After a study has been completed, values for each of these factors exist and the power of the study can be estimated. This is important in TER, especially when the decision has been made not to reject the null (78).

Jacob Cohen (74, 79) was an early proponent of reexamining research in a particular field to discover the power of research reported in a particular discipline. Of the three factors determining power, effect size is probably the least known. An effect size is the degree to which a phenomenon of interest is present in the population (67). In other words, it is an index of the degree of departure from the null hypothesis and is mathematically related to the noncentrality parameter of most test statistics. Cohen (79) arbitrarily defined small, medium, and large effect sizes as .2, .5, and 1.0 standard deviation units (the large effect size was later reduced to .80). That is, a small effect size means that the experimental group was .2 of a standard deviation unit different from the comparison group. He found that in abnormal and social psychology research (70 studies) the statistical power for small, medium, and large effects were .18, .48, and .83, respectively.

Perhaps these results are unique to the social sciences. Levenson (80) found in analyzing 56 studies from two gerontology journals that the power was .37, .88, and .96 for small, medium, and large effect sizes. Reed and Slaichert (78) found power values of .14, .39, and .61 for 355 articles in medicine, whereas Jones and Brewer (81) found power values of .13, .50, and .78 in the *Research Quarterly*, a journal dedicated to exercise science. In fact, Lipsey (4) found, in surveying 14 different disciplines, that research designed to investigate small and medium effects was generally underpowered and that only research designed to detect large effects had sufficient power to detect true differences.

Perhaps small and medium effects are too trivial. After all, .2 of a standard deviation is equivalent to accounting for only 1% of the total variance. However,

the .2 standard deviation unit also represents a 10% difference in success rate between the treatment and comparison groups. Thus, a training program aimed at adherence to increase the training habit might have a 55% success rate compared to another program with only a 45% success rate. Most exercise specialists would consider an additional 10% adherence rate meaningful.

Therefore, it is unlikely that small- and medium-effect-size studies are considered trivial by researchers; of 186 metanalyses reported in Lipsey (4), 77% had effect sizes of greater than .2, whereas only 36% were greater than .5, and only 12% were greater than .8 standard deviation. Because these effect sizes are averaged across many studies, they are probably reasonable estimates of true population effect sizes. Thus, if only large-effect-size studies have sufficient power to show a true difference if one exists, but only 12% of studies examine large effects, then a high percentage of null results would be expected. However, an early review of the psychology literature indicated that only 9% of published articles were null results (82). If only positive results are published, does this support critics of TOSS, who claim that statistical significance is merely a function of sample size, or are journals filled with studies showing Type I errors (83)? On the other hand, the absence of power might suggest that poor design rather than an absence of effect might be the problem.

Power Analysis

All of the authors cited thus far have suggested that researchers conduct a power analysis prior to data collection to avoid underpowered studies. By assuming an appropriate value for power (Cohen suggested .8) and a traditional value of alpha (e.g., .05), and determining or estimating an effect size, sample size can be determined. Sedlmeier and Gigerenzer (84) followed up on the abnormal and social psychology literature 24 years after Cohen's recommendation that researchers conduct power analyses prior to data collection. They found that the median power for a medium effect reported in the *Journal of Abnormal Psychology* had actually dropped from .46 to .37 in the 24 years since Cohen's seminal work. They suggested that this state of affairs was created by a failure to recognize the differences between Fisher's null hypothesis testing and Neyman-Pearson's decision theory. The result, they concluded, has been to combine these two opposing views of data analysis and mix the emphasis on Type I errors (Fisher) with reject–accept decisions (Neyman-Pearson). The typical social research study had a Type II error 11 to 14 times greater than the Type I error. In effect, these studies were underpowered because Type II errors were ignored. The result has been a high percentage of null results being mistakenly accepted as showing no treatment effect.

The similarity of power analyses across disciplines suggests that exercise physiology research is also underpowered and incorrect conclusions, especially negative results, are reached more often than we would like. Sedlmeier and Gigerenzer (84) suggested that this state of affairs will continue until journal editors require estimates of power when significance testing is used. These authors also suggested that focusing decisions solely on statistical significance has taken attention away from other, potentially more important, principles. Specifically, more attention should be given to controlling error before data collection and planning studies to detect a specific effect size.

Thus, power is a function of the effect-size estimator, sample size, and alpha and is indirectly affected by other factors (e.g., reliability of the dependent measure, type of design, procedural variation). The most effective way to increase power, however, is to increase the effect size or increase the sample size. The operating characteristics (85) of effect size and sample size indicate that increases are most effective for low effect sizes (< .8) and low sample size (< 100). Some researchers (86) have suggested increasing alpha to gain power, but this is not very effective. If effect size equals .50 (medium effect size), sample size is 50, and power is .95, then alpha would have to be set to .40 to achieve a sensitive design. This level of alpha would be unacceptable to journal editors. Although altering the probability of a Type I error can have an effect on the power of the statistical test, care should be exercised, because the researcher can choose a level of significance independent of the parameter estimators or sample size, and thus manufacture statistical significance. Some researchers (73) have argued that the Type I error rate should never be raised, but rather an analysis of the importance of Type I and Type II errors should be used to determine power. Although increasing the Type I error rate to a higher level is the least effective method for increasing power (4), the incidence of alpha-adjusted procedures has increased dramatically in recent years (84). This has diverted attention away from more cost-effective strategies for increasing power.

The typical TER study is one with an effect size of .40, a level of significance equal to .05, a sample size (each cell or group) of 40, and power equal to .42. Given this state of affairs, many potentially effective treatments are going undetected. If a fitness study were designed based on these typical figures, and the assumption that Type II errors were just as serious as Type I errors (power equal to .95) were made, then 165 subjects would be needed in both the experimental and the control group to achieve a sensitive design. If Type I errors were considered 4 times as important as Type II errors (alpha = .05 and power = .80), then 100 subjects would be needed in each group. The typical strategy by most researchers is to increase sample size to gain power, but these projected sample sizes are large for a fitness study. If the effect size could be increased to .8 (large effect), then 45 subjects would be needed if power = .95, and 25 subjects for power = .80. With the measurement and monitoring that takes place in a fitness study, 25 subjects per group would be the more desirable situation.

Factors Affecting Design Sensitivity (Power)

Lipsey (4) has identified six factors that affect design sensitivity: effect size, measurement sensitivity, subject heterogeneity, sample size, procedural variation, and the inherent power of the data-analysis procedures employed. Having an appropriate level of power is important in the planning of effective hypothesis-testing procedures. The following sections will deal with these factors and strategies that can be used to optimize design sensitivity.

Effect Size

The power of a statistical test is influenced by the effect-size parameter. In the case of an experimental and control group, the difference in the sample means provides an estimate of the unstandardized effect-size parameter. Because this value would be dependent on the measurement scale of the dependent variable, a standardized effect-size estimate is preferred. Additionally, experimental effects (unstandardized) cannot be compared across studies or even across main effects within a single study (87) unless an index is created. Unfortunately there are many choices of the appropriate metric for effect-size estimates (29, 88).

Cohen (79) was one of the first to use an effect-size estimate. He calculated delta after a study had been completed to determine the power of the statistical test. Glass (89) recommended that delta be used to integrate literature. Although these were landmark studies, Hedges (90) demonstrated that these estimators were biased and that a lack of attention had been given to the distinction between sample estimates and population parameters. For our purposes we will consider the difference between the experimental and control group means divided by the pooled sample standard deviation as an estimate of the population effect size,

$$\Delta = \frac{\mu_t - \mu_c}{\sigma_p}, \tag{1}$$

where Δ is the population effect size, μ_t is the population treatment mean, μ_c is the population control mean, and σ_p is the pooled population standard deviation.

Because the population parameters are not available, sample estimates must be used to calculate a sample effect-size estimate. Specifically,

$$ES_{ai} = \frac{M_t - M_c}{S_p} \qquad (2)$$

where ES_{ai} is the sample, zero-order effect size for independent groups ANOVA; M_t is the sample treatment mean; M_c is the sample control mean; and S_p is the pooled sample standard deviation.

What effect size should be planned for in a study? This is essentially a question of practical significance. How much of an increase in strength or aerobic power, or decrease in total cholesterol or body fat, would be a meaningful change? A variety of approaches has been suggested to arrive at an acceptable value. The three most prominent approaches are the actuarial approach, the statistical translation approach, and the criterion-group contrast approach (4).

The actuarial approach uses the accumulative evidence from similar studies that are available on a topic. The most popular method for this is a metanalysis. Lipsey (4) found that the average effect size for 102 published metanalyses on TER was .45 standard deviation units. This distribution was slightly skewed, but the midpoint of the lower third was .15, the middle third .45, and the upper third .90. These values are close approximations of Cohen's (67) recommendation for small (.2), medium (.5), and large (.8) effect sizes.

Effect sizes in standard deviation units may lack interpretability for some people, or they may seem trivial, as in .2 of a standard deviation. The statistical translation approach converts standardized effect sizes into more interpretable forms. Some researchers may prefer to work with uncorrected units, as Tran did (91) in reporting cholesterol values as unstandardized effect sizes. Thus a 10 mg $\cdot$ dL^{-1} decrease in total cholesterol as a result of exercise is directly understandable. For others a conversion may be necessary; fortunately, effect-size estimators have relatively direct mathematical transformations to other indicators. Many researchers are familiar with the concept of percent variance accounted for. The conversion between effect size and percent variance is quite simple, namely:

$$PV = \frac{ES^2}{ES^2 + 4} \qquad (3)$$

where PV is the percent variance accounted for, and ES is the sample effect size. The effect size can also be estimated from a known percent variance estimator, specifically:

$$ES = \sqrt{\frac{4(PV)}{(1 - PV)}} \qquad (4)$$

Thus a medium effect size, .5, corresponds to 6% of the variance in the outcome variable being accounted for by the treatment. The apparently modest effect size of .5 appears to be a miniscule 6% of the variance. Percent variance seemed to underestimate the effectiveness of TER, and this convinced Rosenthal and Rubin (92) to look for other indicators of meaningful effects. Their approach was to provide an estimate of success rate (also, cure rate, improvement rate, etc.). They developed a binomial effect-size display (BESD), which showed the improved success rate of the treatment group relative to the grand median. When the effect size (.5) that accounted for 6% of the variance in the previous example is converted to a BESD, a 24% difference in success rate (treatment = .62 vs. control = .38) is revealed.

The third approach recommended by Lipsey (4) was the criterion-group contrast approach, which utilizes two groups that are known to differ on a variable of interest. A group of fit athletes could be compared to a normal population, or preseason fitness levels could be compared to end-of-season fitness levels, to estimate effect size.

Measurement Sensitivity

The sensitivity of outcome measures can also affect effect-size estimates. Often there is a choice among different measures. Both the selection of the measure and the administration of the measure can affect effect size. Factors such as the measurement scale, type of instrument construction (norm-referenced or criterion-referenced), sensitivity to measuring change, reliability, uniformity of administration, and motivational strategies will all affect effect size (4). These measurement factors bring about their effects by altering the variability of the study.

The effect-size parameter is influenced by the dependent measure used in TER. Some aspects of the measurement process affect the numerator of the effect-size parameter and other aspects affect the denominator (see Equation 2). It is important to understand which aspect is affected so that strategies can be employed to increase the operative effect size of a study.

The ideal dependent measure is one that is maximally responsive to changes attributable to the treatment and minimally responsive to everything else. This quality in a measure is called sensitivity (4). In addition, measures must be valid (93) but, more importantly, capable of validly measuring change. Finally, outcome measures must be reliable (94).

To ensure that the outcome variables are sensitive, valid, and reliable, the following four steps should be observed: (a) identify the expected changes; (b) identify the potential outcome measures; (c) conduct a measurement assessment study; and (d) select the optimal measure or measures (4).

Prior to collecting data for a study, a measurement assessment study (95) should be conducted. The purpose of a measurement assessment study is to select the most appropriate measure or to identify adjustments that will optimize the operative effect size. A pilot study using a criterion-group contrast could be used to measure potential outcome variables. In some cases multiple measures (e.g., Wingate anaerobic test, Margaria-Kalamen, vertical jump) could be used, and in other cases multiple criterion scores or outcome scores from the same test may be possible (e.g., liters, milliliters per kilogram, milliliters per kilogram of lean body mass). By measuring two groups on all alternatives and comparing the effect size obtained, the most effective criterion measure can be selected.

In some cases alternative methods have been suggested to collect data, such as the force to be used in the Wingate Anaerobic Test. Although the standard procedure is to use 0.075 kp · kg^{-1}, values up to 0.10 kp · kg^{-1} have been investigated (96). Testing subjects comparable to those to be investigated in the study will allow an effect size to be generated, and the protocol producing the largest effect size can be selected.

The sensitivity of the measure can also be affected by the scaling of the measure. Categorically scaled measures have less power than graduated tests, and measurement artifacts such as ceilings or floors can limit the sensitivity of outcome measures.

In addition to the selection or modification of the outcome variable to optimize the operative effect size, the psychometric properties of the criterion measure can influence the power of the statistical test. Concern should be directed toward both the validity and the reliability of the outcome measure. Although the validity of a measure is the most important property of an outcome measure in TER (97), a valid measure of change is a more important concept (4). Validity is a function of both reliability and relevance (98). Relevance is concerned with the degree of agreement between what a test measures and the function it is intended to measure. Reliability, on the other hand, reflects the degree of measurement error. Errors in measurement are a product of inconsistency in performance. In assessments of changes in behavior as a result of a training program, variations in scores can result from differences between people (subject heterogeneity) or variations due to characteristics unrelated to the phenomena of interest (measurement error). It is important to identify which source of variation is responsible for variation in scores.

Measurement error or noise in the data can be the result of random variation due to the subjects, situational factors, the evaluator, or the instrument (94). Individual variation on multiple trials of a fitness test might be due to changes in motivation or concentration. Situational factors might include the psychological climate created to produce maximal efforts or the physical climate of the testing facility. Poorly or improperly trained technicians and poor record keeping can be sources of random error variation, which is attributable to the evaluator. Last, electronic and mechanical equipment can behave erratically and contribute to random errors due to instruments. Identifying these different sources of error and their relative contribution to the unreliability of measurements is the purpose of generalizability theory (99). By understanding the types of errors inherent in a particular measurement, attempts can be made to minimize the error, select among a number of alternative measures the one with the least error, or alter one's decisions in light of the error (100).

Variation in measures can also be attributed to subject heterogeneity. With respect to fitness parameters, people are inherently different on these measures. It is useful to know if the variations in your data are a function of subject heterogeneity or measurement error. The strategies that might be used to reduce score variation depend on knowing to which source to attribute the variation. Variation between subjects is maximized in test construction when norm-referenced measurement models are used, whereas criterion-referenced models maximize the measurement of change (4). Thus, in the selection or construction of a fitness measure, some attention must be given to the underlying measurement model and the purpose of the assessment.

The reliability of your measurements will influence the effect-size estimator and thus the power of your statistical test. In general, when reliability is reduced, the power of the statistical test is decreased. However, some controversy exists concerning the apparent paradoxical relationship between reliability and power (101-103). This issue is especially relevant to physical fitness assessment, because often multiple trials are used to collect data and only a subset of the scores are used in the data analysis, without consideration for the effect on reliability. Another problem is the fact that in many investigations, reliability information about the tests used is not reported. Thus, it is important to understand how reliability affects the statistical power of a test and what are the best strategies for maximizing reliability. (For example, if multiple trials are used to measure handgrip strength, should you use the best value or an average? Or when multiple measurements are taken to determine an underwater weight, how should the criterion score be determined?)

Understanding the relationship between reliability and power requires understanding the relationship between significance tests and classical test theory (104). Most of the current measures of fitness parameters were developed using classical test theory, or psychometrics. That is, decisions concerning testing protocol were made based on a need to maximize differences between people. Under this measurement theory, reliability is defined as the ratio of true score variance to observed score variance. The individual-difference model of classical test theory can be expressed as

$$\sigma_X^2 = \sigma_T^2 + \sigma_E^2 \qquad (5)$$

where σ_X^2 is the observed score variance, σ_T^2 is the true score variance, and σ_E^2 is the error score variance. With this model, reliability is defined as

$$\rho_{tt} = \frac{\sigma_T^2}{\sigma_X^2} \text{ or } \frac{\sigma_T^2}{\sigma_T^2 + \sigma_E^2} \qquad (6)$$

where ρ_{tt} is the reliability coefficient. Thus, any factor (e.g., subject, situation) that adds error to the outcome measure will increase the denominator of the reliability coefficient relative to the true score variance and therefore decrease the reliability coefficient.

The power of a statistical test, however, is a decreasing function of the observed score variance (104). In significance testing, if subjects within a group all differ initially on the outcome measure and do not respond to the treatment in exactly the same manner, this fact is treated as error. This increased error becomes part of the denominator of the standardized effect-size estimator (see Equation 2) and thus decreases power. Because observed score variance is the sum of both true score variance and error score variance, either can reduce power. However, these two sources have different effects on reliability.

If it were assumed that the true score variance is constant, then the power of a statistical test is an increasing function of the reliability of the test, because the error component becomes smaller. Whereas, if the error variance of a test is assumed constant (same tester, same time of day, etc.), then power is a decreasing function of reliability, because the true score must increase, thus increasing subject heterogeneity (104). For this reason it is important to identify the source of variation in potential outcome measures (4).

The issue of reliability becomes especially important in the typical TER study that utilizes a pretest–posttest control group design. The measurement of change and the additive effect of measurement errors has a long (105) and continuing history (106) in the field. It is also somewhat controversial (107, 108). The consensus, however, is that unreliable measures accumulate errors when change scores are analyzed. Thus, researchers should try to select measures with high reliability or maximize the reliability of the measures they are using.

An extension of classical test theory is generalizability theory, which can be used to identify the sources of variation in outcome measurements. Although the foundational work for generalizability theory (109, 110)

has existed for nearly 30 years, there has been a noticeable lack of its application in motor behavior research. Simplified introductions can be found to guide the novice researcher (99, 100, 111).

One application of generalizability theory that is appropriate to the topic of this paper concerns the sources of error in taking skinfold measurements. Skinfolds are generally regarded as being less reliable and less valid than hydrostatic weighing. Thus all attempts should be made to minimize sources of error when obtaining skinfold measures. Three potential sources for error are testers, instruments, and number of trials. To assess the relative contribution of these factors to measurement error, Morrow, Fridye, and Monaghen (112) conducted a generalizability study.

Morrow, Fridye, and Monaghen (112) utilized the *AAHPERD Health Related Physical Fitness Test Manual* (181) procedures to measure the skinfold thicknesses of boys and girls from a single middle school. They measured both subscapular and triceps sites on the boys and triceps only on the girls. They were interested in the facets of testers, instruments, and trials, and in the interactions of these three facets. The tester facet was composed of two inexperienced testers, who had read the manual and had 20 min of training, and one experienced tester. Two relatively expensive calipers and one inexpensive caliper represented the instrument facet. Finally, all measures were taken three times, thus resulting in 54 measures on the boys and 27 on the girls. The sources of variation were reported by gender and site.

By far the greatest proportion of variance was accounted for by subject heterogeneity. The girls' triceps measures accounted for 66.2% of the variance, for the lowest value, and the boys' subscapular measures were highest at 83.2%. Thus, in the measurement of skinfold thicknesses, subject heterogeneity will be the largest source of variation in outcome measures. The testers accounted for between 0.5% and 12.4%, the instruments accounted for 7.1% to 14.2%, and trials were virtually zero for all conditions. The interactions collectively accounted for 5.9% to 9.0% of the total variation. It can be concluded from this study that measurement error, relative to subject heterogeneity, is a relatively minor issue in the measurement of skinfold thicknesses. However, in the measurement of girls' triceps skinfolds, testers, instruments, and the tester-by-instrument interaction can collectively account for 30% of the total variation. Thus, errors in measurement will be held to a minimum by using a single tester, and by using the same calipers for both the pretest and the posttest measurements. Assuming a constant true score, this reduction in errors of measurement will increase reliability and, by reducing observed score variance, increase power.

The implication of this study is that similar generalizability studies need to be completed on other measurement techniques for fitness parameters. Additionally, there may be facets other than testers, instruments, and trials that need to be explored when measuring fitness parameters. For instance, in the measurement of maximal aerobic power, what proportion of the total variation is due to different protocols? What proportion is due to variation across days or occasions? What proportion is due to procedural variations, such as 1-min versus 2-min stages, 1° versus 2° increments in elevation, or verbal encouragement versus none? Quantitative data concerning these issues could help in determining what facets of tests would be likely candidates for modification. If modification is not possible, special concern should be given to ensure that standardized protocols are followed. When generalizability and measurement assessment studies are conducted to determine the most sensitive measures the operative effect size of TER can be enhanced.

If the appropriate measurement studies are conducted, the source of variation can be identified as being due to subject heterogeneity (true score) or measurement error. Subject heterogeneity can be reduced by using criterion-referenced tests, which minimize individual differences but maximize within-individual change, or by removing differences statistically by blocking, analysis of covariance, or repeated measures. These procedures will be described in the next section. Reducing measurement error is principally a function of procedural control. Thus, the uniform administration of tests can reduce measurement error. Additionally, averaging scores will enhance reliability (103, 113, 114). The effect will be to increase the operative effect size of a study and thus increase power.

Subject Heterogeneity

In many cases the largest source of variation in the outcome measures will be due to subject heterogeneity. In these cases statistical control is generally the best way to increase the operative effect size. Because the denominator of the effect-size estimator (observed variance from reliability theory) is composed of variation due to both subjects and measurement error (see Equation 6), this section will focus on eliminating sources of variability that might be systematic, therefore contained in true score variance, but irrelevant to the treatment. Several examples common to fitness research can be suggested. Many training studies in the fitness area include both men and women in the treatment and control groups. Additionally, many training studies have a rather wide range of ages within a study, even though age may be correlated to the outcome measure of interest. The variables of gender and age are being used only

as illustrations of what irrelevant or nuisance variables can do to the power of a study. Researchers doing TER must be ever vigilant for extraneous variables that can compromise the expected effect size of a study by creating variation due to subject heterogeneity.

If the hypothetical study mentioned in the previous paragraph had been completed in a field setting, perhaps at a fitness center, it would not be unusual to have both men and women in the study. Suppose our interest is in the effectiveness of the training programs in enhancing oxygen uptake—the gender of the participants would be irrelevant to the purpose of the study. An appropriate method to control for the extraneous variable of gender would be to block on gender.

Because we do not want to miss an effective treatment if one exists, assume that a Type II error is just as detrimental as a Type I error. Therefore, the desired level of power will be set at .95, with alpha equal to .05. If the zero-order effect size were .40, then 160 subjects would be needed in each group of the study. Sparling (115) found, in a meta-analysis of 15 studies that examined the issue of gender and oxygen uptake, that the point biserial correlation between gender and oxygen uptake expressed relative to body weight was .70. On the average, males had maximum oxygen uptake values that were 28% higher than females, and thus gender accounted for 49% of the variance in oxygen uptake.

It can be shown that the effect size for the blocking design can be corrected for the variance accounted for by the gender factor. Specifically,

$$ES_{ab} = \frac{M_t - M_c}{S_p\sqrt{1 - PV_b}} = \frac{ES_{ai}}{\sqrt{1 - PV_b}} \qquad (7)$$

where ES_{ab} is the effect size, ANOVA, blocking variable; and, PV_b is the percent of variance accounted for by the blocking variable. Thus, the zero-order effect size is .40, but the adjusted effect size is .56. Using the same parameters as before, the redesigned study would require only 90 subjects in each treatment group. If the sample size had remained at 40, then power would have approached .70. Although 90 subjects is still a considerable number, it is a reasonably large reduction for very little cost. Depending on the distribution of male and female clients coming to the fitness center, a modest number of subjects will have to be excluded from the study until the number of males and females is equal in both groups. Also, for each blocking variable, 1 degree of freedom is lost from the error term.

If an extraneous variable is identified that is a continuous variable, then the more effective strategy of controlling variance, analysis of covariance, can be used. An analysis of covariance has been shown to be the most effective method of controlling variance if data on the concomitant variable exists for all subjects and if the relationship of the concomitant variable to the outcome variable is linear (116).

An example of a continuous variable that correlates with oxygen uptake is age. The relationship is linear when viewed over a period of years. Brooks and Fahey (52) reported the correlations to be −.77 in trained men and −.42 in sedentary men between the ages of 35 and 70. It is not uncommon to have a range of 10 or 20 years in a TER study. The correction in the operative effect size for a covariate is very similar to a blocking variable. Specifically,

$$ES_{ac} = \frac{M_t - M_c}{S_p\sqrt{1 - r^2}} = \frac{ES_{ai}}{\sqrt{1 - r_{co}^2}} \qquad (8)$$

where ES_{ac} is the effect size, ANOVA, covariate; and r_{co}^2 is the coefficient of determination between the covariate and the outcome variable. Assuming a best-case scenario, $r = -.77$, the operative effect size would be increased from .40 to .63. In this situation, fewer than 70 subjects would be needed in each group. Or if there were 40 subjects in both groups, the power of the test would be .79 or approximately equal to Cohen's (67) recommended minimal level. The gain in operative effect size is offset by the loss of 1 degree of freedom for each covariate and the fact that only the linear component of the concomitant variable and dependent variable relationship is accounted for.

If both methods of control could be used, even greater rewards could be obtained. Using a hypothetical but more realistic example, assume that gender correlated .7 with milliliters of oxygen consumed per kilogram of body weight and, in a more restricted age range, the linear correlation between age and oxygen consumption was −.6. The operative effect size of the 2 × 2 ANCOVA would be .79. In this case only 42 subjects would be needed in each group. In this hypothetical example, with relatively little work, the typical TER study ($ES = .40$, alpha = .05, sample size = 40) can be redesigned to enhance power to .95 to permit the discovery of a true treatment effect if one exists. If power equal to .80 were deemed sufficient, then only 25 subjects would be needed in each group.

Typically the hypothetical study described above would be a pretest–posttest control group design, and ANCOVA would generally be the recommended analysis (117). Additional details on this analysis will be covered in a later section.

The ultimate strategy for controlling variation due to subject heterogeneity would be to let each subject serve as her or his own control (4). However, in a training study this would not be feasible, due to asymmetric transfer effects (118, 119). The next best thing would be to match subjects on one or more variables to produce homogeneous groups of subjects. The advantage gained by matched pairs or the subject's serving as his or her own control is that blocking occurs on many dimensions. With matched pairs, the issue is covariance and not the ability to predict the variance in the dependent variable accounted for by the independent variable (120). Therefore, the operative effect size is:

$$ES_{ap} = \frac{M_t - M_c}{S_p\sqrt{1 - r}} = \frac{ES_{ai}}{\sqrt{1 - r}} \qquad (9)$$

where ES_{ap} is the effect size, ANOVA, matched pair variable; and r is the correlation between matched pairs on the outcome variable of interest. Thus, in the case of repeated-measures designs, the correlation between treatment conditions becomes the coefficient of determination (4). Therefore a correlation of .8, typical of repeated measures or matched pairs, converts the operative effect size from .4 to .9.

Controlling variance due to subject heterogeneity is an often-overlooked strategy in TER. Because increasing effect size is the most cost-effective method of increasing power, more attention should be given to identifying concomitant variables and design alternatives that can increase the effect-size estimator.

Sample Size

Most researchers try to increase the power of their statistical tests by increasing sample size. However, this strategy can be very expensive. Because the typical TER study has a modest effect size, 100 or more subjects may be needed in each group of a study. The resources needed to test and monitor all of these subjects can be enormous. The researcher would be better off trying to increase power by selecting appropriate measurements, controlling variance, and preserving the integrity of the treatments (4). This will result in reasonably large effect sizes and thus modest sample-size requirements to attain appropriate levels of power.

Procedural Variation

Because the focus of this textbook has been on the measurement and interpretation of physical fitness parameters, only a few comments will be made concerning the treatment dimension of TER. The power of the statistical test will be affected by the dose-response function, the timing of the assessment, the strength and integrity of the treatment implementation, and the type of comparison created.

To determine whether a particular treatment program can bring about a change in fitness, some knowledge of the expected change must exist. This is called the dose-response function (4). This function depends on adequate operationalization of constructs. In other words, what particular aspect of fitness is the treatment likely to affect? And what dimensions of the treatment effect the response? Finally, what is the nature of the relationship expected between the treatment and the physical fitness parameter (dose-response function)? A negatively accelerated function would show substantial changes fairly early in a treatment, whereas a positively accelerated function would require a strong treatment over a longer period of time. A step function would require that the dose be strong enough to reach the threshold for change or a false conclusion could be reached. This points to the importance of working from a conceptual framework, as discussed earlier in this paper.

Two problems concerning procedural variation confront the researcher trying to do TER in the domain of physical fitness. First, generally not enough is known about the dose-response function to make intelligent design decisions when investigating new training systems. The researcher is confronted with the need to optimize decisions to maximize power while doing research to determine the optimal conditions. Second, most fitness research will involve multiple indicators of fitness behavior, each with its own dose-response function. Thus design decisions can only be a compromise.

Much of the physical fitness research is conducted in field settings, and thus the strength and integrity of the treatments will greatly affect the power of the statistical tests (121). Strength of treatment is the a priori likelihood that appropriate treatment dimensions are manipulated to bring about change (experienced exercise specialist vs. novice, 16 weeks vs. 8 weeks, etc.), whereas integrity is whether the treatment is implemented as intended (122). Decisions about strength of treatment are made prior to research and do not vary once the study begins. The integrity of the treatment, however, is another matter.

Nonuniform implementation of treatment creates another source of variation in the subjects. Even when treatment is uniformly implemented, individual differences in subject responses are expected and treated as error. Therefore a lack of standardization in treatment implementations will increase subject heterogeneity, increase error, and lower power. Cook and Poole (121) have suggested that the degree of treatment implementation be measured and included in the study, possibly as a covariate. However, this strategy has been criticized by Mark (123). Although it may increase power, it is also likely to decrease internal validity.

The power of a statistical test is a function of alpha, sample size, and effect size. The greater the variation created in the treatment contrast, the larger the expected difference between sample means. Kerlinger (9) was an early proponent of maximizing the differences between the treatment and control conditions. As an example, if

we were interested in the influence of frequency of training on a specific fitness parameter, we might choose to compare 5 or 6 days per week against none. Certainly this will maximize the variance of the substantive variable and ensure maximal power. However, knowing that exercising nearly every day is better than not exercising is of little practical value. Thus, the researcher must balance the need for power (4) with the need to subject hypotheses to theoretical risks (25). In other words, power is maximized as the treatment and comparison are more unlike one another, but generally knowledge increases as the treatment is placed in greatest jeopardy of refutation.

The largest effect size can be expected when a no-treatment control group is used. An alternative would be to use a traditional training program plus an additional feature. Another design configuration would be to compare a new or innovative program to a traditional training program. The last two designs would have smaller effect sizes and thus require larger samples to achieve acceptable power.

Statistical Design

The five factors we described for increasing power can all be incorporated into the statistical data-analysis techniques. In a simple two-group study comparing differences in sample means, an independent t ratio would be used to test for differences:

$$t_{(a, df)} = \frac{M_t - M_c}{S_p \sqrt{1/n_t + 1/n_c}} \qquad (10)$$

As the differences between the group means increases (uncorrected effect size), the size of the t ratio increases, assuming a constant denominator. Conversely, as the standard error of the mean difference increases (subject heterogeneity, procedural variation), assuming a constant numerator, the t ratio decreases. With a little mathematical manipulation, it can be shown that

$$t_{(\alpha, df)} = \frac{\dfrac{M_t - M_c}{S_p}}{\sqrt{\dfrac{1}{n_t} + \dfrac{1}{n_c}}} \text{ or } \frac{ES_{ai}}{\sqrt{\dfrac{1}{n_t} + \dfrac{1}{n_c}}} \qquad (11)$$

In other words, the size of the t ratio is directly proportional to the effect-size estimate, and as sample size increases the denominator decreases, thus increasing the size of the t ratio and enhancing the probability of exceeding the critical t value (4).

Therefore, sensitive designs can be achieved by increasing the effect size, increasing sample size, or altering alpha (one-tail rather than two-tail test). Each of these strategies is suggested by the revised formulation of the *t* ratio. Additionally, because the effect-size estimator is a ratio of between-group variability to within-group variability, other strategies for enhancing the power of a statistical test should be evident.

Summary

The preceding pages have described the factors related to design sensitivity. Many of the strategies that were suggested to maximize power concerned design issues (e.g., enhancing effect size, choosing sensitive measures, standardizing procedures), but the role of the data-analysis procedure cannot be ignored. Therefore the concepts of design sensitivity and statistical conclusion validity are highly related and overlapping. The role of hypothesis testing is critical to both of these concepts (4, 124). However, the appropriate analysis of a sensitive design is not an end in itself. The conclusions or inferences that you make based on the data from a study, require that you are able to say that *X* and *Y* covary (statistical-conclusion validity) or that you have sufficient power to show a difference if one truly exists (design sensitivity). TOSS rule out few plausible rival hypotheses and merely give you permission to try to exclude other explanations (125). In other words, once you are sure you have statistical conclusion validity, you must move on to internal validity, construct validity, population validity, and ecological validity before finalizing your conclusions.

INTERNAL AND EXTERNAL VALIDITY

A concern for all researchers is the appropriateness of the scientific inferences that they are making based on their data. In fact, the ultimate goal of research is to persuade the reader that the findings of a study are believable (126). To do this, alternative plausible rival hypotheses must be eliminated so that the researcher's scientific hypothesis is clearly the best explanation for the data. A variety of sources of invalid inferences were first identified by Donald Campbell (127) and then popularized in a monograph published by Campbell and Stanley (6). The validity of inferences was initially judged by two criteria: internal and external validity. The appropriateness of inferences (internal validity) is first judged by asking whether the treatment made a difference in the outcome variable, whereas external validity is concerned with generalizing results to other populations, settings, and variables.

Campbell and Stanley (6) considered internal validity to be the sine qua non of research and external validity

to be never completely answerable. In addition to identifying these broad categories by which experimental and quasi-experimental inferences could be misinterpreted, they identified 12 threats to valid inferences and demonstrated how each potentially affected 16 experimental designs. The majority (8) of these threats jeopardized the internal validity of these designs. This apparent underrepresentation of external validity stimulated Bracht and Glass (128) to identify 12 threats to external validity. Their attempt was not to criticize but merely to extend the earlier work of Campbell and Stanley (6). Nor were Bracht and Glass alone.

Campbell (124, 129, 130) also worked to extend his earlier work. In part, this work was in response to the increased use of quasi experimentation. Campbell added the threat of instability as a source of internal invalidity, in large part as a response to critics of significance testing. By instability, Campbell meant drawing false conclusions concerning population parameters from unstable sample data. In addition, Campbell (124) added three more sources of external invalidity. Campbell (130) also turned his attention toward strategies for eliminating various threats to valid inferences. As the list of possible threats increased, the complexity of identifying how they adversely affected various designs also increased.

Due to this complexity, researchers began to partition the sources of invalidity into smaller components. Kerlinger (9) (having received a prepublication copy of Campbell and Stanley's classic monograph) partitioned external validity into variable representativeness, sample generalizability, and ecological representativeness. Bracht and Glass (128) had also partitioned external validity into population validity and ecological validity. But perhaps the most refined attempt to partition validity into more specific components was the work of Cook and Campbell (47).

They used Campbell and Stanley's original concept of internal validity and partitioned it into statistical conclusion validity and internal validity. They then partitioned external validity into construct validity and external validity. An excellent example of how threats to TER might appear in a typical research article is provided by Mahoney (5).

Statistical Conclusion Validity

This threat is concerned with whether the treatment and outcome covary and is highly related to design sensitivity. Statistical evidence is needed to make inferences about covariation, and the major threats to invalidity are low statistical power, unreliable outcome measures, and heterogeneity of respondents. Each of these topics was covered in earlier sections of this paper, and strategies to overcome these weaknesses were offered.

Internal Validity

The interpretation of a study can go wrong if the presence or absence of covariation is falsely interpreted. However, once the existence of covariation is accurately established, the next step is to demonstrate that the operationally defined treatment was the cause of the operationally defined outcome. In essence this means that the existence of plausible rival hypotheses, that is, the existence of third variables, must be ruled out. Cook and Campbell (47) referred to establishing causal relationships and their direction as internal validity. The existence of plausible third variables is normally thought to result in false positive conclusions, that is, incorrectly interpreting covariation in the outcome variable to the treatment. But false negative conclusions can also occur, as when a third variable has an opposite but equal effect on the outcome variable relative to the treatment. Collectively, statistical conclusion validity (7 threats) and internal validity (12 threats) correspond to Campbell and Stanley's (6) conceptualization of internal validity.

Most threats to internal validity can be accounted for by randomization (47). However, threats such as imitation of treatment, compensatory equalization or rivalry by respondents, and resentful demoralization cannot be eliminated by randomization. Many fitness-training studies are likely to be quasi-experimental research because subjects are not randomly assigned to treatments or, even with random assignment, subjects are likely to drop out of long training studies. Therefore, the most serious threats to the internal validity of fitness research are differential selection of subjects and subject attrition. Additionally, because of the pretest–posttest nature of the typical fitness study and the intensive reliance on electronic equipment, history, testing, and instrumentation are other likely sources of threats to valid inferences.

Construct Validity

Kerlinger (9) was an early proponent of the concept of variable representativeness. Two issues are involved here. First, to what other treatments or measures of the outcome can we generalize our results? Second, to what theoretical construct can we generalize?

Although internal validity is concerned with establishing causal relationships with operationally defined variables, construct validity is concerned with the fit between these operationally defined variables and the constructs they are meant to represent. Cook and Campbell (47) referred to this source of invalidity as construct validity.

Specific threats to construct validity generally result from construct underrepresentation or surplus construct irrelevancies. Construct underrepresentation results when operationally defined variables fail to incorporate all dimensions of a construct. Surplus construct irrelevancies result from the inclusion of irrelevant dimensions in operationally defined variables. The result of construct invalidity is confounding. That is, although the investigator might propose that theoretical construct A caused theoretical construct B, another person might propose that X caused B, or A caused Y, or even that X caused Y. A classical example of a threat to construct validity is the placebo effect. Does a treatment work because of the exercise specialist's concern, the program's effect, or the client's belief that the program will work? There are a number of other threats to construct validity that cannot all be discussed in this chapter.

Population Validity

Perhaps the threat to valid inference easiest to understand is population validity. Bracht and Glass (128) stressed the difference between a target population and an accessible population. The experimentally accessible population is the group of subjects who are available for possible participation in the study, whereas the target population is the group to which the investigator would like to generalize her or his conclusions. When probability sampling has been used, then generalizing from a sample to the accessible population is straightforward. However, generalization to the target population is based on logic and a knowledge of characteristics of both the accessible and the target populations.

Cook and Campbell (47) in their treatment of external validity stressed the difference between generalizing to and generalizing across a target population. Generalizing to a target population depends on identifying a population, appropriately sampling experimental units, and then accounting for sampling error before making conclusions. Generalizing across a target population is concerned with subpopulations (e.g., gender, age groups, fitness levels) that might be disproportionate in your sample. Thus, will a training program that is effective for males be effective for females? Will what works for fit subjects work for the unfit? These questions refer to the second threat, namely, aptitude-treatment interaction.

Ecological Validity

Because research is often conducted in rather artificial settings, the issue of generalizing across settings often arises. The experimental environment can raise issues concerning the experimenter, the setting, and the time of measurement. For these reasons, Bracht and Glass (128) referred to this threat as ecological validity. In fitness research the most likely sources of ecological invalidity are failure to describe the treatment so that it can be replicated, reactive effects (e.g., Hawthorne effect, placebo effect), experimenter effects, and sensitization effects.

Summary

Although it may be useful to partition threats to valid inferences into smaller components, it is perhaps easier to return to Campbell and Stanley's (6) original formulation to understand the relationship between internal and external validity. Just as Type I and Type II errors oppose one another, internal and external validity appear to be on opposite ends of a seesaw. Strategies that will maximize the internal validity of an experiment (increase control) will be a detriment to external validity. Thus, whereas statistical conclusion validity and internal validity are concerned with establishing causal relationships, construct and external validity specify the contingencies on which these causal relationships depend (47).

Although these categories of valid inferences have a countervailing relationship with one another, it is necessary to assign a priority. The type of research, basic or applied, will be a factor in assigning priority. But by the very nature of the purpose of experiments—investigating causal hypotheses—priority must be given to internal validity. Cook and Campbell (47) hypothesized that the theoretical researcher would order the validity types as internal, construct, statistical conclusion, and external validity. On the other hand, the applied researcher would order them internal, external, construct for the effect, statistical conclusion, and construct for the cause. The importance of internal validity is clear, as it appears first no matter what type of research is conducted. Also, the reduced priority given statistical conclusion validity is very apparent. These validity distinctions are not always supported by all researchers. In fact, proponents of these major threats to valid inferences have shifted terminology and the placement of particular threats over the years. New and related concepts have also been developed.

The effectiveness of a particular treatment for enhancing physical fitness will enhance internal validity if subjects are randomly assigned to groups and groups are treated similarly except for the treatment for the experimental group. Construct validity will be less of an issue if careful thought is given to the operationalization of the treatment and if the outcome variables adequately represent the construct of interest. Finally, external validity will exist if careful thought is given

to sampling and to what settings and times are to be generalized. Yet the research needs to be sensitive before issues of validity can be considered.

STATISTICAL ISSUES

Any one chapter on statistical procedures in fitness assessment cannot hope to cover all topics. Because this chapter is focused on design sensitivity and validity of inferences, a few important issues have been left out. First, because the typical TER study in the fitness field will probably involve a pretest–posttest control group design, we would like to raise some issues concerning the appropriate analysis of such designs. Second, most conceptions of fitness regard fitness as multidimensional. Thus the issue of univariate versus multivariate analysis is likely to be raised. Third, assessments of the bioequivalence of different interventions have inappropriately relied on standard significance testing procedures, and alternative strategies are offered. Finally, during the last 3 decades there has been a growing dissatisfaction with hypothesis testing. Alternatives, such as estimating the magnitude of an effect and confidence intervals, have been suggested. Supporters of these alternative strategies have argued that practical significance is a greater concern than statistical significance. Therefore, a few brief comments will be made concerning the role of hypothesis testing in TER.

Analyzing Pretest–Posttest Designs

The simplest pretest–posttest control group design would be a treatment and control group as the between-subject factor and a pretest and posttest as the within-subject factor (see Figure 14.1). There would also be an interaction of group and time, according to most conceptions of the general linear model (131, p. 519). However, this generally accepted model is flawed (117). Subjects are typically assigned to groups after the pretest but before the treatment. The treatment cannot interact with the pretest, but when the variance components for the main effect of treatment are decomposed, the treatment effect is "spread out" over the two trials (pretest and posttest). The result is that the main effect for treatment is too conservative and results in an inflated Type II error.

Another confusing aspect of the pretest–posttest analysis is that it is actually the interaction between the groups and time that reflects the effectiveness of the treatment. If the subjects are randomly assigned to groups, then there should be no initial differences. A test of posttest scores should reflect only treatment differences. However, Hendrix, Carter, and Hintze (132) warned that this analysis would be inappropriate for factors in which random assignment did not occur or could not occur.

The realization that the interaction *F* ratio is the substantive component of the analysis does not solve all of the problems. Most researchers follow up significant interactions with tests of simple main effects or pairwise post hoc procedures. Unfortunately both strategies are likely to result in misinterpretations (117). There are at least three options for completing tests of simple main effects. Many researchers simply do all tests and thus inflate the experimentwise error rate. Another issue related to Type I errors is whether to adjust the post hoc tests because multiple tests are performed. Finally, Levin and Marascuilo (133) coined the term *Type IV error* to refer to the use of inappropriate analyses or explanations following a correctly rejected hypothesis. The appropriate analysis should involve the differential effect (134) and not pairs of means. However, Games (135) has criticized Levin and Marascuilo's arguments, and there does not seem to be a consensus. Type IV errors may be the reason why traditional follow-up tests often fail to detect significance from a correctly rejected interaction term. The appropriate analysis and interpretation of interaction effects has recently been revitalized in the literature (136).

There are situations when the researcher might want to measure the fitness parameters on more than one occasion. Instead of a typical pretest–posttest design, the researcher might take measures at 4-week intervals over a 16-week training program. In this situation special attention must be given to the special assumptions of repeated-measures designs (137). In the past there has been a tendency for researchers to ignore or fail to test for these assumptions. In many cases this can result in false positive results.

These problems could be avoided if more researchers realized that the interaction *F* ratio and an analysis of gain scores were mathematically equivalent (117, 132). In addition, the gain score analysis would avoid the issue of post hoc tests because there would be only two groups. Jennings (138) has supported Huck and McLean's conclusion, although taking a regression approach to the problem.

An alternative to the gain score analysis would be an ANCOVA with the pretest as a covariate. In most cases the ANCOVA analysis will be more sensitive (higher power) than the gain score analysis (4, 117). The gain score analysis and ANCOVA are mathematically equivalent if the regression slopes between the pretest scores and the posttest scores equal 1. Because of regression toward the mean, this will rarely occur, and thus the ANCOVA is more sensitive because of a smaller error term. Pretest and posttest correlations often approach test-retest reliabilities (4), and thus the operative effect size can be greatly affected by the percent variance accounted for in the dependent variable by the covariate (see Equation 8).

Those who are proponents of the gain score analysis because of its simplicity should realize that the same assumptions (e.g., homogeneity of regression slopes) apply to gain score analysis and ANCOVA. The preferred method of analysis is ANCOVA, because failure to meet assumptions can be corrected in ANCOVA but not in gain score analysis (117). Additionally, ANCOVA takes into consideration the actual slopes of the regression lines and does not assume a value of 1.

The standard ANCOVA involves an interpretation of the adjusted posttest means. Hendrix, Carter, and Hintze (132) in a variation on the traditional ANCOVA analysis suggest a gain score analysis with the pretest as a covariate. This analysis produces an equivalent solution to the standard ANCOVA but allows for interpretation of adjusted gains.

Univariate Versus Multivariate Analysis

Most TER concerned with physical fitness will deal with multiple outcome measures because of the multidimensionality of fitness. A sample TER study and introduction to multivariate methods is provided by Donner and Cunningham (139). Our purpose in this section is to briefly discuss the issues involved in deciding whether to use univariate or multivariate data-analysis techniques. We also will outline a general overview of MANOVA techniques and how to interpret significant effects. Last, we will give some special considerations for analyzing repeated measures with multivariate techniques.

The debate about whether to use multiple ANOVAs or a multivariate analysis of variance has a long history with multiple issues. A recent review of the major issues and recommendations is provided by Huberty and Morris (140). In a survey of six behavioral science journals, involving 222 studies, 40% of the studies used the illogical and inappropriate strategy of following the primary MANOVA with multiple ANOVAs.

Huberty and Morris (140) recommended four situations when multiple ANOVAs might be appropriate: when (a) the outcome variables are conceptually independent; (b) the research is considered exploratory; (c) there is a previous history of univariate analysis in similar studies; or (d) comparability of a number of descriptors of a comparison group is being established. They then suggested three problems for which a MANOVA would be appropriate: (a) the variable selection problem, (b) the variable ordering problem, and (c) when identifying system structures. The first problem is concerned with finding a subset of variables that account for group separation. The second issue, variable ordering, is concerned with determining the relative contributions of each variable to group separation. The last problem is concerned with naming an underlying construct. The decision rule of whether to use multiple ANOVAs or MANOVA depends a great deal on the conceptual orientation of the researcher. A poor or weak theoretical foundation concerning physical fitness can undermine a researcher's understanding of what constitutes an effective training program. This may be the result of an inappropriate analysis. A unidimensional, global physical fitness construct would probably be most appropriately analyzed with a MANOVA, whereas a multidimensional construct would entail multiple ANOVAs. A combination analysis would be needed for a hierarchical fitness model.

Obviously the techniques for conducting a multivariate analysis of variance and interpreting the outcome are beyond the scope of this chapter. An excellent introduction to multivariate analysis is provided by Tabachnick and Fidell (141), and Schutz, Smoll, and Gessaroli (142) provide an introductory paper on when to use MANOVA. Once an overall significant MANOVA is uncovered, identifying the reason for significance is the primary concern of the researcher. Unlike univariate analyses, this process is not very straightforward nor do the experts agree on how to proceed with it. Some good recommendations are provided by Bray and Maxwell (143), Huberty (144), and Share (145).

The typical TER study will probably involve multiple outcome variables in addition to repeated measures. The most popular analysis for multiple variables and repeated measures has been the doubly multivariate analysis of variance. Suggestions can be found in O'Brien and Kaiser (146) and Schutz and Gessaroli (147).

"Proving" the Null

A common tactic used by researchers to eliminate or at least make less plausible rival hypotheses is to demonstrate the equivalence of the groups (control and experimental) on these alternative explanations (75, 148). However, attempts to establish the bioequivalence of groups are plagued by philosophical (149-151), logical (1, 152-155), and mathematical problems (156). If a researcher adopts the Yule, Karl Pearson, and Fisher significance test approach to hypothesis testing, then accepting the null hypothesis is philosophically incorrect. However, if a researcher adopts the Neyman-Pearson and Wald decision theory approach, then accepting the null is possible.

Drawing conclusions based on the data collected from an experiment requires inductive reasoning. When hypothesis testing is used as part of this inferential process, certain problems become evident. One of the major criticisms of hypothesis testing is that the inductive process is asymmetrical (68). The asymmetry of the hypothesis-testing process ultimately inspired the development of the concepts of power and Type II errors by Neyman and Pearson (153-155). These concepts also pointed out problems of misinterpreting nonsignificant results. In fact, Reed and Slaichert (78) reported that between 50% and 73% of medical studies had statistical errors in them. The majority of these errors, they concluded, concerned inferences about accepting the null hypothesis.

Sir Ronald A. Fisher introduced many statistical techniques, most notably analysis of variance. When testing the relative effectiveness of two training programs for developing physical fitness, the Fisherian approach would be to establish a point null hypothesis. Specifically, the hypothesis would be that the two programs were equally effective in enhancing physical fitness. The alternative hypothesis, implied in the Fisherian approach, would be any non-zero value, that is, a composite hypothesis of nonequality. Thus, in the Fisherian approach, the asymmetry in logic occurs because a point null hypothesis is tested against a composite alternative and the point null hypothesis can be rejected but not accepted.

An alternative strategy for avoiding asymmetry is to specify a point alternative. This is the approach taken by Neyman-Pearson (68). If a specific value for the alternative hypothesis is provided, then a Type II error, and hence power, can be estimated. The specific alternative value depends on estimating an anticipated effect size. The procedures for determining an estimated effect size were covered in a previous section of this chapter.

The failure to reject is often equated with accepting the null, that is, establishing no difference. When the researcher wants to reject the null, based on her or his research hypothesis, the conservative approach is to avoid committing a Type I error. Thus it would not be unusual to set alpha at .01 or even .001. In accepting the null, however, the conservative approach is to avoid Type II errors (75). Thus, researchers who want to act as though they have accepted the null must implicitly adopt the Neyman-Pearson approach to hypothesis testing and try to minimize Type II errors. A failure to reject the null can easily occur by designing a study poorly, underpowering the study, using insensitive measures, or using treatments that lack integrity. Thus, the test for accepting the null must be more stringent than simply failing to reject the null (157).

A variety of strategies for "proving" the null hypothesis have been suggested; some are still quite controversial. From the researcher's point of view, the easiest strategy is to adjust the alpha value. Obviously, substantial differences between groups could still exist if the significance level just failed significance at .06. Just a few more subjects and the conclusion would have been to reject the null. Therefore, Blackwelder (157) suggested using an alpha value of .5, whereas Julnes and Mohr (75) suggested the more liberal value of .25 and Rosemier (158) suggested an exaggerated value of .90. Researchers can then either reject the null, suspend judgment, or act as if they are accepting the null.

Greenwald (45) has suggested a four-point procedure for accepting the null hypothesis. The essence of this approach is to rely on a Bayesian posterior probability procedure before accepting the null. As mentioned previously in this paper, Bayesian procedures do allow statements about the probability that the null hypothesis is true. These procedures are not universally accepted, however.

Blackwelder (157) has suggested that a specified difference be part of the null hypothesis. It has also been suggested that confidence intervals (75, 157) and power analyses (75) can be used to provide evidence for the null. However, statistical evidence alone cannot establish the truth of the null hypothesis (148).

The procedures outlined in this section have value in establishing the equivalence of groups and thus eliminating rival hypotheses. As always the researcher is concerned with convincing the consumer that her or his explanation is the appropriate explanation. This often requires that other alternative explanations be eliminated.

Tests of Statistical Significance Versus Effect-Size Estimators

The value of TOSS in advancing knowledge has long been a matter of controversy. Excellent summaries of the most salient issues are provided by Morrison and Henkel (16) and Oakes (17). A good summary of the early history of the development of TOSS is provided by Clark (13).

Many researchers have taken the position that TOSS just do not provide enough information. For this reason some researchers prefer to use regression analysis because they can obtain measures of strength of association that are not readily available with traditional ANOVA analyses. However, it has long been known (159) that multiple regression (with dummy coding) and fixed-effect analysis of variance are merely different approaches to the general linear model. Therefore, it would seem logical that the same summary values could be obtained from both analyses. In fact, Knapp (160) has suggested that virtually all of the parametric TOSS are special cases of canonical correlation analysis. Thus

the real differences between these analyses are concerned with the ease of setting up the computer analysis and the form of the output.

Because TOSS represent only the first step (not the last) in scientific inferences, some researchers have recommended additional strategies to replace, supplement, or follow up TOSS. One of the more popular supplements has been to report estimates of the magnitude of an effect (161). Others have offered calculating confidence intervals (162) or graphical analyses (163) as alternatives or supplements to TOSS. Each of these data-analytic systems has its weaknesses, however.

Recently, journals such as the *Research Quarterly for Exercise and Sport* have editorialized the importance of providing both TOSS and magnitude-of-effect (ME) estimates (164, 165). The recent interest in synthesizing research findings has also resulted in the development of effect-size estimators. In fact, effect size, magnitude of effect, and strength of association are all related concepts.

As mentioned previously, TOSS are perhaps misnamed because they cannot be used to judge the significance, importance, or meaningfulness of the relationships they are used to investigate. TOSS can only inform about the direction and rareness of a relationship (29). For this reason, researchers have employed a variety of techniques to reflect the magnitude or size of an effect. Whereas TOSS are known to be affected by sample size, ME estimates were developed because they are not (27, 161). However, this is a controversial point (166, 167).

The most familiar ME estimators are eta squared (168), epilson squared (169), omega squared (170), and the intraclass correlation coefficient squared. Recent developments in meta-analysis have focused attention on delta (89) and the standardized mean difference (90). Although these procedures were all developed from different perspectives, Friedman (171) showed their relationship and an easy method for estimating the ME. Eta squared was developed initially in a regression context and is a descriptive index equal to the sample coefficient of determination (161). Epilson- and omega-squared estimates were developed independently and attempted to eliminate bias in estimating the proportional reduction in error by knowing group membership (161). Both of these inferential statistics are to be used with fixed-effect analysis of variance designs. The intraclass correlation coefficient squared is to be used in random-effect analysis of variance designs (87). Because most studies are fixed-effect designs, researchers generally must choose between eta, epsilon, and omega if a percent variance measure is wanted. The largest values will be produced by eta squared and the smallest by omega squared.

These statistics have been misinterpreted just as much as the TOSS they are intended to replace or supplement.

These statistics are thought to be independent of sample size and the complexity of the design. Although intended as indicators of practical significance or importance, they have been inappropriately interpreted for a variety of measurement, methodological, and theoretical reasons (172).

Most of the problems with ME estimators originate from the failure to realize that they are sample statistics and from the false assumption that they are independent of sample size (166). However, sample size does affect nondirectional ME estimators such as eta and omega squared, whereas directional estimators like delta and the coefficient of determination are unaffected by sample size (167).

Common ME estimators like eta squared and omega squared reflect the proportion of the total variance that can be accounted for by a treatment (161). The percent variance accounted for is often used as an indicator of practical significance. However, if the researcher is interested in estimating whether the magnitude of the treatment effect is large or not, then some critical value on the sampling distribution must be exceeded. That is, to answer the question of what constitutes a large (big) effect, a criterion for bigness must exist.

Murray and Dosser (166) have shown that eta squared is dependent on the beta sampling distribution. This distribution is a function of the number of treatment levels, the total number of observations, and the noncentrality parameter. Thus the size of eta squared must be interpreted in terms of these factors. These authors have shown that eta squared and the F statistic provide the same conclusions concerning the significance of a treatment. Therefore, neither is a satisfactory indicator of practical significance or importance.

The fact that the complexity of a design influences ME estimators has been known for some time. Many researchers (173, 174) have suggested that partial and semipartial estimators may be better indicators of the ME. Because design complexity affects the size of ME estimates, Murray and Dosser (166) have recommended that combining ME estimates from studies of different sizes may be inappropriate. This procedure has been followed in meta-analysis.

Another problem with ME estimators is the fact that as point estimates they may be overinterpreted. The sampling errors can often be quite large, and thus it is recommended that confidence intervals be calculated (175) and a range of values reported. Tolson (176) suggested that an omega-squared value of .10 might be a minimal level of interest to the exercise specialist, although 95% confidence intervals should be reported.

In addition to these statistical issues, ME estimators also suffer from methodological and conceptual problems. Unless the levels of the treatment are selected randomly, it does not make sense to generalize to the population of possible treatment conditions (177). However, most researchers use fixed-effects designs but interpret the ME as estimates of the population. This issue is similar to the problem of calculating a correlation coefficient on a restricted range of values and then generalizing to the entire population of values.

The size of a ME estimator is also affected by the reliability of the measures used to measure the outcome variable (172). Because all measures lack perfect reliability, the interpretation of the ME is compromised. As mentioned in an earlier section, reliabilities are rarely reported in physical fitness studies, and thus the effect on the ME estimator is unknown.

Finally, the size of the ME is influenced by several rather arbitrary decisions made by the researcher. Because experimental research tends to employ weaker independent variables than would occur in reality (because of a need for control), smaller differences between means generally result (166). The result is to produce a smaller ME (172). Narrowly defining the population to study can also reduce the size of the ME (172). Also, within-subject designs tend to produce larger ME estimates than between-group designs (172).

In conclusion, the importance or practical significance of a treatment effect is not a statistical issue (161). Importance is a question of validity. Statistical results indicate only whether a difference between sample means *needs* explanation. Many of the same criticisms that have been directed toward TOSS apply to ME. There is value in using ME as a summary statistic but, like TOSS, it should not be confused as an indicator of importance. Most of the criticisms directed toward ME and TOSS are usually the result of misapplication or misinterpretation of the statistics. The consumer must realize that the techniques covered in this chapter are merely tools to be used by the exercise specialist. Like all tools, they must be used correctly to be of value.

SUMMARY

The electronic and print media seem to be bombarding the public with infomercials and advertisements praising all sorts of training programs and exercise equipment. As professionals dedicated to healthy lifestyles we have an obligation to determine the effectiveness of these exercise programs and training devices. Whether as research consumers or because of a desire to be competent researchers, we need to understand the fundamental principles of how sound scientific studies are conducted. This chapter integrated principles of measurement, research design, and data analysis as they applied to evaluating training programs and exercise equipment. A much more extensive treatment of the integration of measurement, design, and analysis principles can be found in a book by Pedhazur and Schmelkin (178).

The initial portion of this chapter reviewed the basic principles of conducting Treatment Effectiveness Research (TER), with a special emphasis on the role of hypothesis testing as a means of providing the evidence to judge the truth or falsity of the researcher's hypothesis. Because tests of statistical significance (TOSS) are often misunderstood and, therefore, misused, special emphasis was given to some common myths concerning the interpretation of these tests. It was pointed out that TOSS merely indicate statistical rareness of the data and communicate to the researcher the need to explain this finding. Because the otucomes of TOSS have been used as evidence in support of the researcher's hypothesis, this has perpetuated the confirmation bias popular in the logical positivist approach to research. The issues related to this fallacious form of logic were discussed.

The second section of this chapter was concerned with design sensitivity or power. Most research studies in the biological and behavioral sciences have been underpowered. Because of the expense needed to monitor and test subjects in training studies, the traditional method of increasing power—increasing sample size—is not a viable option for most exercise scientists. Thus, other strategies are needed for increasing power. This chapter provided a review of how to conduct a power analysis and a discussion of factors that influence power. Special attention was given to measurement and design factors. The often confusing influence of reliability on power and the need to conduct measurement assessment and generalizability studies were also covered. The confusion with reliability is caused by the fact that if true scores are assumed to be constant, then any factor that decreases error variance will increase power. However, if error variance is assumed to be constant, then any factor that increases true score variance will lower power. This indicates that researchers must know the sources of error (generalizability studies) when measuring fitness parameters in order to maximize power. Power can also be increased by reducing subject heterogeneity through data analysis. The effectiveness of blocking, matching, using a covariate, and allowing subjects to serve as their own controls are effective means of increasing the operative power of a study.

The third section of this chapter covered threats to valid inferences. Sources of invalid inferences included threats to statistical conclusion validity, internal validity, construct validity, population validity, and ecological validity. The most common threats to each form of validity in TER were covered, and design alterations were suggested to avoid these threats.

The last section of the chapter dealt with selected data-analysis problems. Because most training studies will probably be analyzed with repeated-measures designs, the alternative strategies for handling these designs were covered. An ANCOVA analysis was recommended for most cases, but data analysts still debate this issue (see Schutz and Gessaroli [179] for an alternative recommendation). Second, we presented a multidimensional model of fitness and suggested that the investigator's theoretical conception of fitness would dictate the most appropriate method of analysis. A third statistical issue covered was the misinterpretation of TOSS for the purpose of establishing equivalency. Many fitness studies will involve intact groups. Moreover, subject attrition from research groups is likely to occur. Therefore, there will be a need to establish the equivalency of the groups before an intervention is introduced. We recommended that equivalency not be declared unless the associate probability (p-value) of the statistical test is greater than 0.5. Finally, we encouraged the use of magnitude-of-effect estimators as supplements to TOSS to ensure that studies have practical significance as well as statistical significance.

It is important for the exercise scientist to understand and utilize measurement, design, and analysis concepts effectively. It is all too common for exercise scientists to ignore measurement while performing fancy statistical tests, or to select a data-analysis procedure without regard for the theoretical foundation of the construct under study. Research must consist of a balance of tensions between the experimental question and how the question is to be answered.

REFERENCES

1. Fisher, R.A. (1971). *The design of experiments* (8th ed.). New York: Hafner Press.
2. Coleman, W. (1987). Experimental physiology and statistical inference: The therapeutic trial in nineteenth-century Germany. In L. Kruger, G. Gigerenzer, & M.S. Morgan (Eds.), *The probabilistic revolution* (pp. 201-226). Cambridge, MA: MIT Press.
3. Gigerenzer, G. (1991). From tools to theories: A heuristic of discovery in cognitive psychology. *Psychological Review*, **98**, 254-267.
4. Lipsey, M.W. (1990). *Design sensitivity: Statistical power for experimental research*. Newbury Park, CA: Sage.
5. Mahoney, M.J. (1978). Experimental methods and outcome evaluation. *Journal of Consulting and Clinical Psychology,* **46**, 660-672.
6. Campbell, D.T., & Stanley, J.C. (1966). *Experimental and quasi-experimental designs for research*. Chicago: Rand McNally.
7. Spector, P. E. (1981). *Research designs*. Beverly Hills, CA: Sage.

8. Kenny, D.A. (1975). A quasi-experimental approach to assessing treatment effects in the nonequivalent control group design. *Psychological Bulletin, 82,* 345-362.

9. Kerlinger, F.N. (1964). *Foundations of behavioral research.* New York: Holt, Rinehart & Winston.

10. Manicas, P.T., & Secord, P.F. (1983). Implications for psychology of the new philosophy of science. *American Psychologist, 38,* 399-413.

11. Chow, S.L. (1989). Significance tests and deduction: Reply to Folger (1989). *Psychological Bulletin, 106,* 161-165.

12. Popper, K.R. (1968). *The logic of scientific discovery* (rev. ed.). London: Hutchinson.

13. Clark, C.A. (1963). Hypothesis testing in relation to statistical methodology. *Review of Educational Research, 33,* 455-473.

14. Spielman, S. (1974). The logic of tests of significance. *Philosophy of Science, 41,* 211-226.

15. Carver, R.P. (1978). The case against statistical significance testing. *Harvard Educational Review, 48,* 378-399.

16. Morrison, D.E., & Henkel, R.E. (1970). *The significance test controversy—A reader.* Chicago: Aldine.

17. Oakes, M. (1986). *Statistical inference: A commentary for the social and behavioural sciences.* Chichester, England: Wiley.

18. Birnbaum, A. (1962). On the foundations of statistical inference. *Journal of the American Statistical Association, 57,* 269-306.

19. Gibbons, J.D., & Pratt, J.W. (1975). P-values: Interpretation and methodology. *The American Statistician, 29,* 20-25.

20. Pollard, P., & Richardson, J.T.E. (1987). On the probability of making type I errors. *Psychological Bulletin, 102,* 159-163.

21. Mohr, L.B. (1990). *Understanding significance testing.* Newbury Park, CA: Sage.

22. Cohen, J. (1990). Things I have learned (so far). *American Psychologist, 45,* 1304-1312.

23. Kish, L. (1959). Some statistical problems in research design. *American Sociological Review, 24,* 328-338.

24. Meehl, P.E. (1967). Theory testing in psychology and physics: A methodological paradox. *Philosophy of Science, 34,* 103-115.

25. Meehl, P.E. (1978). Theoretical risks and tabular asterisks: Sir Karl, Sir Ronald, and the slow progress of soft psychology. *Journal of Consulting and Clinical Psychology, 46,* 806-834.

26. Weitzman, R.A. (1984). Seven treacherous pitfalls of statistics, illustrated. *Psychological Reports, 54,* 355-363.

27. Chow, S.L. (1988). Significance test or effect size? *Psychological Bulletin, 103,* 105-110.

28. Gigerenzer, G., & Murray, D.J. (1987). *Cognition as intuitive statistics.* Hillsdale, NJ: Erlbaum.

29. Cooper, H.M. (1981). On the significance of effects and the effects of significance. *Journal of Personality and Social Psychology, 41,* 1013-1018.

30. Edwards, W., Lindman, H., & Savage, L.J. (1963). Bayesian statistical inference for psychological research. *Psychological Review, 70,* 193-242.

31. Rosnow, R.L., & Rosenthal, R. (1989). Statistical procedures and the justification of knowledge in psychological science. *American Psychologist, 44,* 1276-1284.

32. Sterling, T.D. (1959). Publication decisions and their possible effects on inferences drawn from tests of significance—Or vice versa. *Journal of the American Statistical Association, 54,* 30-34.

33. Schwartz, S., & Dalgleish, L. (1982). Statistical inference in personality research. *Journal of Research in Personality, 16,* 290-302.

34. Bolles, R.C. (1962). The difference between statistical hypotheses and scientific hypotheses. *Psychological Reports, 11,* 639-645.

35. Goodman, S. N., & Royall, R. (1988). Evidence and scientific research. *American Journal of Public Health, 78,* 1568-1574.

36. Dominowski, R.L. (1989). Method, theory, and drawing inferences. *American Psychologist, 44,* 1078.

37. Folger, R. (1989). Significance tests and the duplicity of binary decisions. *Psychological Bulletin, 106,* 155-160.

38. Klayman, J., & Ha, Y.W. (1987). Confirmation, disconfirmation, and information in hypothesis testing. *Psychological Review, 94,* 211-228.

39. Lakatos, I. (1970). Falsification and the methodology of scientific research programmes. In I. Lakatos & A. Musgrave (Eds.), *Criticism and the growth of knowledge* (pp. 91-195). London: Cambridge University Press.

40. Platt, J.R. (1964). Strong inference. *Science, 146,* 347-353.

41. Bakan, D. (1966). The test of significance in psychological research. *Psychological Bulletin, 66,* 423-437.

42. Rozeboom, W.W. (1960). The fallacy of the null-hypothesis significance test. *Psychological Bulletin, 57,* 416-428.

43. Oakes, W. F. (1975). On the alleged falsity of the null hypothesis. *The Psychological Record, 25,* 265-272.

44. Swoyer, C., & Monson, T.C. (1975). Theory confirmation in psychology. *Philosophy of Science, 42,* 487-502.

45. Greenwald, A.G. (1975). Consequences of prejudice against the null hypothesis. *Psychological Bulletin, 82,* 1-20.

46. Mahoney, M.J. (1977). Publication prejudices: An experimental study of confirmatory bias in the peer review system. *Cognitive Therapy and Research, 1,* 161-175.

47. Cook, T.D., & Campbell, D.T. (1979). *Quasi-experimentation: Design & analysis issues for field settings.* Chicago: Rand McNally.

48. Vogel, S. (1988). *Life's devices.* Princeton, NJ: Princeton University Press.

49. Lachman, R. (1960). The model in theory construction. *Psychological Review, 67,* 113-129.

50. Bompa, T.O. (1990). *Theory and methodology of training: The key to athletic performance* (2nd ed.). Dubuque, IA: Kendall/Hunt.

51. Brooks, G.A. (1987). The exercise physiology paradigm in contemporary biology: To molbiol or not to molbiol—that is the question. *Quest, 39,* 231-242.

52. Brooks, G. A., & Fahey, T.D. (1984). *Exercise physiology: Human bioenergetics and its applications.* New York: Wiley.

53. Gardiner, P.R. (1986). Exercise physiology in the 1990's: Mechanistically defining the exercise model. *Canadian Journal of Applied Sport Sciences, 11*(1), 1-10.

54. Johnson, R.E., & Lavay, B. (1989). Fitness testing for children with special needs—An alternative approach. *Journal of Physical Education, Recreation and Dance, 60*(6), 50-53.

55. Matveyev, L. (1977). *Fundamentals of sports training.* Moscow: Progress.

56. Selye, H. (1956). *The stress of life.* New York: McGraw-Hill.

57. Whitehead, J.R. (1989). Fitness assessment results—Some concepts and analogies. *Journal of Physical Education, Recreation and Dance, 60*(6), 39-43.

58. Butts, N.K. (1985). The elite athlete. In N.K. Butts, T.T. Gushiken, & B. Zarins (Eds.), *Profiles of elite athletes: Physical and physiological characteristics* (pp. 183-208). New York: Medical & Scientific Books.

59. Grandjean, A.C. (1985). Profile of nutritional beliefs and practices of the elite athlete. In N.K. Butts, T.T. Gushiken, & B. Zarins (Eds.), *Profiles of elite athletes: Physical and physiological characteristics* (pp. 239-248). New York: Medical & Scientific Books.

60. Nichols, J.A. (1984). The value of sports profiling. *Clinics in Sports Medicine, 3,* 3-9.

61. Puhl, J.L., Van Handel, P.J., Williams, L.L., Bradley, P.W., & Harms, S.J. (1985). Iron status training. In N.K. Butts, T.T. Gushiken, & B. Zarins (Eds.), *Profiles of elite athletes: Physical and physiological characteristics* (pp. 209-238). New York: Medical & Scientific Books.

62. Sobolski, J.C., Kolesar, J.J., Kornitzer, M.D., De Backer, G.G., Mikes, Z., Dramaix, M.M., Degre, S.G., & Denolin, H.F. (1988). Physical fitness does not reflect physical activity patterns in middle-aged workers. *Medicine and Science in Sports and Exercise, 20,* 6-13.

63. Calvert, T.W., Banister, E.W., Savage, M.V., & Bach, T. (1976). A systems model of the effects of training on physical performance. *IEEE Transactions on Systems, Man, and Cybernetics, 6*(2), 94-102.

64. Walberg, J.L., Ruiz, V.K., Tarlton, S.L., Hinkle, D.E., & Thye, F.W. (1988). Exercise capacity and nitrogen loss during a high or low carbohydrate diet. *Medicine and Science in Sports and Exercise, 20,* 34-43.

65. Fox, E.L. (1979). *Sports physiology.* Philadelphia: W. B. Saunders.

66. Glassford, R.G. (1987). Methodological reconsiderations: The shifting paradigms. *Quest, 39,* 295-312.

67. Cohen, J. (1988). *Statistical power analysis for the behavioral sciences* (2nd ed., revised). Hillsdale, NJ: Erlbaum.

68. Chase, L.J., & Tucker, R.K. (1976). Statistical power: Derivation, development, and data-analytic implications. *The Psychological Record, 26,* 473-486.

69. Cowles, M., & Davis, C. (1982). On the origins of the .05 level of statistical significance. *American Psychologist, 37,* 553-558.

70. Franks, B.D., & Huck, S.W. (1986). Why does everyone use the .05 significance level? *Research Quarterly for Exercise and Sport, 57,* 245-249.

71. Labovitz, S. (1968). Criteria for selecting a significance level: A note on the sacredness of .05. *The American Sociologist, 3,* 220-222.

72. Nelson, N., Rosenthal, R., & Rosnow, R.L. (1986). Interpretation of significance levels and effect sizes by psychological researchers. *American Psychologist, 41,* 1299-1301.

73. Ryan, T.A. (1985). ''Ensemble-adjusted *p* values'': How are they to be weighted? *Psychological Bulletin, 97,* 521-526.

74. Cohen, J. (1965). Some statistical issues in psychological research. In B.B. Wolman (Ed.), *Handbook of clinical psychology* (pp. 95-121). New York: McGraw-Hill.

75. Julnes, G., & Mohr, L.B. (1989). Analysis on no-difference findings in evaluation research. *Evaluation Review, 13,* 628-655.

76. Cohen, J. (1970). Approximate power and sample size determination for common one-sample and

two-sample hypothesis tests. *Educational and Psychological Measurement, 30*, 811-831.

77. Kraemer, H.C., & Thiemann, S. (1987). *How many subjects? Statistical power analysis in research.* Newbury Park, CA: Sage.

78. Reed, J.F., III , & Slaichert, W. (1981). Statistical proof in inconclusive 'negative' trials. *Archives of Internal Medicine, 141*, 1307-1310.

79. Cohen, J. (1962). The statistical power of abnormal-social psychological research: A review. *Journal of Abnormal and Social Psychology, 65*, 145-153.

80. Levenson, R.L., Jr. (1980). Statistical power analysis: Implications for researchers, planners, and practitioners in gerontology. *The Gerontologist, 20*, 494-498.

81. Jones, B.J., & Brewer, J.K. (1972). An analysis of the power of statistical tests reported in the *Research Quarterly. Research Quarterly, 43*, 23-30.

82. Smart, R.G. (1964). The importance of negative results in psychological research. *The Canadian Psychologist, 5*, 225-232.

83. Rosenthal, R. (1979). The "file drawer problem" and tolerance for null results. *Psychological Bulletin, 86*, 638-641.

84. Sedlmeier, P., & Gigerenzer, G. (1989). Do studies of statistical power have an effect on the power of studies? *Psychological Bulletin, 105*, 309-316.

85. Freiman, J.A., Chalmers, T.C., Smith, H., Jr., & Kuebler, R.R. (1978). The importance of beta, the type II error and sample size in the design and interpretation of the randomized control trial: Survey of 71 "negative" trials. *The New England Journal of Medicine, 299*, 690-694.

86. Cascio, W.F., & Zedeck, S. (1983). Open a new window in rational research planning: Adjust alpha to maximize statistical power. *Personnel Psychology, 36*, 517-526.

87. Sechrest, L., & Yeaton, W.H. (1982). Magnitudes of experimental effects in social science research. *Evaluation Review, 6*, 579-600.

88. McGaw, B., & Glass, G.V. (1980). Choice of the metric for effect size in meta-analysis. *American Educational Research Journal, 17*, 325-337.

89. Glass, G. V. (1976). Primary, secondary, and meta-analysis of research. *Educational Researcher, 5*(10), 3-8.

90. Hedges, L. V. (1982). Estimation of effect size from a series of independent experiments. *Psychological Bulletin, 92*, 490-499.

91. Tran, V.T., Weltman, A., Glass, G., & Mood, D.P. (1983). The effects of exercise on blood lipids and lipoproteins: A meta-analysis of studies. *Medicine and Science in Sports and Exercise, 15*, 393-402.

92. Rosenthal, R., & Rubin, D.B. (1982). A simple, general purpose display of magnitude of experimental effect. *Journal of Educational Psychology, 74*, 166-169.

93. Messick, S. (1989). Validity. In R.L. Linn (Ed.), *Educational measurement* (pp. 13-103). New York: Macmillan.

94. Feldt, L.S., & Brennan, R.L. (1989). Reliability. In R.L. Linn (Ed.), *Educational measurement* (pp. 105-146). New York: Macmillan.

95. Lipsey, M.W. (1983). A scheme for assessing measurement sensitivity in program evaluation and other applied research. *Psychological Bulletin, 94*, 152-165.

96. Bar-Or, O. (1987). The Wingate anaerobic test: An update on methodology, reliability and validity. *Sports Medicine, 4*, 381-394.

97. American Educational Research Association, American Psychological Association, & National Council on Measurement in Education. (1985). *Standards for educational and psychological testing.* Washington, DC: American Psychological Association.

98. Wood, T.M. (1989). The changing nature of norm-referenced validity. In M.J. Safrit & T.M. Wood (Eds.), *Measurement concepts in physical education and exercise science* (pp. 23-44). Champaign, IL: Human Kinetics.

99. Shavelson, R.J., Webb, N.M., & Rowley, G.L. (1989). Generalizability theory. *American Psychologist, 44*, 922-932.

100. Mazzeo, J., & Seeley, G.W. (1984). A general framework for evaluating the reliability of medical measurement systems. *Evaluation & the Health Professions, 7*, 379-411.

101. Nicewander, W.A., & Price, J.M. (1978). Dependent variable reliability and the power of significance tests. *Psychological Bulletin, 85*, 405-409.

102. Nicewander, W.A., & Price, J.M. (1983). Reliability of measurement and the power of statistical tests: Some new results. *Psychological Bulletin, 94*, 524-533.

103. Sutcliffe, J.P. (1980). On the relationship of reliability to statistical power. *Psychological Bulletin, 88*, 509-515.

104. Zimmerman, D.W., & Williams, R.H. (1986). Note on the reliability of experimental measures and the power of significance tests. *Psychological Bulletin, 100*, 123-124.

105. Lord, F.M. (1963). Elementary models for measuring change. In C.W. Harris (Ed.), *Problems in measuring change* (pp. 21-38). Madison, WI: University of Wisconsin Press.

106. Schutz, R.W. (1989). Analyzing change. In M.J. Safrit & T.M. Wood (Eds.), *Measurement*

concepts in physical education and exercise science (pp. 207-228). Champaign, IL: Human Kinetics.

107. Fleiss, J.L. (1976). Comment on Overall and Woodward's asserted paradox concerning the measurement of change. *Psychological Bulletin,* **83**, 774-775.

108. Overall, J.E., & Woodward, J.A. (1976). Reassertion of the paradoxical power of tests of significance based on unreliable difference scores. *Psychological Bulletin,* **83**, 776-777.

109. Cronbach, L.J., Rajaratnam, N., & Gleser, G.C. (1963). Theory of generalizability: A liberalization of reliability theory. *The British Journal of Statistical Psychology,* **16**(Pt. 2), 137-163.

110. Gleser, G.C., Cronbach, L.J., & Rajaratnam, N. (1965). Generalizability of scores influenced by multiple sources of variance. *Psychometrika,* **30**, 395-418.

111. Morrow, J.R., Jr. (1989). Generalizability theory. In M.J. Safrit & T.M. Wood (Eds.), *Measurement concepts in physical education and exercise science* (pp. 73-96). Champaign, IL: Human Kinetics.

112. Morrow, J.R., Jr., Fridye, T., & Monaghen, S.D. (1986). Generalizability of the AAHPERD health related skinfold test. *Research Quarterly for Exercise and Sport,* **57**, 187-195.

113. Henry, F.M. (1967). "Best" versus "average" individual scores. *Research Quarterly,* **38**, 317-320.

114. Kroll, W. (1967). Reliability theory and research decision in selection of a criterion score. *Research Quarterly,* **38**, 412-419.

115. Sparling, P.B. (1980). A meta-analysis of studies comparing maximal oxygen uptake in men and women. *Research Quarterly for Exercise and Sport,* **51**, 542-552.

116. Maxwell, S.E., Delaney, H.D., & Dill, C.A. (1984). Another look at ANCOVA versus blocking. *Psychological Bulletin,* **95**, 136-147.

117. Huck, S.W., & McLean, R.A. (1975). Using a repeated measures ANOVA to analyze the data from a pretest-posttest design: A potentially confusing task. *Psychological Bulletin,* **82**, 511-518.

118. Greenwald, A.G. (1976). Within-subjects designs: To use or not to use? *Psychological Bulletin,* **83**, 314-320.

119. Morris, H.H. (1981). Experimental considerations in the analysis of repeated measures. In R.H. Cox & R.C. Serfass (Eds.), *AAHPERD research consortium symposium papers: Analysis of repeated measures and identifying causal relationships in physical education research 1981* (pp. 25-44). Reston, VA: AAHPERD.

120. Ozer, D.J. (1985). Correlation and the coefficient of determination. *Psychological Bulletin,* **97**, 307-315.

121. Cook, T.J., & Poole, W.K. (1982). Treatment implementation and statistical power: A research note. *Evaluation Review,* **6**, 425-430.

122. Yeaton, W.H., & Sechrest, L. (1981). Critical dimensions in the choice and maintenance of successful treatments: Strength, integrity, and effectiveness. *Journal of Consulting and Clinical Psychology,* **49**, 156-167.

123. Mark, M.M. (1983). Treatment implementation, statistical power, and internal validity. *Evaluation Review,* **7**, 543-549.

124. Campbell, D.T. (1969). Reforms as experiments. *American Psychologist,* **24**, 409-429.

125. Winch, R.F., & Campbell, D.T. (1969). Proof? No. Evidence? Yes. The significance of tests of significance. *The American Sociologist,* **4**, 140-143.

126. Yeaton, W.H., & Sechrest, L. (1987). Assessing factors influencing acceptance of no-difference research. *Evaluation Review,* **11**, 131-142.

127. Campbell, D.T. (1957). Factors relevant to the validity of experiments in social settings. *Psychological Bulletin,* **54**, 297-312.

128. Bracht, G.H., & Glass, G.V. (1968). The external validity of experiments. *American Educational Research Journal,* **5**, 437-474.

129. Campbell, D.T. (1963). Problems in measuring change. In C.W. Harris (Ed.), *From description to experimentation: Interpreting trends as quasi-experiments* (pp. 212-242). Madison, WI: University of Wisconsin Press.

130. Campbell, D.T. (1969). Prospective: Artifact and control. In R. Rosenthal & R.L. Rosnow (Eds.), *Artifact in behavioral research* (pp. 351-382). New York: Academic Press.

131. Winer, B.J. (1971). *Statistical principles in experimental design* (2nd ed.). New York: McGraw-Hill.

132. Hendrix, L.J., Carter, M.W., & Hintze, J.L. (1978/79). A comparison of five statistical methods for analyzing pretest-posttest designs. *Journal of Experimental Education,* **47**, 96-102.

133. Levin, J.R., & Marascuilo, L.A. (1972). Type IV errors and interactions. *Psychological Bulletin,* **78**, 368-374.

134. Levin, J.R., & Marascuilo, L.A. (1977). Post hoc analysis of repeated measures interactions and gain scores: Whither the inconsistency? *Psychological Bulletin,* **84**, 247-248.

135. Games, P.A. (1973). Type IV errors revisited. *Psychological Bulletin,* **80**, 301-307.

136. Rosnow, R.L., & Rosenthal, R. (1989). Definition and interpretation of interaction effects. *Psychological Bulletin,* **105**, 143-146.

137. Vasey, M.W., & Thayer, J.F. (1987). The continuing problem of false positives in repeated

measures ANOVA in psychophysiology: A multivariate solution. *Psychophysiology,* **24,** 479-486.

138. Jennings, E. (1988). Models for pretest-posttest data: Repeated measures ANOVA revisited. *Journal of Educational Statistics,* **13,** 273-280.

139. Donner, A.P., & Cunningham, D.A. (1983). The use of multivariate analysis of variance in physiological research: The two-group case. *Medicine and Science in Sports and Exercise,* **15,** 545-548.

140. Huberty, C.J., & Morris, J.D. (1989). Multivariate analysis versus multiple univariate analyses. *Psychological Bulletin,* **105,** 302-308.

141. Tabachnick, B.G., & Fidell, L.S. (1989). *Using multivariate statistics* (2nd ed.). New York: Harper & Row.

142. Schutz, R.W., Smoll, F.L., & Gessaroli, M.E. (1983). Multivariate statistics: A self-test and guide to their utilization. *Research Quarterly for Exercise and Sport,* **54,** 255-263.

143. Bray, J.H., & Maxwell, S.E. (1982). Analyzing and interpreting significant MANOVAs. *Review of Educational Research,* **52,** 340-367.

144. Huberty, C.J. (1984). Issues in the use and interpretation of discriminant analysis. *Psychological Bulletin,* **95,** 156-171.

145. Share, D.L. (1984). Interpreting the output of multivariate analyses: A discussion of current approaches. *British Journal of Psychology,* **75,** 349-362.

146. O'Brien, R.G., & Kaiser, M.K. (1985). MANOVA method for analyzing repeated measures designs: An extensive primer. *Psychological Bulletin,* **97,** 316-333.

147. Schutz, R.W., & Gessaroli, M.E. (1987). The analysis of repeated measures designs involving multiple dependent variables. *Research Quarterly for Exercise and Sport,* **58,** 132-149.

148. Yeaton, W.H., & Sechrest, L. (1986). Use and misuse of no-difference findings in eliminating threats to validity. *Evaluation Review,* **10,** 836-852.

149. Binder, A. (1963). Further considerations on testing the null hypothesis and the strategy and tactics of investigating theoretical models. *Psychological Review,* **70,** 107-115.

150. Cook, T.D., Gruder, C.L., Hennigan, K.M., & Flay, B.R. (1979). History of the sleeper effect: Some logical pitfalls in accepting the null hypothesis. *Psychological Bulletin,* **86,** 662-679.

151. Grant, D.A. (1962). Testing the null hypothesis and the strategy and tactics of investigating theoretical models. *Psychological Review,* **69,** 54-61.

152. Fisher, R.A. (1955). Statistical methods and scientific induction. *Journal of the Royal Statistical Society Series B (Methodological),* **17,** 69-78.

153. Neyman, J., & Pearson, E.S. (1928). On the use and interpretation of certain test criteria for purposes of statistical inference. Part I. *Biometrika,* **20A,** 175-240.

154. Neyman, J., & Pearson, E.S. (1928). On the use and interpretation of certain test criteria for purposes of statistical inference. Part II. *Biometrika,* **20A,** 263-294.

155. Neyman, J., & Pearson, E.S. (1933). On the problem of the most efficient tests of statistical hypotheses. *Philosophical Transactions of the Royal Society (Series A),* **231,** 289-337.

156. Londeree, B.R., Speckman, P.L., & Clapp, D. (1990). Testing for hypothesized equality. *Research Quarterly for Exercise and Sport,* **61,** 275-279.

157. Blackwelder, W.C. (1982). "Proving the null hypothesis" in clinical trials. *Controlled Clinical Trials,* **3,** 345-353.

158. Rosemier, R.A. (1968). The use of an exaggerated alpha in a test for the initial equality of groups. *Research Quarterly,* **39,** 829-830.

159. Cohen, J. (1968). Multiple regression as a general data-analytic system. *Psychological Bulletin,* **70,** 426-443.

160. Knapp, T.R. (1978). Canonical correlation analysis: A general parametric significance-testing system. *Psychological Bulletin,* **85,** 410-416.

161. Maxwell, S.E., Camp, C.J., & Arvey, R.D. (1981). Measures of strength of association: A comparative examination. *Journal of Applied Psychology,* **66,** 525-534.

162. Natrella, M.G. (1960). The relation between confidence intervals and tests of significance: A teaching aid. *The American Statistician,* **14**(1), 20-22.

163. Wainer, H., & Thissen, D. (1981). Graphical data analysis. *Annual Review of Psychology,* **32,** 191-241.

164. Thomas, J.R. (1983). Editor's viewpoint. *Research Quarterly for Exercise and Sport,* **54,** ii.

165. Thomas, J.R., Salazar, W., & Landers, D.M. (1991). What is missing in $p < .05$? Effect size. *Research Quarterly for Exercise and Sport,* **62,** 344-348.

166. Murray, L.W., & Dosser, D.A., Jr. (1987). How significant is a significant difference? Problems with the measurement of magnitude of effect. *Journal of Counseling Psychology,* **34,** 68-72.

167. Strube, M.J. (1988). Some comments on the use of magnitude-of-effect estimates. *Journal of Counseling Psychology,* **35,** 342-345.

168. Fisher, R.A. (1922). The goodness of fit of regression formulae, and the distribution of regression coefficients. *Journal of the Royal Statistical Society,* **85,** 597-612.

169. Kelley, T.L. (1935). An unbiased correlation ratio measure. *Proceedings of the National Academy of Sciences, 21*, 554-559.

170. Hays, W.L. (1963). *Statistics*. New York: Holt, Rinehart & Winston.

171. Friedman, H. (1968). Magnitude of experimental effect and a table for its rapid estimation. *Psychological Bulletin, 70*, 245-251.

172. O'Grady, K.E. (1982). Measures of explained variance: Cautions and limitations. *Psychological Bulletin, 92*, 766-777.

173. Cohen, J. (1973). Eta-squared and partial eta-squared in fixed factor ANOVA designs. *Educational and Psychological Measurement, 33*, 107-112.

174. Keren, G., & Lewis, C. (1979). Partial omega squared for ANOVA designs. *Educational and Psychological Measurement, 39*, 119-128.

175. Fleishman, A.I. (1980). Confidence intervals for correlation ratios. *Educational and Psychological Measurement, 40*, 659-670.

176. Tolson, H. (1980). An adjunct to statistical significance: ω^2. *Research Quarterly for Exercise and Sport, 51*, 580-584.

177. Glass, F.V., & Hakstian, A.R. (1969). Measures of association in comparative experiments: Their development and interpretation. *American Educational Research Journal, 6*, 403-414.

178. Pedhazur, E.J., & Schmelkin, L.P. (1991). *Measurement, design, and analysis: An integrated approach*. Hillsdale, NJ: Lawrence Erlbaum.

179. Schutz, R.W., & Gessaroli, M.E. (1993). Use, misuse, and disuse of psychometrics in sport psychology research. In R.N. Singer, M. Murphey, & L.K. Tennant (Eds.), *Handbook of research in sport psychology* (pp. 901-917). New York: Macmillan.

Index

Contributors

Lynn E. Ahlquist has been director of exercise physiology at the Exercise Physiology and Nutrition Center in Shrewsbury, MA, and an assistant professor of medicine at the University of Massachusetts Medical School for the past four years. She received her MS and PhD degrees in exercise physiology from the University of Wisconsin–Madison. Dr. Ahlquist has since moved to Connecticut and currently is focusing her energies on her new baby daughter.

Miriam Y. Cortez-Cooper is an instructor in the cooperative physical therapy program between the University of Texas Medical Branch at Galveston and the University of Texas at El Paso. She received her degree in physical therapy at Boston University and her master's degree in exercise physiology at the University of Texas at Austin. She teaches a number of clinical courses, and her interests include orthopaedics and muscle physiology.

David L. Costill holds the Janice and John Fisher Endowed Chair in Exercise Science and is director of the Human Performance Laboratory at Ball State University, Muncie, IN. He received his PhD from The Ohio State University in 1965 and came to Ball State to head up the Human Performance Lab in 1966. Since then he has done a variety of studies with runners, cyclists, and swimmers, looking at muscle physiology, sports nutrition, and environmental adaptations. His interests are wide-ranging, from computers and photography to the restoration of classic cars.

Jack Daniels is head men's and women's cross-country and track coach and professor of physical education at the State University of New York at Cortland. Before earning his PhD from the University of Wisconsin at Madison, Jack was a two-time Olympic medal winner in modern pentathlon. His research interests have focused mainly on elite athletes in the sports of swimming, paddling, and running. As a coach he has produced numerous national champions and national championship teams, and over 100 collegiate All-Americans. His scientifically based approach to training is used throughout the world.

James A. Davis is professor and director of the Laboratory of Applied Physiology at California State University, Long Beach. He received his PhD in physiology from the University of California, Davis, in 1975. His research interests include acid/base balance during exercise, and lung mechanics.

William J. Fink is assistant to the director and laboratory technician for the Human Performance Laboratory at Ball State University, Muncie, IN. For over 20 years he has overseen the analysis of blood and muscle for a variety of projects in muscle physiology and sports nutrition. He claims to have done more muscle glycogen analyses on human muscle than anyone in the world.

Carl Foster has a PhD in exercise physiology from the University of Texas and did postdoctoral work at Ball State University. He has been at Sinai Samaritan Medical Center in Milwaukee throughout his working career and is presently director of cardiac rehabilitation and exercise testing at the Milwaukee Heart Institute of Sinai Samaritan Medical Center, where he is also an associate professor of medicine in the University of Wisconsin Medical School. He has published over 150 scientific papers or chapters, several hundred lay articles and 5 books/monographs including *ACSM's Standards and Guidelines for Health and Fitness Facilities*. Dr. Foster was a member of the Board of Trustees and Vice President of the American College of Sports Medicine during the period of 1983-1987, and since 1989 has been an associate editor for *Medicine and Science in Sports and Exercise*. Outside of work, he is an enthusiastic participant in an ever-growing list of sports including distance running, old timers' soccer, speed skating, and taekwondo.

Andrew C. Fry is an assistant professor in the Department of Human Movement Sciences and Education at The University of Memphis. He received his PhD in exercise physiology from Penn State University in 1993, followed by two years of postdoctoral study at Ohio University. Currently chair of the Sport Science and Medical Committee of the U.S. Weightlifting Federation, Andrew also serves on the Research Committee of the National Strength and Conditioning Association. His current research interests include skeletal muscle and endocrine adaptations to heavy resistance exercise.

Linda Garzarella is lab coordinator for the Center for Exercise Science, Departments of Medicine and Exercise Science, University of Florida, Gainesville. She received her BS in nutrition science from Drexel University (Philadelphia, PA) and MS in exercise physiology from the University of Florida. Her thesis project, "Predicting Body Composition of Healthy Females by B-Mode Ultrasound: Comparison with Anthropometry and Bioelectrical Impedance" was conducted under the guidance of Drs. M.L. Pollock and J.E. Graves. She is currently working part-time towards a PhD in exercise physiology with a minor in nutrition science at the University of Florida.

James E. Graves is associate professor and chair of the health and physical education program at Syracuse University. He earned his PhD in exercise science at the University of Massachusetts in 1985. His research interests include exercise and aging, exercise training for the prevention and rehabilitation of orthopaedic injury to the lumbar spine and knee, body composition analysis, and microcomputer applications in biomedical research.

Everett Harman heads the biomechanics laboratory at the U.S. Army Research Institute of Environmental Medicine, where he conducts research into the biomechanics and physiology of physically demanding work and sport activities. He received his PhD in exercise science from the University of Massachusetts at Amherst in 1984. He taught at Boston University and has produced many articles and presentations on the science of human physical performance. Recently, he completed a 3-year term as Vice President for Research of the National Strength and Conditioning Association.

Lisa L. Hector has a master's degree in adult fitness/cardiac rehabilitation from Northeastern Illinois University. She is currently doing research with renal transplant patients in the Department of Physiologic Nursing at the University of California—San Francisco School of Nursing. Her other interests include weight training and wilderness camping.

William J. Kraemer, PhD, is the director of research in the Center for Sports Medicine, and an associate professor of applied physiology at The Pennsylvania State University. He also holds appointments in the Intercollege Program in Physiology, the Exercise and Sport Science Department, the Gerontology Center and is associate director for the Center for Cell Research. Dr. Kraemer is a fellow in the American College of Sports Medicine (ACSM) and has served on the ACSM's Board of Trustees and Administrative Council. He is a past president of the National Strength and Conditioning Association (NSCA) and serves as editor-in-chief of the *Journal of Strength and Conditioning Research*. He has published over 100 manuscripts and two books in the areas of strength training, sports medicine, physiology, exercise and sport science.

Norman Lamarra is a systems engineer whose technical career has spanned radar, communications, simulation, and software development; he is currently at Caltech's Jet Propulsion Lab in Pasadena, CA. He holds BSc and MSc degrees from the University of Birmingham, UK, in mathematical physics (1973) and electronic engineering (1974) respectively, and a PhD in system science from UCLA (1982). His interest in human exercise performance began in 1978 at UCLA where he developed and refined the use of microcomputers in calibration, measurement, analysis, simulation and modelling of respiratory control, and he has written and presented on the application of analytical methods to physiological research since then. He was appointed adjunct assistant professor of anesthesiology at UCLA in 1990.

Robert M. Malina is a professor in the Department of Kinesiology and Health Education and the Department of Anthropology at the University of Texas at Austin. He has PhD degrees in physical education from the University of Wisconsin at Madison in 1963 and in anthropology from the University of Pennsylvania in Philadelphia in 1968. In addition, he has an honorary degree from the Institute of Physical Education of the Faculty of Biomedical Sciences of the Katholieke Universiteit Leuven, Belgium, in 1989. His academic interests focus on the growth, maturation and performance of children and youth.

Peter J. Maud is a professor in the Kinesiology and Sports Studies Program at the University of Texas at El Paso. His primary area of expertise is exercise physiology and he has taught this and related subjects in a number of college and universities at both the undergraduate and graduate levels. Born and raised in England, Peter attended Loughborough and Chester Colleges, received his bachelor's degree from the University of Oregon and his master's and doctoral degrees from the University of New Mexico. He has played rugby for thirty-five years, and has enjoyed squash, fives, handball and badminton. More recently he has competed in several triathlons but now is returning his interests to kayaking, a difficult pursuit in the desert.

Kerry McDonald has a PhD in biology from Marquette University. He presently is a postdoctoral fellow in the Department of Physiology at the University of Wisconsin Medical School, Madison, where he studies muscle mechanics in cardiac muscle.

Michael L. Pollock is director, Center for Exercise Science, Departments of Medicine and Exercise Science, University of Florida, Gainesville. He received his BS from the University of Arizona and MS and PhD degrees from the University of Illinois. He has been director of research at the Institute for Aerobics Research, Dallas, Texas, and director of cardiac rehabilitation at Mount Sinai Medical Center, Milwaukee, WI. Dr. Pollock is a Past President of the American College of Sports Medicine and has over 250 publications and four books and monographs.

William A. Sands is an associate professor in the Department of Exercise and Sport Science at the University of Utah and teaches classes in biomechanics, kinesiology, and training theory. He is a former All-American gymnast and during his 21-year coaching career, coached 3 Olympians, 5 world championship team members, and 8 national team members. Dr. Sands has published 8 books, 8 chapters in books, and over 50 articles in refereed journals. He has made over 150 presentations at professional conferences and talks with coaches and athletes.

Matthew Schrager has a master's degree in physical education from the University of Indiana—Bloomington. He is currently in medical school. He was a collegiate soccer player and long jumper, and when his studies allow, is learning the finer points of sprint cycling.

Barry B. Shultz is the director of graduate studies and the director of the Motor Behavior Research Laboratory at the University of Utah in the Department of Exercise and Sport Science. He teaches classes in motor learning, research design, and experimental analysis. He has been a data analysis consultant for many grants and has published over 50 papers on topics in motor learning, data analysis, sport psychology, and exercise physiology.

Ann C. Snyder, PhD, is an associate professor and chair of the Department of Human Kinetics at the University of Wisconsin–Milwaukee, and is also director of the university's Exercise Physiology Laboratory. She has published numerous research articles dealing with enhancing exercise performance and nutrition, particularly in the areas of carbohydrate ingestion just prior to exercise and the influence of the consumption of vegetarian diets on health and exercise performance. Dr. Snyder was recently a Fulbright Scholar and performed research in the Netherlands examining the influence of carbohydrate ingestion on the incidence of overtraining.

Ann Ward currently teaches courses in exercise physiology in the Department of Kinesiology at the University of Wisconsin–Madison. She received a PhD in physical education with an emphasis in exercise physiology from the University of Wisconsin–Madison in 1984. Her research interests include assessment of fitness and physical activity and the role of exercise in health, particularly the role of exercise in the treatment of hypertension and obesity.

Brian Whipp is professor and chairment of the Department of Physiology at St. George's Hospital Medical School, University of London, UK. He has a PhD in physiology from Stanford University, a DSc from Loughborough University and is a fellow of the American College of Sports Medicine. His research interests are focused on the integrative aspects of human bioenergetics and the control of pulmonary ventilation. He has had a life-long interest in physical activity (former Welsh champion at decathlon and high hurdles) and remains active, when time permits, as a squash player.